Brachial Plexus Injuries

Brachial Plexus Injuries

Robert D. Leffert, M.D.

Associate Professor of Orthopaedic Surgery
Harvard Medical School
Chief of the Surgical Upper Extremity Rehabilitation Unit
and of the Department of Rehabilitation Medicine
Massachusetts General Hospital
Boston, Massachusetts

Churchill Livingstone
New York, Edinburgh, London, and Melbourne 1985

Acquisitions Editor: Toni M. Tracy
Copy Editor: Margot Otway
Production Designer: Karen Goldsmith Montanez
Production Supervisor: Sharon Tuder
Compositor: Progressive Typographers, Inc.
Printer/Binder: Halliday Lithograph

Accurate indications, adverse reactions, and dosage schedules for drugs are provided in this book, but it is possible that they may change. The reader is urged to review the package information data of the manufacturers of the medications mentioned.

The Publisher has made every effort to locate the source of borrowed material. If credit has been inadvertently omitted, please notify the Publisher.

Distributed in the United Kingdom by Churchill Livingstone, Robert Stevenson House, 1–3 Baxter's Place, Leith Walk, Edinburgh EH1 3AF and by associated companies, branches and representatives throughout the world.

First published in 1985

Printed in U.S.A.

ISBN 0-443-08026-7

9 8 7 6 5 4 3 2 1

Library of Congress Cataloging in Publication Data

Leffert, Robert D.
Brachial plexus injuries.

Includes bibliographies and index.
1. Brachial plexus—Wounds and injuries. I. Title.
[DNLM: 1. Brachial Plexus—injuries. WL 400 L493b]
RD595.L35 1985 617′.483 85-13319
ISBN 0-443-08026-7

Manufactured in the United States of America

In Memoriam

This work is dedicated to the memory of my father,
Jacob Leffert, M.D., physician and teacher,
who showed me the way. . . .

Preface

In a sense, writing this monograph was like putting a message in a bottle and setting it adrift—I wondered who would read it, and under what circumstances. Because I knew only in general terms the demographics and needs of my readers, I had to present my material in a form useful to a variety of care-providers and specialists interested in brachial plexus injuries. When to this requirement was added the complexity and controversial nature of this evolving field, I was presented with what appeared to be an impossible task.

These difficulties crossed my mind when Tim Hailstone, then of Churchill Livingstone, asked me to write this book. Nevertheless, I agreed. I have had a long and intense interest in the brachial plexus, going back to my introduction to the subject in 1964 by Sir Herbert Seddon, Donal Brooks, and Philip Yeoman at the Royal National Orthopaedic Hospital in London. Their devotion to the study and care of patients with brachial palsy was both inspiring and infectious, and I still regard this work as something of a mission.

In essence, my task has been to synthesize my ongoing experience, which encompasses the care of between 50 and 100 brachial plexus injuries per year, with the work of others in the field. Over the six years that I have spent researching and writing this book, the field has continued to evolve, and the compulsion to constantly revise the manuscript has been balanced by the liability of never calling a halt. Ultimately, with full knowledge of the consequences, one must do just that and hope that obsolescence will not come swiftly.

Very early in the process of writing, it became clear that because of the wide divergences of opinion that have characterized the management of brachial plexus lesions, it would be necessary to trace in detail the controversial history of surgical management. Even the anatomy of the brachial plexus has been the subject of great debate, going back to the 19th century. And, since significant contributions to our knowledge have been made by French-speaking anatomists and surgeons, I had to translate their works, an enjoyable but time-consuming task.

Because I realized that the book was more likely to be consulted piecemeal, to research specific topics, than to be read cover to cover, I designed the chapters to be largely independent of one another. Some duplication of material was therefore unavoidable.

I must acknowledge with thanks the assistance of French surgeons, Drs. Alnot, Allieu, and Gilbert, who provided me with their publications. Furthermore, the opportunity to discuss and sometimes debate with Drs. Narakas of Lausanne and Millesi of Vienna has been extremely valuable, as have been my conversations with Sir Sidney Sutherland, who provides an overall perspective that is unique.

This work would not have been possible without a great deal of support. My wife Linda's career as a trial lawyer and the demands of my work make our time together very precious, yet she did not begrudge the many occasions when I simply had to work on the manuscript. Her encouragement was all-important to me.

The research staffs of the Countway Library at the Harvard Medical School and the Treadwell Library of the Massachusetts General Hospital were extremely courteous and efficient in obtaining the many references. The technical expertise of Sidney Rosenthal of Arrco Medical Photographers of Boston and Alan Lucas, then of the Audio-Visual Department of the Massachusetts Eye and Ear Infirmary, made the preparation of the illustrations a manageable task and added tremendously to their quality.

The section on radiologic diagnosis was read by Dr. Paul New of the Department of Radiology of the Massachusetts General Hospital, and I appreciate his constructive criticism and suggestions. The chapter on radiation neuropathy was read by Dr. Henry Mankin, Chief of Orthopaedics at the Massachusetts General Hospital, who has been my colleague for 19 years and who urged me to write the book now rather than in my dotage.

My introduction to the problems of the brachial plexus at the Royal National Orthopaedic Hospital in London would not have been possible without the support provided by the Frauenthal Travel Fellowship of the Hospital for Joint Diseases in New York.

Since the writing and revising have gone on during an extremely busy period when patient care, teaching, and administrative duties have been ever-present, I simply could not have honored all these commitments and produced the manuscript without the help of four dedicated and efficient women who help me in my professional life at the hospital: Dolores Palumbo, Christine McAdam, Carol Danner, and Robin Morello.

Most authors are expected to say something nice about their publisher. Lew Reines, former president of Churchill Livingstone, got me into this thing, and in the past six years, he has become my friend. Even when my chagrin at being three years overdue with the manuscript made me very uncomfortable, he was never anything but warmly encouraging. For his kind and astute direction, I am very grateful.

Finally, the task of editing the manuscript was done with great patience, acumen, and tolerance for my literary voice by Margot Otway. One could not ask for more. Those errors that exist are mine.

Robert D. Leffert, M.D.

Contents

1

The Anatomy of the Brachial Plexus

Qu'ils n'oublient jamais que sans anatomie il n'y a point de physiologie, point de chirurgie, point de medecine.

J. CRUVEILHIER
Traité d'Anatomie Descriptive, 1834

To begin a treatise about brachial plexus injuries other than with a chapter on the pertinent anatomy might spare you, the reader, an uncomfortable flashback to the anxieties that most of us experienced when first we encountered the subject as students. However, I can think of no area of medical interest more thoroughly dependent on anatomical considerations than this one, and no words that express the dependency better than those of Cruveilhier, with which Emanuel Kaplan[18] began his classic book on the anatomy of the hand. To be sure, the anatomic literature devoted to the brachial plexus is vast and spans several hundred years and numerous languages. How fortunate that the present-day would-be surgeon of this biological work of art can have access to the record of a time past when careful study of morphology was an end in itself! The purpose of this chapter, then, must be threefold: to serve as an outline upon which to build a logical concept of diagnosis and treatment, to supply a source of references for in-depth study, and finally, to indicate wherever possible those areas that demand the application of contemporary methods of investigation to answer questions that could not have been addressed without them. No attempt will be made to be encyclopedic beyond these aims; it is a task beyond the scope of this monograph.

GENERAL MORPHOLOGY OF THE BRACHIAL PLEXUS

There are many detailed descriptions of the basic anatomy of the brachial plexus, as well as descriptions intended for the beginning student of anatomy or the casual reader who would just as soon have an unvarying and easily managed diagram of the nerves (Fig. 1.1). I have borrowed liberally from the works of Hovelacque,[17] Kerr,[20] Hollinshead,[16] Gray,[12] and Walsh[33] as well as many others for these descriptions. My preference for the most complete general picture (as well as an exhaustive reference) is the treatise by Hovelacque, published in French in 1927, and encompassing 128 pages devoted solely to the plexus and its variations. The section on the general morphology is particularly useful.

Prefixed and Postfixed Plexus

The brachial plexus is usually said to be formed by the anterior primary rami of the last four cervical nerve roots as well as that of the first thoracic root. Often there is a contribution from the C4 root to C5, and, less frequently, one from T2 to T1 and the plexus. Kerr[20] found that 62% of 175 plexuses received a contribution of C4 to C5 that varied from a small twig to a branch the size of the suprascapular nerve (Fig. 1.2). Thirty percent received no fibers from C4 but received all of the anterior ramus of C5 (Fig. 1.3). There may also be a contribution from the second thoracic nerve to the plexus, but this is often quite small. Where there is a rudimentary first thoracic rib, there is usually a large T2 contribution.

Although the terms "prefixed," "cephalic," or "high" have been applied when C4 joins C5, and

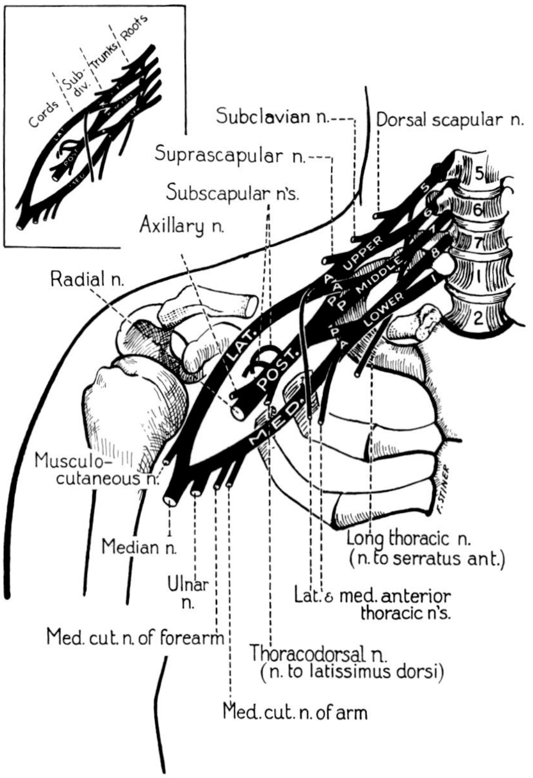

Fig. 1.1. The brachial plexus. (Reprinted from Haymaker W, Woodhall B: Peripheral Nerve Injuries. 2nd Ed. Saunders, Philadelphia, 1956.)

"postfixed," "caudal," or "low" to describe the contribution of T2, the practical consequences of these situations have been the subject of great debate.

There are two possible interpretations that can be made: the first implies that there is an actual physical shift of the plexus along the axis of the body, with a preservation of the expected total number of roots plus one, so that if C4 contributes significantly to C5 and the plexus, T2 does not (prefixed) (Fig. 1.4). If T2 contributes to T1 and the plexus, then C4 does not (postfixed) (Fig. 1.5). Even though Kerr's studies did not define the nature of the T2 connections and the caudal limit of the plexus in most cases, he rejected the above formulation, and considered the additional root contributions as expansions or contractions of the plexus, rather than a shift along the cord. The other criterion used by some anatomists to define the plexus as prefixed or postfixed is the position in the plexus of the strongest elements, or the nerves with the greatest diameters. Kerr found that the largest nerve to enter the plexus was the seventh or eighth cervical in 19 of 27—over 70%. The seventh was largest in seven, the eighth in six, and the seventh and eighth equally large in six. After taking all these things into consideration, he concluded that the method of classifying plexuses as prefixed or postfixed, based on the size of the nerve, is of doubtful value.

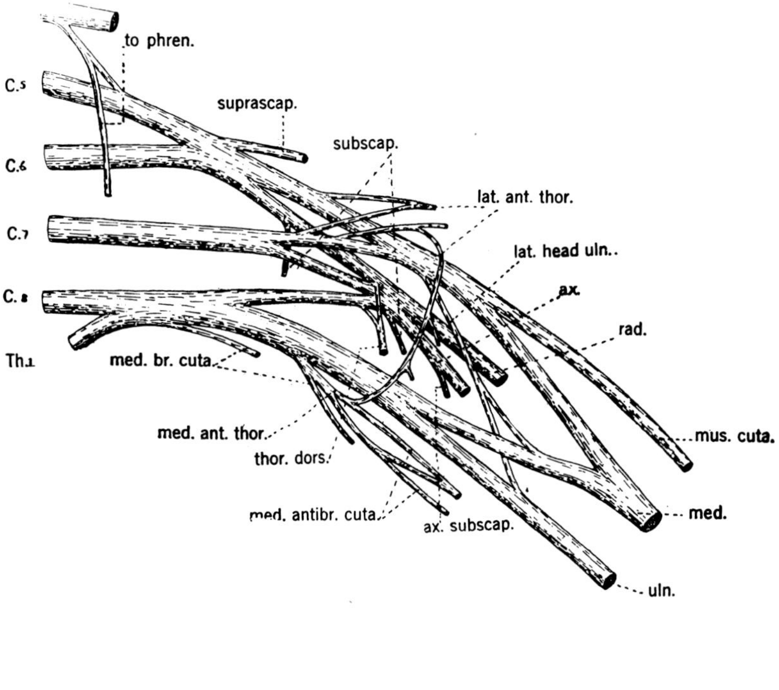

Fig. 1.2. Brachial plexus. (Reprinted from Kerr AT: The brachial plexus of nerves in man, the variations in its formation and its branches. Am J Anat 23:285, 1918.)

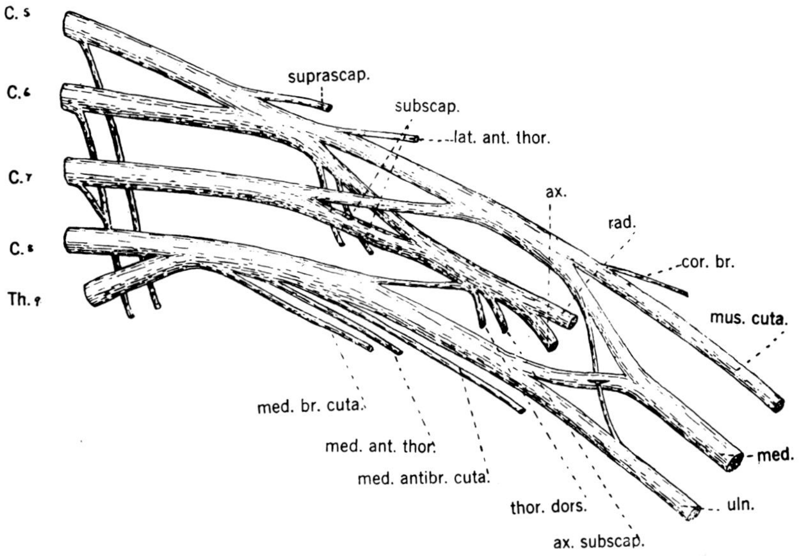

Fig. 1.3. Brachial plexus. (Reprinted from Kerr AT: The brachial plexus of nerves in man, the variations in its formation and its branches. Am J Anat 23:285, 1918.)

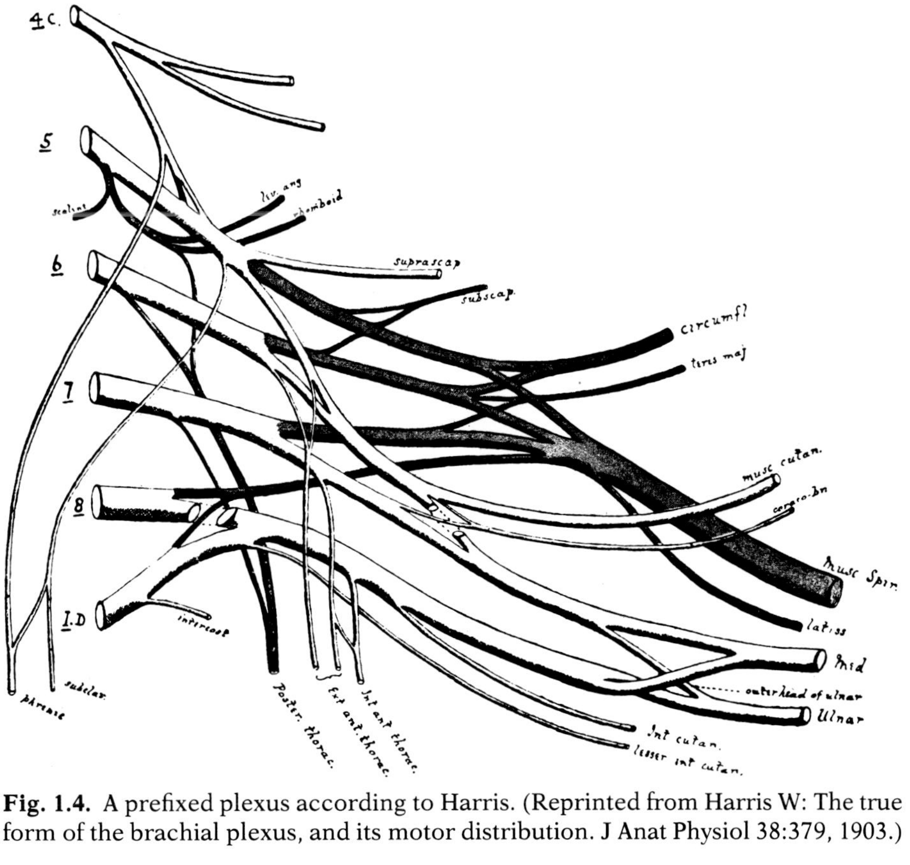

Fig. 1.4. A prefixed plexus according to Harris. (Reprinted from Harris W: The true form of the brachial plexus, and its motor distribution. J Anat Physiol 38:379, 1903.)

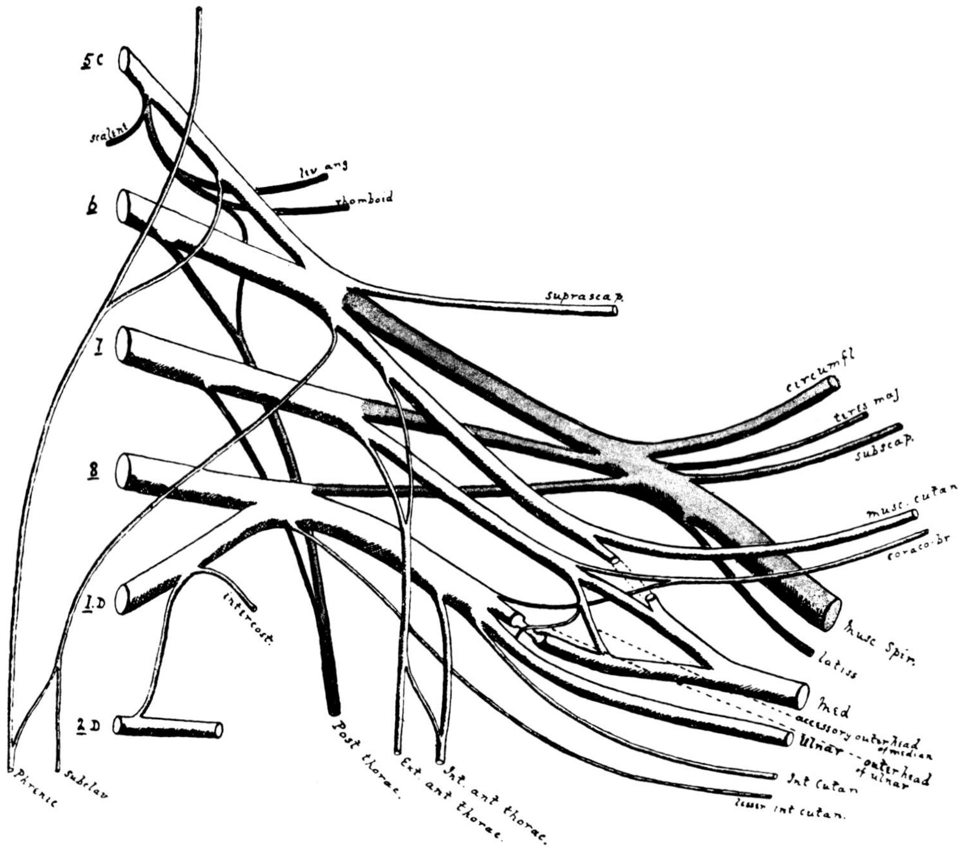

Fig. 1.5. A postfixed plexus according to Harris. (Reprinted from Harris W: The true form of the brachial plexus, and its motor distribution. J Anat Physiol 38:379, 1903.)

Where this question becomes of considerable significance is in the process of evaluating clinical cases of partial paralysis due to traction injury by indirect methods, particularly myelography and electromyography, and their correlation in calculations to determine root level of injury. Often these methods of evaluation fail to agree by one root level. It would appear, then, that functional axial shifts, rather than expansions or contractions, would better explain the discrepancies. It should be noted, however, that, at most, the difference between the high plexus and the low one is only one root, and since the number of cervical vertebrae is remarkably constant at seven, at least this facet of the anatomic picture is stable and predictable. Nevertheless, Kerr found in a series of 63 bilateral cadaver dissections that the brachial plexus was asymmetrical in 24 bodies.

The Problem of Defining the "True Form of the Brachial Plexus"

Before proceeding, it is most important that the reader gain insight into the difficulties involved in obtaining an accurate or uniform picture of the morphology of the human brachial plexus. Not only have the differences in what has been recorded as observed been widely debated, but they continue to serve as a source of frustration to the serious student of the subject.

In 1877 J. F. Walsh of Philadelphia,[33] in a masterful treatise on the plexus, bemoaned the tremendous variations to be found between one author's description and another's, commenting that what one characterized as the standard arrangement, the next would label an anomaly. He gave numerous examples of these discrepancies (Fig. 1.6A,B) and

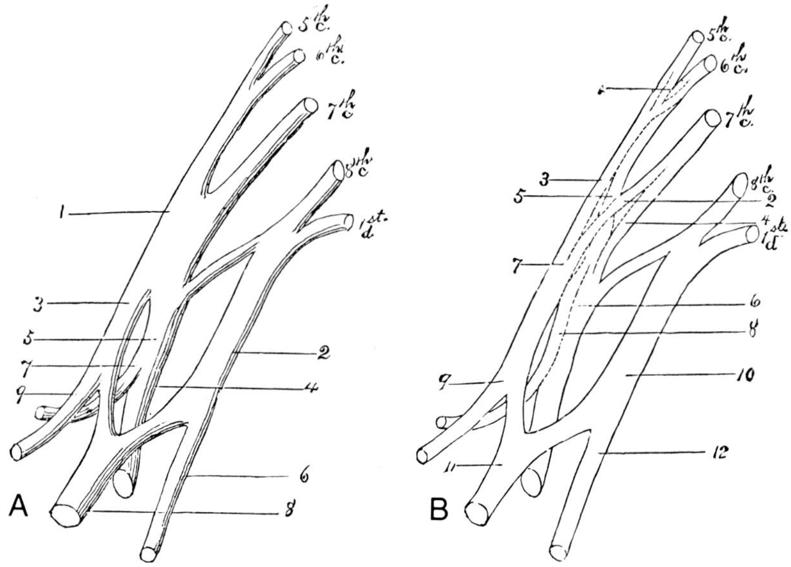

Fig. 1.6. A: An arrangement produced by leaving undisturbed the enveloping fascia in the upper portion of the plexus. (Reprinted from Walsh JF: The anatomy of the brachial plexus. Am J Med Sci 74:387, 1877.)

1. Apparently a common trunk formed by the fifth, sixth, and seventh cervicals and a branch from the eighth cervical and first dorsal
2. Inner cord
3. Outer cord
4. Musculospiral (radial) nerve
5. Apparently a trunk common to circumflex (axillary) and musculospiral (radial) nerves
6. Ulnar nerve
7. Circumflex nerve (axillary)
8. Median nerve
9. Musculocutaneous nerve

B: The same plexus, showing the arrangement of the nerves within the envelope of fascia

1. Union of fifth and sixth cervicals
2. Superior division of seventh cervical
3. Anterior division of fifth and sixth cervicals
4. Inferior division of fifth and sixth cervicals
5. Posterior division of fifth and sixth cervicals
6. Musculospiral nerve
7. Outer cord
8. Circumflex nerve
9. Musculocutaneous nerve
10. Inner cord
11. Median nerve
12. Ulnar nerve

then, based on 350 personally observed or performed dissections, presented what he considered to be the most usual arrangement (Fig. 1.7). The many variations cited by other authors he considered to be usually artificially produced either by inadequate removal of enveloping fascia or by overzealous division of the nerves to produce spurious separate branches when none existed.

Twenty-seven years later, in 1904, Wilfred Harris wrote "The True Form of the Brachial Plexus, and Its Motor Distribution,"[13] again describing the difficulties of achieving an accurate picture (but then claiming to have so done). His particular focus was motor distribution, and he criticized the work of Sherrington[26] in 1898 and Ferrier and Yeo[8] in 1881. They had attempted to apply the results of experimental stimulation and division of the spinal roots of monkeys to the human brachial plexus. In this objection he was correct, since they are not identical. Although he did not have the opportunity to perform a series of experimental stimulations of the human plexus, he did record the results of stimulation of the nerves of several patients with brachial plexus injuries. His treatise is remarkably clear and well worth reading.

Abram Kerr's[20] study of the brachial plexus,

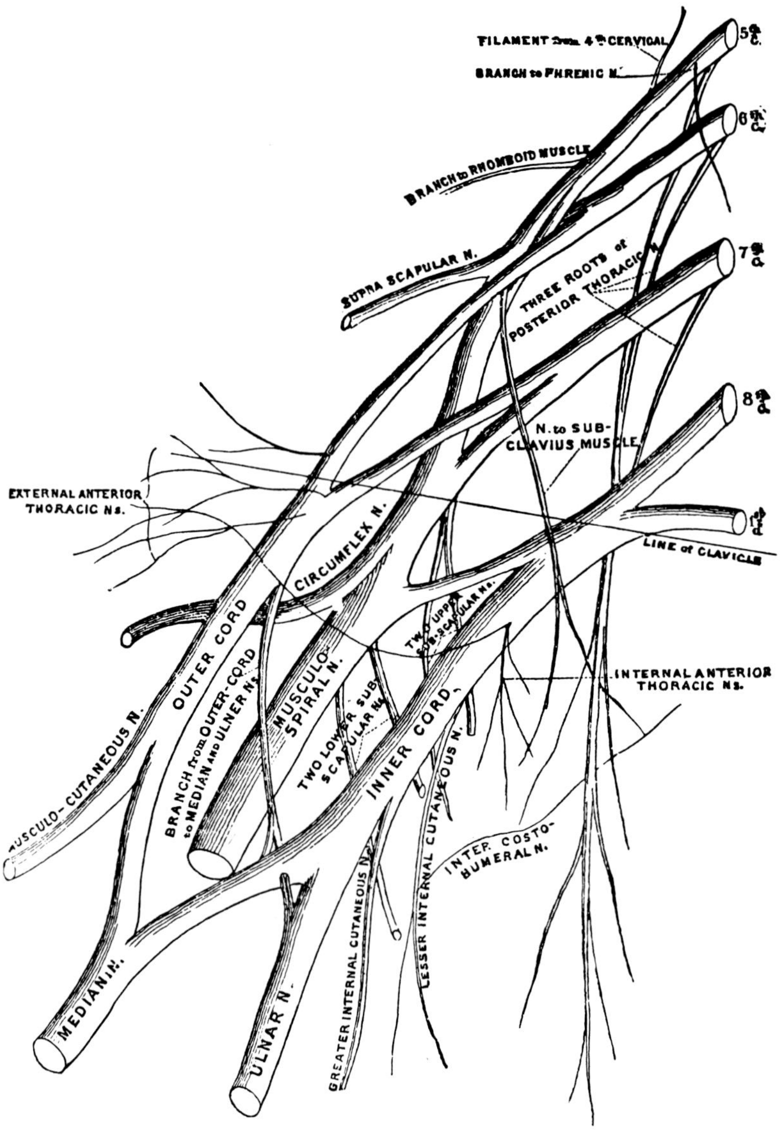

Fig. 1.7. The anatomy of the brachial plexus in its most usual form. (Reprinted from Walsh JF: The anatomy of the brachial plexus. Am J Med Sci 74:387, 1877.)

published in 1918, although a masterpiece of observation and often quoted for its excellent detail, illustrates some of the significant difficulties encountered in attempting a "true picture" of the anatomy of the plexus. It is based on records of dissections from the anatomic laboratories of Johns Hopkins and Cornell medical schools done by medical students from 1895 to 1910. The dissections were supervised by instructors who also checked the accuracy of the records and drawings. Although between 400 and 500 records were preserved, only 175 were selected by the author as having absolute scientific accuracy, and these served as the basis of the report. The cephalic limit of the plexus was verified in all cases, but the caudal portion, if it extended to T2, often was not verified because this root would have been exposed by the dissector of the chest, who was usually different from the student displaying the upper extremity. A number of maceration specimens (Fig. 1.8) were done using nitric acid technique, and these showed the complex way in which the nerve bundles interface and join, and how difficult it is to trace the bundles even without the epineurium. Kerr concluded that the fibers of a given spinal nerve can rarely be traced

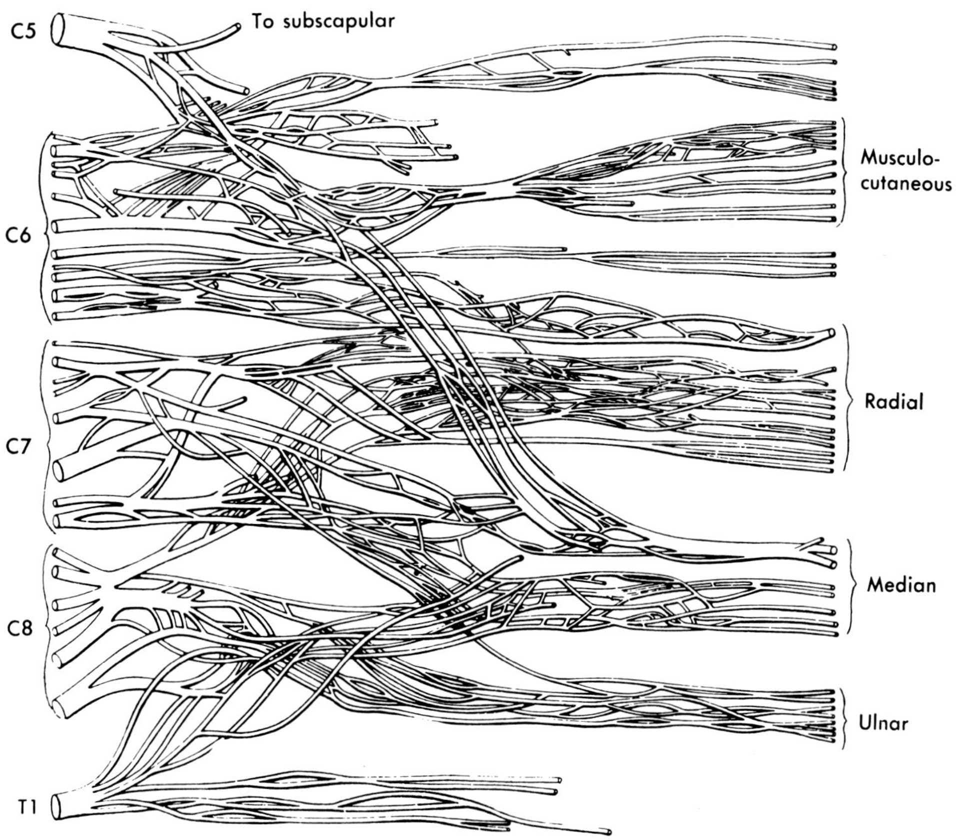

Fig. 1.8. A maceration specimen of the brachial plexus. (From Kerr AT: The brachial plexus of nerves in man, the variations in its formation and its branches. Am J Anat 23:285, 1918.)

by anatomic methods through the plexus to their ultimate destination. In only 6.28% of the 175 plexuses did Kerr find a real anomaly in the formation of the cords. Walsh[33] had reported an anomalous plexus in only 2 of 350 dissections.

The problems thus enumerated have not been solved to this day. Rather than being of purely academic interest, they assume new importance for the surgeon contemplating direct reconstruction of the nerves by suture or graft. The variations relative to the subclavian and axillary arteries must also be understood, not only because they influence segmental innervation, but because they also impose a hazard in dissection during surgery. The work of Ruth Miller,[24] which will be discussed at the end of this chapter, is the basis for our understanding of this facet of the problem. The most difficult area, intraneural topography, has been approached by many authors, most recently by Alnot and Huten[2] and Narakas,[25] some of whose maps of roots of the plexus are reproduced here (Fig. 1.9). Further investigation is necessary, so that not only must we be able to delineate the components of the plexus in the cadaver or anatomical specimen, but also intraneural topography in the living patient at the operating table. Histochemical techniques defining motor from sensory fibers are available, and have been employed by Engel[7] and others at the time of neurorrhaphy in the peripheral nerves. Narakas[25] has pointed out that, although knowledge of intraneural topography is helpful at the time of plexus reconstruction, there is no "universal map" that can be applied to all patients, thus limiting its duplication.

The modern techniques of electrodiagnosis have evolved considerably from the primitive electrical stimulation of the nineteenth century, so that today,

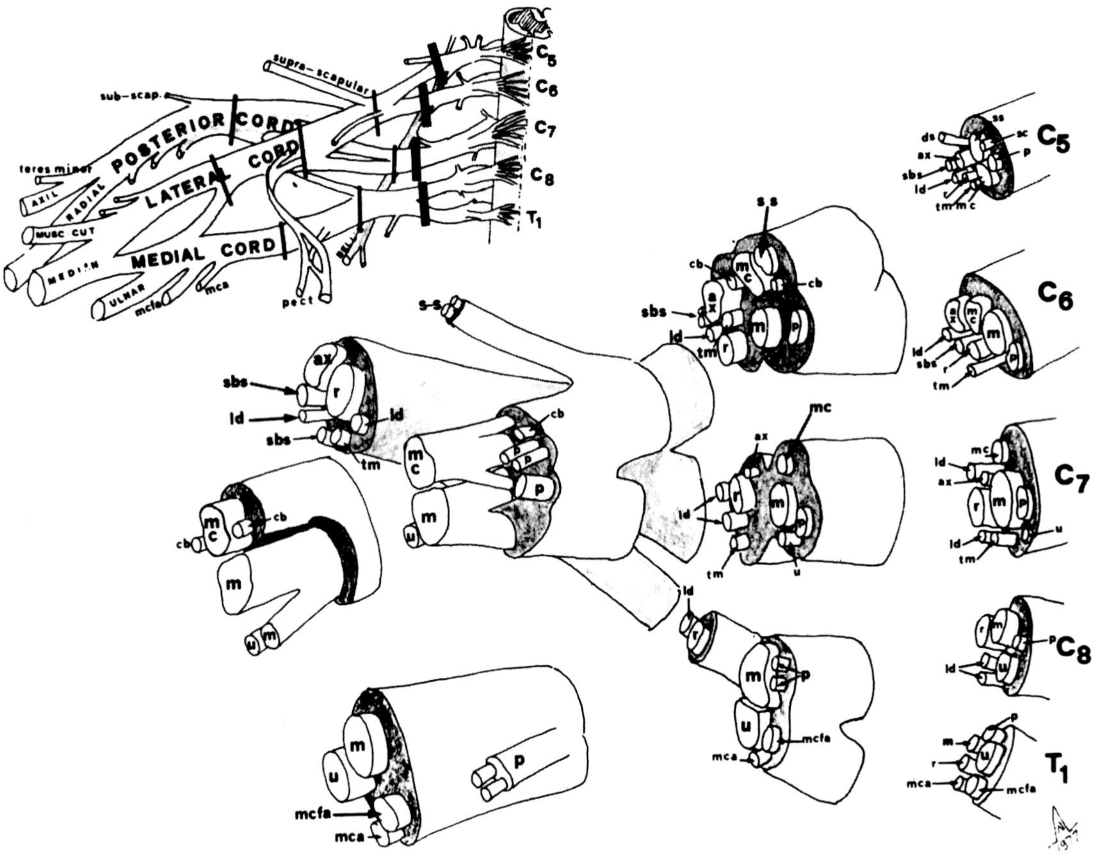

Fig. 1.9. Intraneural topography of the brachial plexus. (Reproduced from Narakas AO: Surgical treatment of traction injuries of the brachial plexus. Clin Orthop 133:71, 1978, with permission.)

electromyography, evoked potentials, and specific refinements of root stimulation hold great promise.[4] These sophisticated procedures can be used intraoperatively, and experience with them has been described by Kline and Judice.[21] Further intensive work is needed in this area to develop the capability and specific resolution of these techniques so that they may be used with confidence to solve anatomic problems in a patient undergoing reconstruction of the plexus. An encouraging report of this type has been published by Landi et al.[22]

THE CERVICAL NERVE ROOTS AND THEIR CONTRIBUTION TO THE BRACHIAL PLEXUS

In order to understand the brachial plexus under normal and pathological conditions, it is necessary to consider a typical spinal nerve and its relationship to the meninges and the intervertebral foramen. Where specific and important individual differences exist between the various levels, these will be described.

The typical spinal nerve root, as depicted in Figure 1.10, results from the confluence of the ventral nerve rootlets originating in the anterior horn cells of the spinal cord and the dorsal nerve rootlets which join the spinal ganglion in the region of the intervertebral foramen. Bowden, Abdullah, and Gooding[3] have shown that there is no clear-cut demarcation between segments of the cord. The posterior rootlets are more irregularly arranged. In addition, there may be communications between bundles of adjacent segmental nerves. Figures 1.11 and 1.12 illustrate the differences in the rootlets. Each nerve root consists of a number of rootlets gathered into a smaller number of bundles which pass through the dorsal and ventral foramina in the dura. The posterior root-

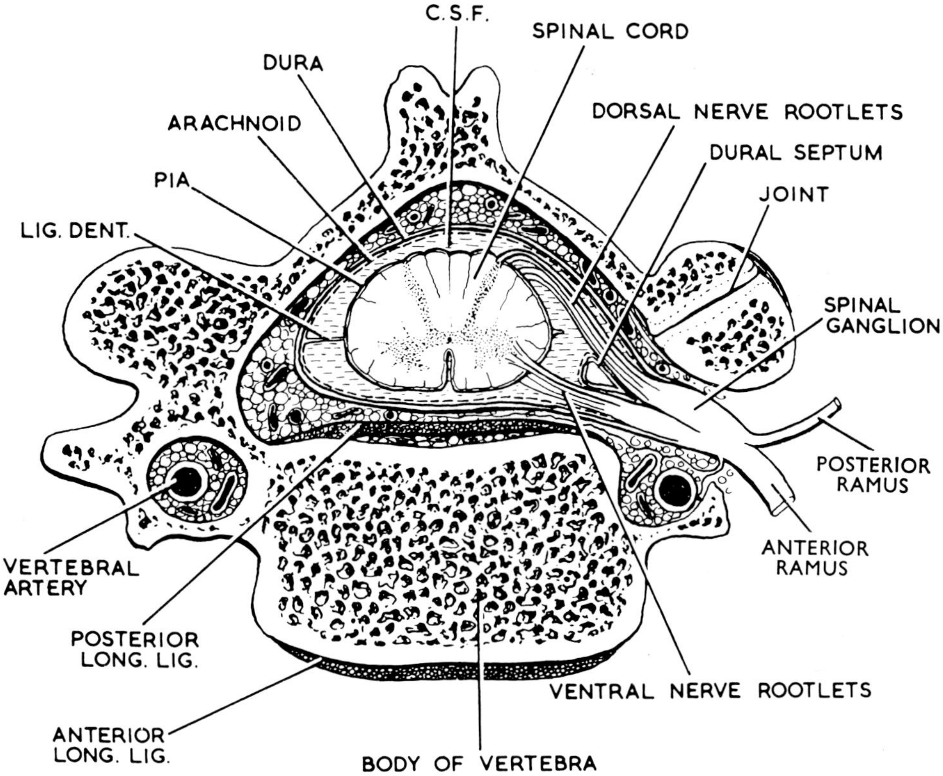

Fig. 1.10. A diagrammatic spinal root and its anatomic relations as shown by an oblique section through a cervical vertebra, membranes, and spinal cord. (Reproduced from Bowden REM, Abdullah S, Gooding MR: Anatomy of the cervical spine, membranes, spinal cord, nerve roots, and brachial plexus. In Lord Brain, Wilkinson M (eds): Cervical Spondylosis and Other Disorders of the Cervical Spine. W.B. Saunders, Philadelphia, 1976.)

lets are more numerous than the anterior, and so a posterior root is thicker than the corresponding anterior root by a factor of about 3 in the cervical region.

It is important to understand that, despite the common designation of both the intraspinal portions of the nerve root complex, which extend to the level of the foramina, and the extraspinal segments that form the trunks, as "roots," these two structures should be differentiated. The latter are really spinal nerves rather than roots, which are intraspinal, and the reason for making this definition will be elaborated upon when the meningeal envelope of the nerve root complex is discussed. Briefly, ventral and dorsal intraspinal nerve roots, which are condensations of their respective rootlets, lack the intimate contact of the meninges, and consequently do not have the protection against traction elongation that the perineurium of the more peripheral spinal nerves possess. It is this anatomic feature that makes them vulnerable to avulsion at the level of the spinal cord.

The position of the dorsal nerve root ganglion in relation to the intervertebral foramina has been studied by Abdullah[1] and is shown in Table 1.1.

The position of the nerve root complexes in the intervertebral foramina may vary according to their level.[28] Usually they pass through the dura in their meningeal sleeves opposite the corresponding foramen, giving them a central position. In the lower cervical and upper thoracic regions the nerve roots commonly descend intradurally to a level that may be as much as 8 mm below the foramen, but they then angle up and over the lower margin of the foramen as they proceed outward (Fig. 1.13). The position of the complex in the foramen changes with the

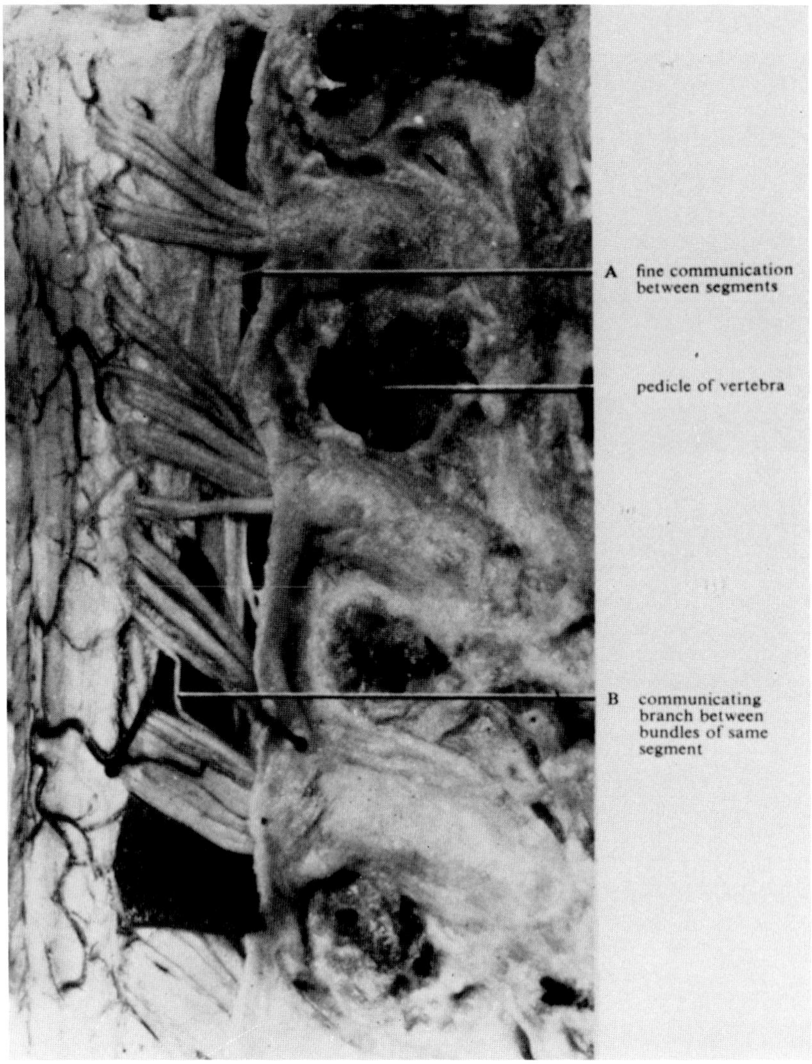

Fig. 1.11. Left side of cervical spinal cord showing orderly continuous series of posterior rootlets of spinal nerve. (Reproduced from Bowden REM, Abdullah S, Gooding MR: Anatomy of the cervical spine, membranes, spinal cord, nerve roots, and brachial plexus. In Lord Brain, Wilkinson M (eds): Cervical Spondylosis and Other Disorders of the Cervical Spine. Saunders, Philadelphia, 1967.)

Table 1.1. Position of Dorsal Root Ganglia in Relation to the Intervertebral Foramina (IVF)

Position at IVF	C3	C4	C5	C6	C7	C8	T1	Total
Mainly within IVF	4	10	8	4	2	—	—	28
Half inside and half outside	—	—	2	6	7	5	2	22
Mainly outside	—	—	—	—	1	5	8	14

From Bowden REM, Abdullah S, Gooding MR: Anatomy of the cervical spine, membranes, spinal cord, nerve roots and brachial plexus. In Lord Brain, Wilkinson M (eds): Cervical Spondylosis and Other Disorders of the Cervical Spine. Saunders, Philadelphia, 1967.

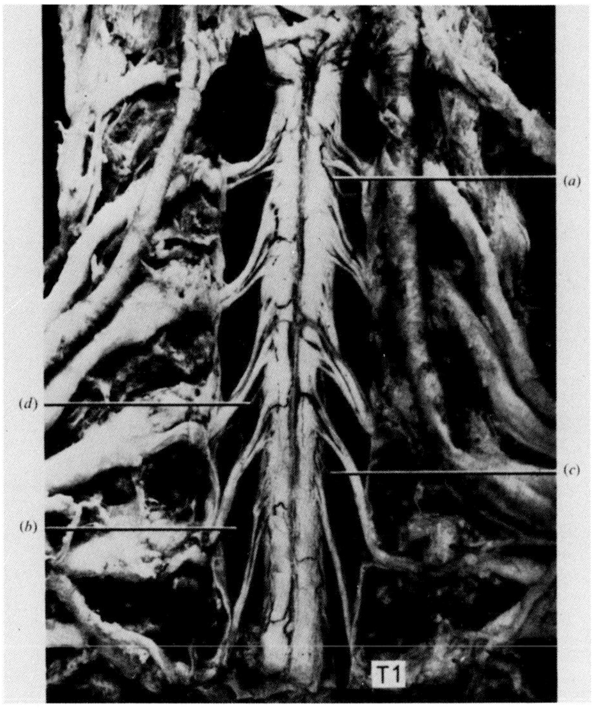

Fig. 1.12. Anterior view of roots of the brachial plexus show intersegmental communication; a, b, c, d indicate intersegmental communications. (Reproduced from Bowden REM, Abdullah S, Gooding MR: Anatomy of the cervical spine, membranes, spinal cord, nerve roots and brachial plexus. In Lord Brain, Wilkinson M (eds): Cervical Spondylosis and Other Disorders of the Cervical Spine. Saunders, Philadelphia, 1967.)

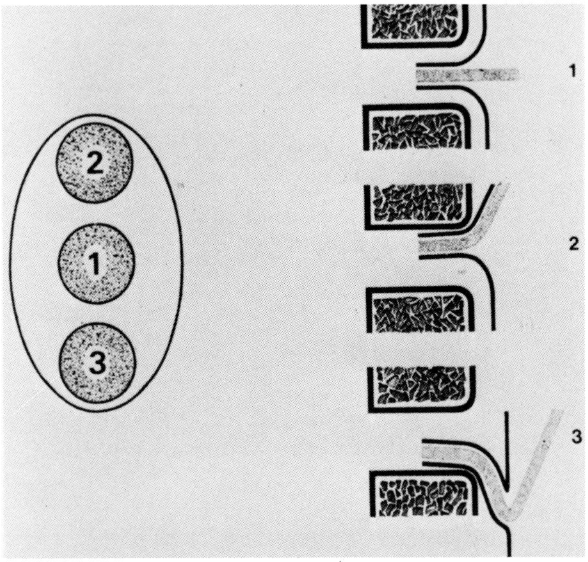

Fig. 1.13. Variations in the position occupied by the nerve complex in the foramen. (Reproduced from Sunderland S: Nerves and Nerve Injuries. 2nd Ed. Churchill Livingstone, Edinburgh, 1978, with permission.)

movements of the head and neck, and the foramina themselves are narrowed by hyperextension, lateral flexion, and rotation of the cervical spine, while forward flexion enlarges them. The spinal nerves, as they emerge from the intervertebral foramina, receive gray rami communicantes from the sympathetic ganglia[27] (Fig. 1.14). Although the first four cervical nerves receive their rami from the superior cervical ganglion, the fifth and sixth are supplied by the middle, and the seventh and eighth cervical nerves from the inferior cervical ganglion. The first ten thoracic nerves receive gray rami from the corresponding ganglia. Each spinal nerve usually receives two or three sympathetic gray rami, which join it just distal to the union between the dorsal and ventral roots.

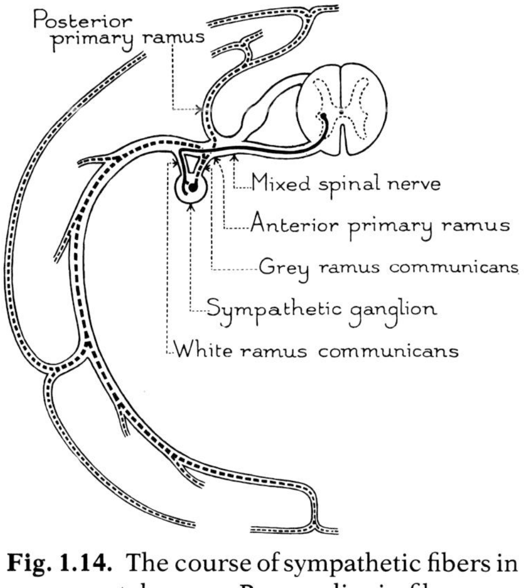

Fig. 1.14. The course of sympathetic fibers in a segmental nerve. Preganglionic fibers are indicated by solid line, postganglionic by broken lines. (Reproduced from Haymaker W, Woodhall B: Peripheral Nerve Injuries. 2nd Ed. Saunders, Philadelphia, 1956, with permission.)

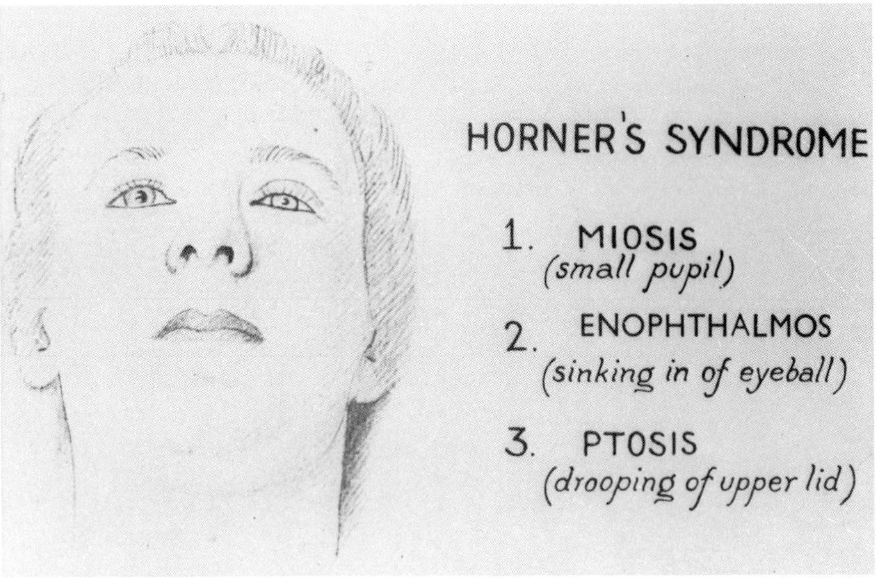

Fig. 1.15. Horner's syndrome.

The white rami communicantes are the branches of the spinal nerve through which the preganglionic fibers from the spinal cord reach the sympathetic chain. They arise from the upper ten segments. The outflow from the head and neck comes from the upper two thoracic segments. The upper limb has an extensive supply, but usually the first thoracic segment does not contribute to it.

The distribution of preganglionic fibers provide a valuable sign in severe traction injuries to the brachial plexus. If the patient has Horner's syndrome (Fig. 1.15) accompanying sensorimotor paralysis of the outflow of the lower roots of the plexus, most likely there is either avulsion of the T1 root or severe traction injury close to the cord, since these preganglionic fibers leave the ventral primary divisions of the spinal nerve soon after they emerge from the intervertebral foramen.

A small meningeal branch is given off by each spinal nerve immediately after its emergence from the foramen. This branch reenters the vertebral canal.

The typical spinal nerve terminates by splitting into two primary divisions, a ventral and a dorsal, immediately after the two roots join. Both divisions receive fibers from both roots.

Figure 1.16 shows in cross section the transition of the nerve roots to peripheral roots and from there to peripheral nerves as well as the attachment of the nerve complex to bone.

The dorsal primary divisions, after they arise from the spinal nerves, are directed dorsad, and then divide into medial and lateral branches to supply the muscles and the skin on the dorsal part of the neck. The segmental arrangement of the innervation of the third and fourth layers of erector spinae musculature has been employed by Bufalini and Pescatori[4] to electromyographically identify the presence of a supraganglionic rupture or avulsion of the spinal root. This test is discussed in Chapter 4.

It is the ventral primary divisions that supply the outflow to the limb plexuses. They are larger than the dorsal divisions, and those of the fifth to eighth cervical and the first thoracic nerves are the origin of the brachial plexus and the nerve supply to the upper limb.

The Meningeal Components of the Spinal Nerve Root Complex

In this section we shall discuss the meningeal components of the spinal nerve root complex.[3,9,10,28] Figure 1.10 illustrates an oblique section through a cervical vertebra, meninges, spinal cord, and nerve roots. The extradural space, within the bony canal, is filled with soft fat through which the vertebral vein plexus ramifies. The dura, the outermost layer of me-

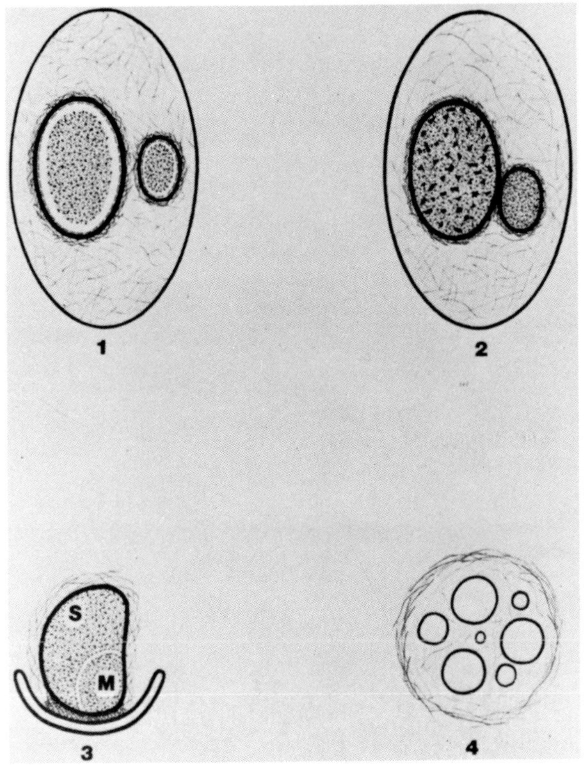

Fig. 1.16. Successive cross sections showing transition from nerve roots (1) to peripheral nerves (4). The only attachment of the nerve complex to bone is in the cervical region where the spinal nerve is adherent to the gutter of the transverse process (3). S = sensory fibers; M = motor fibers. (Reproduced from Sunderland S: Nerves and Nerve Injuries. 2nd Ed. Churchill Livingstone, Edinburgh, 1978, with permission.)

ninges, is a tough and relatively inelastic membrane that extends down from the meningeal layer of the posterior cranial fossa and is tethered above to the margin of the foramen magnum. It is also adherent anteriorly to the posterior longitudinal ligament behind the upper two vertebrae, and below this it is attached to the ligament in the midline. Posteriorly the dural sac lies free in the epidural space, and laterally the paired root sleeves exit through the intervertebral foramina, where they envelop the dorsal ganglia and anterior roots and form an outer fibrous sheath for these structures. This sheath becomes the perineurium, while a condensed layer of epidural tissue is continuous with the epineurium of the spinal nerve (Fig. 1.17). A septum of dura actually forms two separate sleeves proximal to the dorsal root ganglia, but these merge into a single sleeve distal to it. The position of the union may vary considerably, as reported by Abdullah, whose studies in this area have been extremely valuable.

The arachnoid lies within the dura and may be likened to a tube within an automobile tire. It contains more elastic fibers, and it is separated from the dura by a potential space. The pia consists of two fused layers. Between the dorsal and ventral roots, it forms the dentate ligaments, which are attached in continuous lines along the spinal cord.

FACTORS INFLUENCING THE SUSCEPTIBILITY TO TRACTION DEFORMATION OF THE SPINAL NERVE ROOTS

Sir Sidney Sunderland's[28–31] analysis of the factors that influence susceptibility to traction deformation of spinal nerve roots has related specific anatomy to potential traumatic pathology in a manner

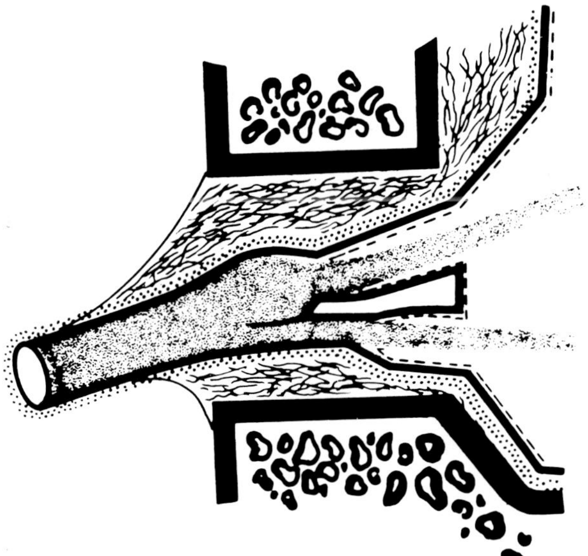

Fig. 1.17. Diagram, not to scale, of meningeal–neural relations in the intervertebral foramen: —, dura becoming the perineurium; ---, arachnoid; · · ·, relative condensation of epidural connective tissue on the external surface of the dura which laterally is continuous with the epineurium of the spinal nerve. (Reproduced from Sunderland S: Nerves and Nerve Injuries. 2nd Ed. Churchill Livingstone, Edinburgh, 1978, with permission.)

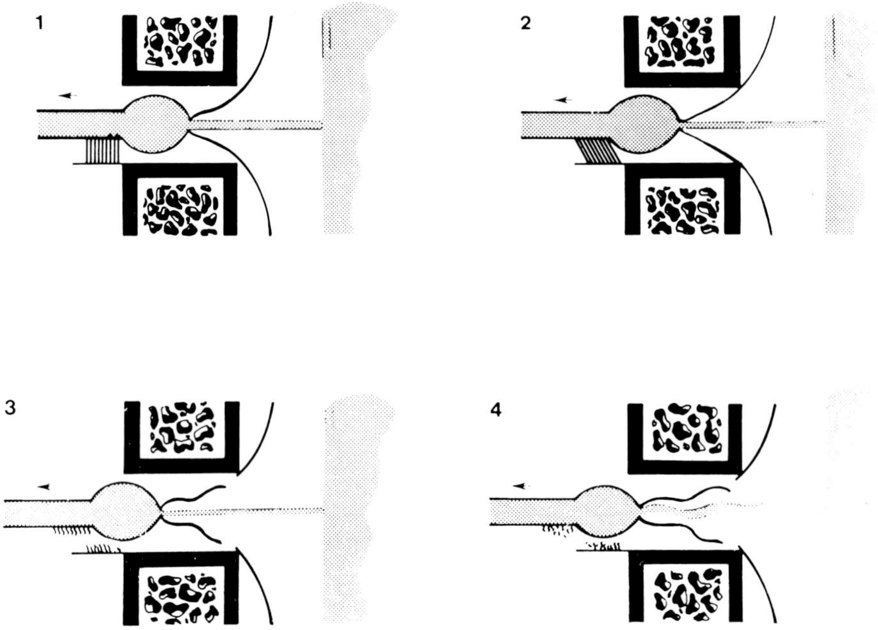

Fig. 1.18. The changes leading to avulsion of nerve roots caused by lateral traction on the spinal nerve. (Reproduced from Sunderland S: Nerves and Nerve Injuries. 2nd Ed. Churchill Livingstone, Edinburgh, 1978, with permission.)

that is fundamental to the understanding of traction injuries of the brachial plexus.

The general configuration of the meninges has already been described. The nerve roots are seen to carry continuations of the various meningeal layers as they exit their respective foramina to become spinal nerves. The subarachnoid space is continued along the nerve root as far as the sensory ganglion and extends farther distally along the posterior than along the anterior root, but not as far as the level of the spinal nerve. The nerve root complexes are actually free to move within the intervertebral foramina, since they are not attached here. As lateral movement in response to traction on the nerves occurs, the local dura and arachnoid are deformed into a funnel shape, the neck of the funnel around the nerve exerting a plugging action as it is pulled into the bony intervertebral foramen.[9] Additional protection against lateral displacement is conveyed by fibrous attachments of the spinal nerves to the cervical transverse processes (Fig. 1.18). The fourth, fifth, sixth, and seventh cervical nerves are securely attached to the vertebral column within the gutters of the transverse processes by epineural sheath, prevertebral fascia, and fibrous slips extending from the transverse process above to the epineurium of the nerve below. In addition, the vertebral artery adventitia blends with the sheath of the nerve. C8 and T1 do not have these additional attachments. This anatomical arrangement explains why the incidence of avulsion injury is much higher in the lower two roots, since they are anatomically predisposed.

The significance of the length of the individual nerve roots is of more than academic interest, since, in general, the shorter the nerve root, the less traction elongation it will tolerate before failure. The cervical spinal nerve roots are relatively short, compared to those further caudad. They have been measured by several authors, and the results differ considerably, among other reasons, according to whether the measurements were made along the upper or lower border of the root.

Table 1.2 is a summary of nerve root length, from Sunderland.

Clinically it is not uncommon, following traction injury, to observe greater motor loss than sensory. This can be explained by the greater resistance of the posterior roots to the effects of trauma, due to several factors. First, the posterior roots are thicker than the anterior. Second, traction on the anterior root is transmitted directly to the spinal cord and anterior horn cell, whereas the interposition of the sensory ganglion on the posterior root allows some additional diffusion of stresses. Finally, the manner in which the rootlets arise from the cord predisposes the anterior rootlets more than the sensory rootlets

Table 1.2. Nerve Root Length in Millimeters

Nerve Root	Testut and Latarjet 1949	Soulie 1899	Hovelacque 1927	Sunderland 1976 Upper/Lower
C3	18	16	10	—
C4	—	18	9	10/8
C5	26	20	10	15/11
C6	—	23	11	15/11
C7	—	25	11	15/11
C8	—	27	14	17/12
T1	33	29	16	25/17

From Sunderland S: Nerves and Nerve Injuries. 2nd Ed. Churchill Livingstone, Edinburgh, 1978, with permission.

to mechanical failure because the latter are generally evenly distributed, while the motor roots are more widely separated.

THE BLOOD SUPPLY OF THE BRACHIAL PLEXUS

The anterior blood supply of the cervical spinal roots and brachial plexus is based largely on the subclavian artery and its branches, with rich anastomoses to the longitudinal vessels of the cord that assure adequate vascularization under most conditions. The vertebral artery, which usually arises from the first part of the subclavian artery, may vary in its origin, symmetry, and path. However, the investigations of Abdullah, Bowden, and Gooding[1,3,11] have demonstrated that it has a major role in supplying the plexus. As the vertebral artery crosses the emergent nerves, it gives off inconstant branches at multiple levels. The anterior branches supply prevertebral and scalene muscles but may also send twigs to nerves and ganglia. The medial branches, which enter the intervertebral foramina, supply the ganglia and roots and anastomose with the longitudinal vessels on the cord. Small posterior branches supply the ganglia. The lateral branches, which also supply the ganglia and spinal nerves, anastomose with spinal branches of the ascending cervical, deep cervical, and superior intercostal arteries. Figure 1.19, taken from the work of Abdullah,[1] illustrates the pattern of arterial supply.

GENERAL CONFIGURATION AND RELATIONS OF THE BRACHIAL PLEXUS

The general shape of the plexus has been depicted by Hovelacque[17] and others as consisting of two triangles joined at their apices. The larger, located in the neck, has as its base the vertebral column; one leg is directed down and laterally, while the other, inferior, corresponds to the thoracic outlet and dome of the pleura. The smaller triangle, also with its apex behind the clavicle, is located within the axilla, where its base corresponds to the terminal branches of the plexus. It should be noted, however, that even at root level, all portions of the plexus are not in the same frontal plane; because of the normal lordosis of the cervical spine, C5 and C6 are actually anterior to C8 and T1, located behind the clavicle. Failure to appreciate these relationships can make dissection in a plexus scarred by traction injury virtually impossible.

Although numerous variations in the formation of the plexus have been reported, the following common schema can be taken as a point of departure: the anterior primary ramus of C5 joins that of C6 to form the upper trunk, while C8 joins T1 in similar fashion to form the lower trunk. C7 continues between the two to constitute the intermediate or middle trunk. Each of these trunks then splits into an anterior and a posterior division. The anterior division of the upper and middle trunks unite to form the lateral cord, which gives off the lateral root of the median nerve and the musculocutaneous nerve. The anterior division of the lower trunk forms the medial cord, which gives rise to the medial root of the median nerve, the ulnar nerve, and both the medial cutaneous nerve of the arm and forearm. The posterior division of the three trunks of this "classic plexus" unites to form the posterior cord, which ultimately provides the radial, axillary, and subscapular nerves (Fig. 1.1).

The relations of the C5, C6, and C7 roots share the following features: as they emerge from the intervertebral foramina and give off their posterior primary rami, they lie in bony troughs of the transverse processes between the vertically oriented intertrans-

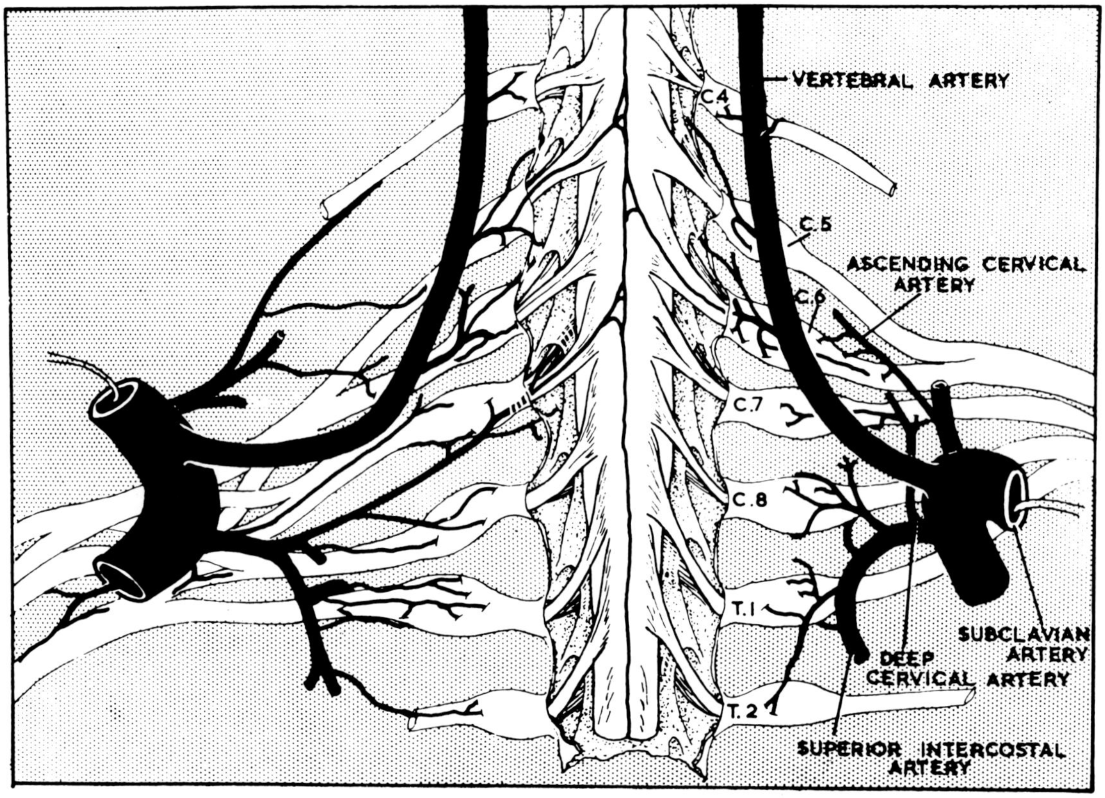

Fig. 1.19. The arterial supply of the brachial plexus. Note anastomosis with the anterior spinal artery. (Reproduced from Abdullah S, Bowden REM: The blood supply of the brachial plexus. Proc R Soc Med 53:203, 1960, with permission.)

versalis muscles. The vertebral artery is located within the foramina transversaria anteromedially (Fig. 1.20). As the now anterior primary rami incline forward and down, they emerge between the anterior and middle scalenes (Fig. 1.21), but C5 and C6 may actually run through the anterior scalene. They then join on the surface of the middle scalene at what has been called "Erb's point," which is located 2–3 cm above the clavicle, covered by the posterior edge of the sternomastoid muscle when the head is facing forward. If C4 is to join C5, it does so proximal to this point.

The two inferior roots occupy a retroclavicular position in a space bounded by the pleura inferiorly, the first two ribs posteriorly, the scalenus minimus or transversopleural ligaments laterally, and the vertebropleural ligaments medially. C8 anterior primary ramus crosses obliquely and down over the neck of the first rib with the inferior cervical or stellate ganglion in front. Then, as it crosses the pleura, it lies between the scalenus posterior and the transversopleural muscle to join the anterior primary ramus of the first thoracic nerve root on the inner border of the first rib. T1 comes from beneath the neck of the first rib through a hiatus in the suprapleural membrane. The rib is thus between the two roots at its neck, and when they join, the lower trunk runs over the surface of the rib more anteriorly. The branch from T2, if present, is usually small, and may join the T1 in a variable fashion. The inferior or lower trunk, as it traverses the surface of the first rib, occupies the interval between the anterior and middle scalene with the subclavian artery anterior to it. Often the two structures are in contact, but they may be separated by as much as 1.5 cm, with either being at a higher or lower level. The lower trunk may actually not be in contact with the bone because of the intervention of the middle scalene muscle attachment. Also, the first

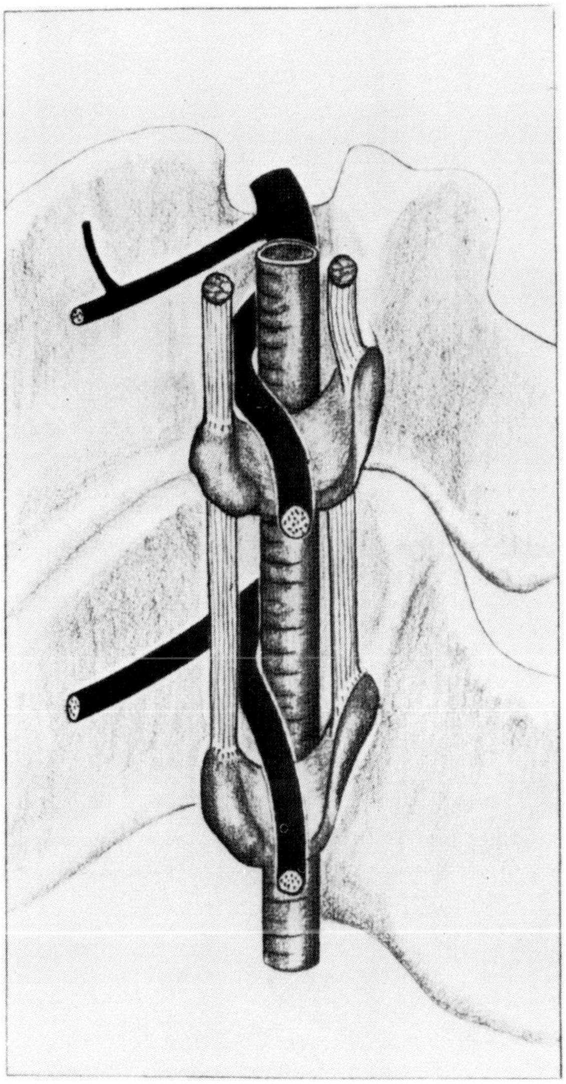

Fig. 1.20. The relationship between the cervical spine nerves, the transverse processes, and the vertebral artery. (Reproduced from Sunderland S: Nerves and Nerve Injuries. 2nd Ed. Churchill Livingstone, Edinburgh, 1978, with permission.)

rib is not usually oriented horizontally, and may be inclined as much as 45 degrees caudally, thus effecting the relationships of the nerves and artery.

The omohyoid muscle (Fig. 1.22), which crosses the plexus just above the clavicle, is a useful reference point which divides the posterior triangle of the neck into two unequal triangles. The upper and larger of the two, the omotrapezial, contains the upper and middle trunks and their divisions, while the lower and smaller omoclavicular triangle and area behind the clavicle conceal the lower trunk and subclavian vessels. The other structure providing ready reference is the external jugular vein, running longitudinally, superficial to the sternocleidomastoid muscle toward its lateral border, and in the line of the upper trunk. In most individuals, the external jugular vein may be observed through the skin. It is covered by the platysma muscle, which is embedded in the deeper layers of the superficial fascia, separated from the deep fascia by a distinct cleft that facilitates the action of the muscle and gives the skin greater mobility. The vein is actually located immediately subjacent in the superficial surface of the investing or deep fascia. This same fascia splits to invest the sternomastoid and trapezius muscles and covers the posterior triangle of the neck as a single sheet. When the lateral border of the sternomastoid is retracted medially to reveal the interscalene interval and the plexus, the latter is covered by a deep or prevertebral layer of deep cervical fascia that encloses the nerves as they emerge from between the scalenes. This distinct fascial layer also covers the subclavian artery and vein as the neurovascular bundle runs under the clavicle, where it is then appreciated as the axillary sheath. The external jugular vein must traverse both layers of deep cervical fascia as it occupies the angle between the sternomastoid and the clavicle on its way to terminate in the subclavian vein.

Two arterial branches, which may both arise from the thyrocervical trunk, traverse the plexus as they cross the posterior triangle of the neck (Fig. 1.23). The higher of these, the transverse cervical, is at the level of the upper and middle trunks, while the more inferior, the suprascapular, relates more to the middle trunk just above the level of the clavicle and behind it as it goes laterally and posteriorly to reach the supraspinous fossa of the scapula.

The divisions of the plexus ramify behind the clavicle, and then the cords surround the axillary artery within the axilla. This space is actually pyramidal in shape, apex superior. Medially, there is the first rib overlaid by the upper digitations of the serratus anterior.

The posterior wall is formed from above down by the subscapularis, teres major, and latissimus dorsi, with the last accounting for the greater part of the lower border. The teres major forms the most lateral part of this lower border. The anterior wall of

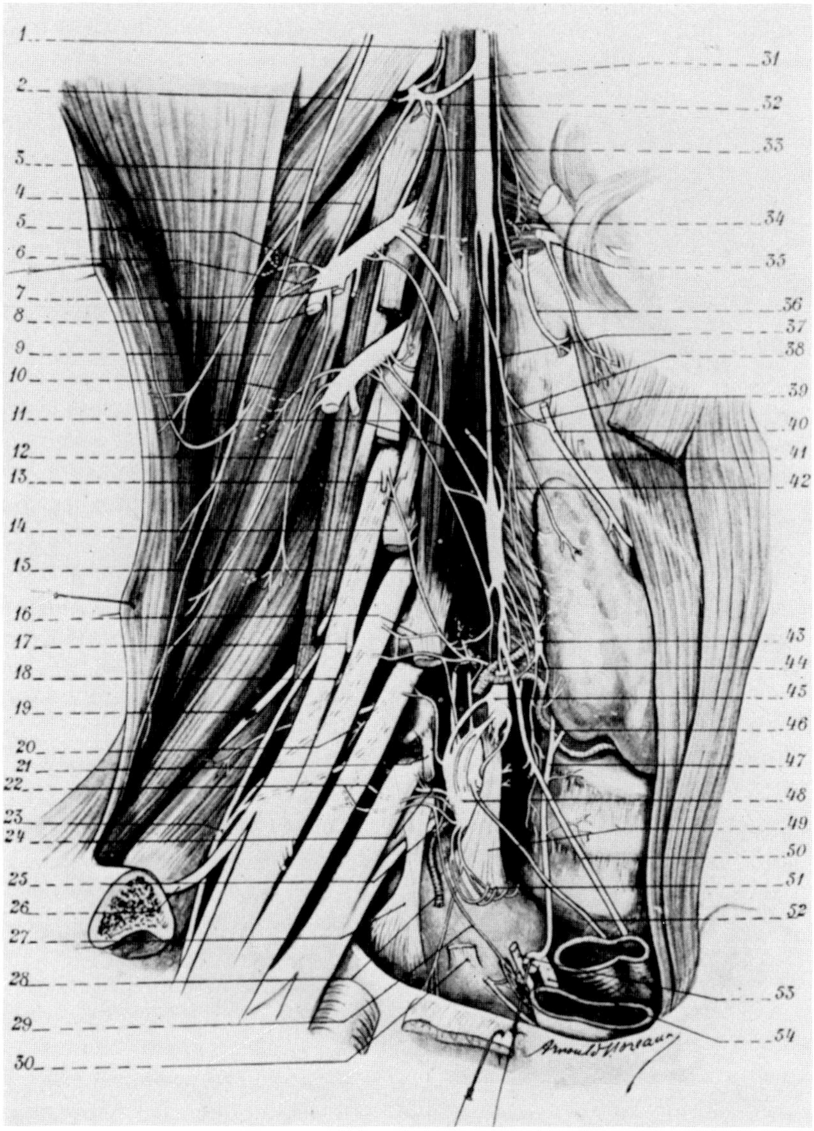

Fig. 1.21. The relationship between the cervical plexus, brachial plexus, and cervical sympathetics. (Reproduced from Hovelacque A: Anatomie des nerfs craniens et rachidiens et du système grand sympathique. Doin, Paris, 1927.)

1. Ansa
2. Nerve to sternomastoid
3. External branch of spinal accessory nerve
4. Juncture of C2 and C3 branches
5. Nerve to levator scapulae
6. Juncture of C3 and external branch of spinal accessory
7. Auricular branch
8. Transverse cervical branch
9. Mastoid branch
10. Branch to trapezius
11. C4 communicating branch
12. Levator scapulae branch
13. Branch to anterior scalene
14. Transected anterior scalene muscle
15. C5 branch to prevertebral muscles
16. C6 communicating branches
17. Nerve to subclavius
18. Nerve to middle scalene
19. Nerve to levator and rhomboid
20. Nerve to middle scalene
21. Sectioned transversopleural ligament
22. Nerves to middle scalene

the axilla is formed by the pectoralis major with the pectoralis minor and subclavius enclosed within the clavipectoral fascia behind it. The lateral wall of the axilla is defined by the convergence of the slanting anterior and posterior walls. The three posterior muscles attach to the lesser tuberosity and the bony crest that descends from it, while the pectoralis major, the anterior wall, inserts on the crest coming from the greater tuberosity. The lateral wall is then the narrow area of bone between these two prominences, the intertubercular sulcus or bicipital groove.

At the level of the first rib, the nerve trunks are in contact with each other as they are separated from the vein by the artery. As they descend and surround the axillary artery beyond the first rib and beneath the tendon of the pectoralis minor, the lateral cord is both lateral and superficial, the medial cord is deep and medial, and the posterior cord, the largest of the three, is much deeper and posterior. The medial and lateral cords each provide a root of the median nerve, and below the level of the pectoralis minor, the terminal branches of the plexus are seen as distinct entities.

COMPOSITION AND VARIATIONS OF THE TRUNKS, CORDS, AND BRANCHES OF THE BRACHIAL PLEXUS

The trunks of the plexus generally conform to the "classical" description given above. Kerr found 157 of 175 (90%) of the specimens had an upper trunk formed by C5 and C6, which then divided into anterior and posterior divisions. In four, the upper trunk was joined by C7 before its division so that C5, C6, and C7 then formed the trunks which then divided into two parts. In 14 cases, the upper trunk did not exist as such, but C5 and C6 each immediately divided into anterior and posterior divisions. The last formulation was also described by Herringham.[15]

Kerr found the C7 to remain single and form the intermediate trunk in all cases, dividing into anterior and posterior branches in 164 or 93.7%. In five instances, the intermediate trunk divided into three parts, one posterior and two anterior branches.

The lower trunk, according to Kerr, was formed by the union of T1 and C8 in 166 of 175 plexuses or 95.4%. In 165 of these, it then divided into anterior and posterior divisions. In six plexuses, C8 divided into posterior and anterior branches. The anterior branch joined T1 to form the medial cord. There was no dorsal branch of T1 and no lower trunk that divided into posterior and anterior divisions. About these last six specimens as well as two others, Kerr raised the possibility of production by inaccurate dissection.

The contribution of T1 to the formation of the posterior cord was the subject of great controversy. Herringham[15] dissected 45 specimens and found only 6 in which the posterior cord received a branch of T1. Cunningham[6] and Testut[32] considered that T1 did not contribute to the posterior cord. To the contrary, Harris[13] found such a contribution in 9 of 14 specimens and believed that it ultimately innervated the extensors of the fingers and thumb.

THE TERMINAL BRANCHES OF THE SUPRACLAVICULAR BRACHIAL PLEXUS

The five terminal branches of the supraclavicular portion of the brachial plexus are (1) dorsal scapular, (2) long thoracic, (3) phrenic, (4) suprascapular, and (5) nerve to the subclavius.

In addition to specific anatomical considerations, which will be detailed below, it will be useful to

23. Long thoracic nerve
24. Rami communicantes for C8
25. Rami communicantes for T1
26. Suprascapular nerve
27. Costopleural ligament
28. Intercostocervical artery
29. Branch to internal mammary artery plexus
30. Inferior portion of transversopleural ligament
31. Communicating branch of C2
33. Communicating branch of C3
35. Hypoglossal nerve
36. Superior laryngeal nerve
37. Superior cardiac nerve (sympathetic)
38. Junction of external laryngeal and superior cardiac nerves
39. A deep communicating branch
40. External laryngeal nerve
45. Middle cervical ganglion
47. Recurrent nerve
48. Stellate ganglion
49. Vertebropleural ligament
53. Phrenic nerve

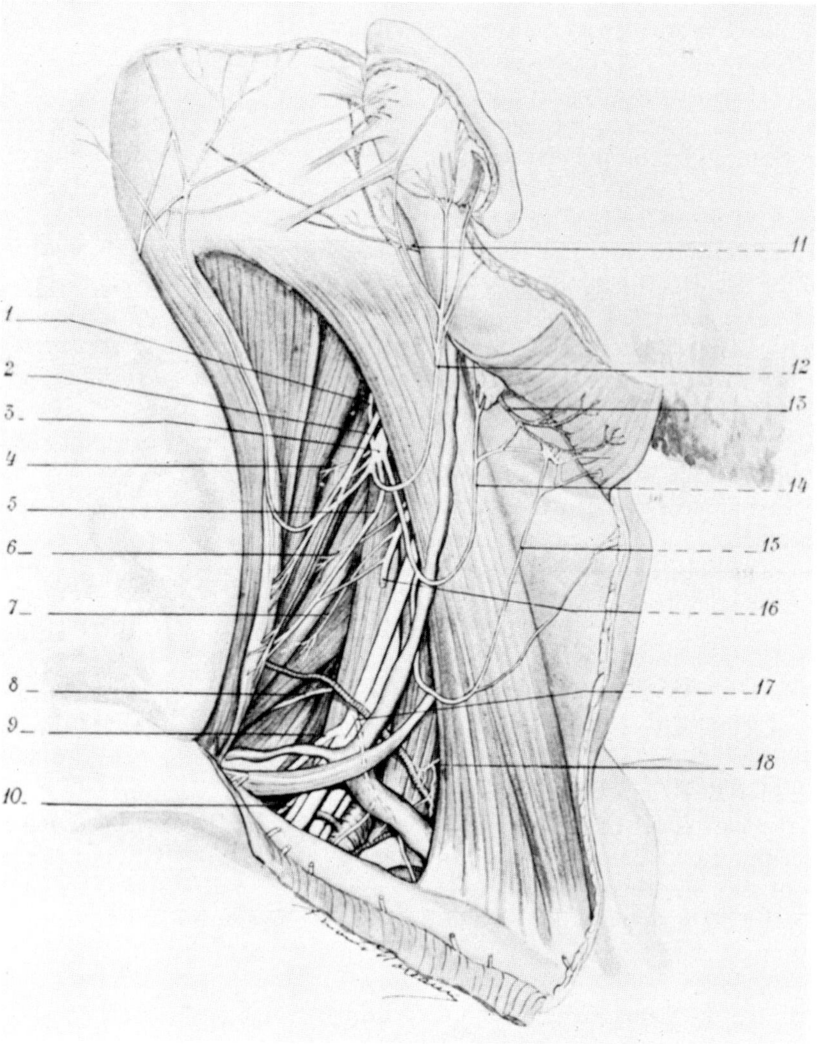

Fig. 1.22. The posterior triangle showing superficial relationships of external jugular vein and cervical and brachial plexus. Arrow indicates omohyoid muscle. (Modified from Hovelacque A: Anatomie des nerfs craniens et rachidiens et du système grand sympathique. Doin, Paris, 1927.)

1. Junction between C2 and C3
2. External branch of spinal accessory nerve
3. Anterior branch of C3
4. Nerve to levator scapulae
5. Branch from cervical plexus to trapezius

6, 7. Nerves to levator scapulae

8. Nerve to levator scapulae and rhomboids
9. Suprascapular nerve
10. Nerve to serratus anterior
11. Posterior auricular branch of facial nerve
12. Auricular branch from cervical plexus
13. Cervicofacial branch of facial nerve
14. Parotid branch of cervical plexus
15. Transverse cervical branch of cervical plexus
16. Supraclavicular branch
17. Nerve to subclavius
18. Sympathetic rami

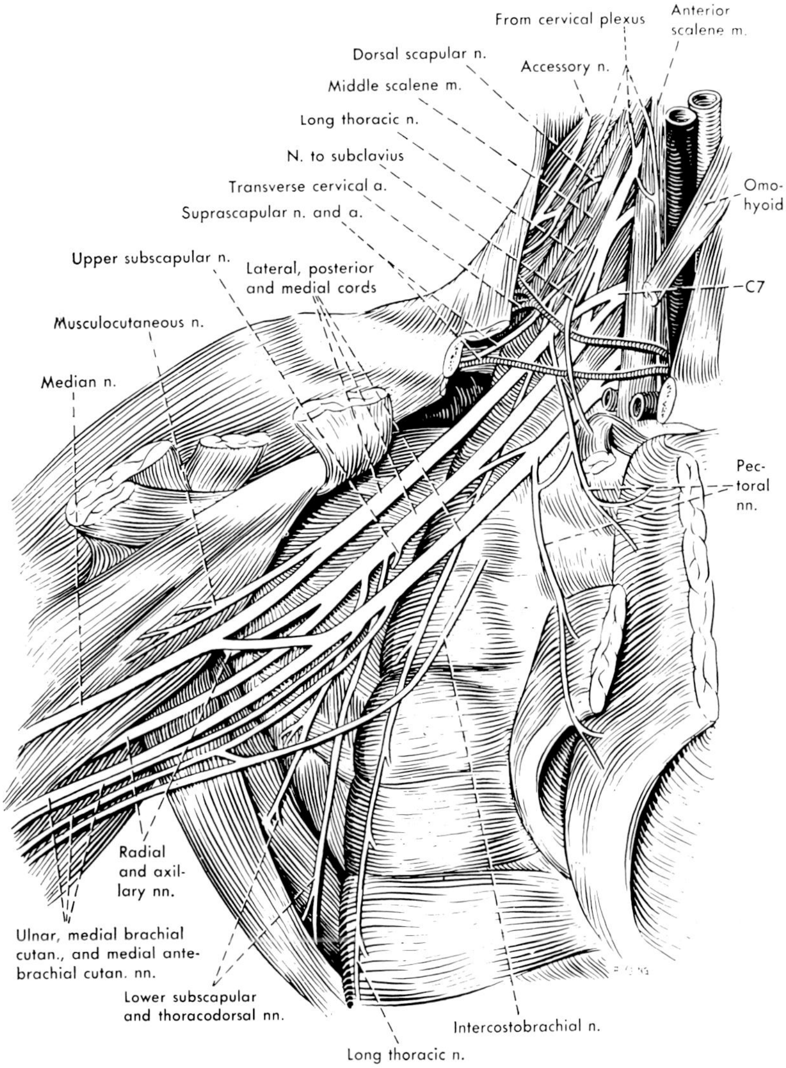

Fig. 1.23. Dissection showing relationships between brachial plexus and transverse arterial branches. (Reproduced from Hollinshead WH: Anatomy for Surgeons. Vol. 3: The Back and Limbs. 2nd Ed. Harper & Row, Hagerstown, MD, 1969, with permission.)

review their general clinical applications to evaluation of the patient with a traction injury to the brachial plexus. Knowledge of the disposition of the supraclavicular branches will often permit the clinician to accurately localize the site and extent of the lesion within the plexus. The phrenic nerve, dorsal scapular, and nerve to the serratus anterior may in almost all cases be considered as "root collaterals," so that evidence of injury to them as shown by denervation of the muscles they supply would favor intraspinal avulsion of their respective roots rather than distal rupture (Fig. 1.24A,B). Clinical examination of diaphragmatic excursion with radiographic confirmation as well as careful manual muscle testing of the scapular musculature is easily done and of great value. If, for example, the rhomboids and serratus are intact and the supraspinatus and infraspinatus paralyzed, then one can accurately pinpoint the lesion to the region of Erb's point. A paralyzed ipsilateral hemidiaphragm is indicative of intraspinal lesion of the C5 root. Further consideration of this deductive process will be given in Chapter 2.

The Dorsal Scapular Nerve

The dorsal scapular, or nerve to the rhomboids, almost always arises from C5 just after its exit from the intervertebral foramen, often with one of the roots of the long thoracic nerve (Figs. 1.21, 1.23). It

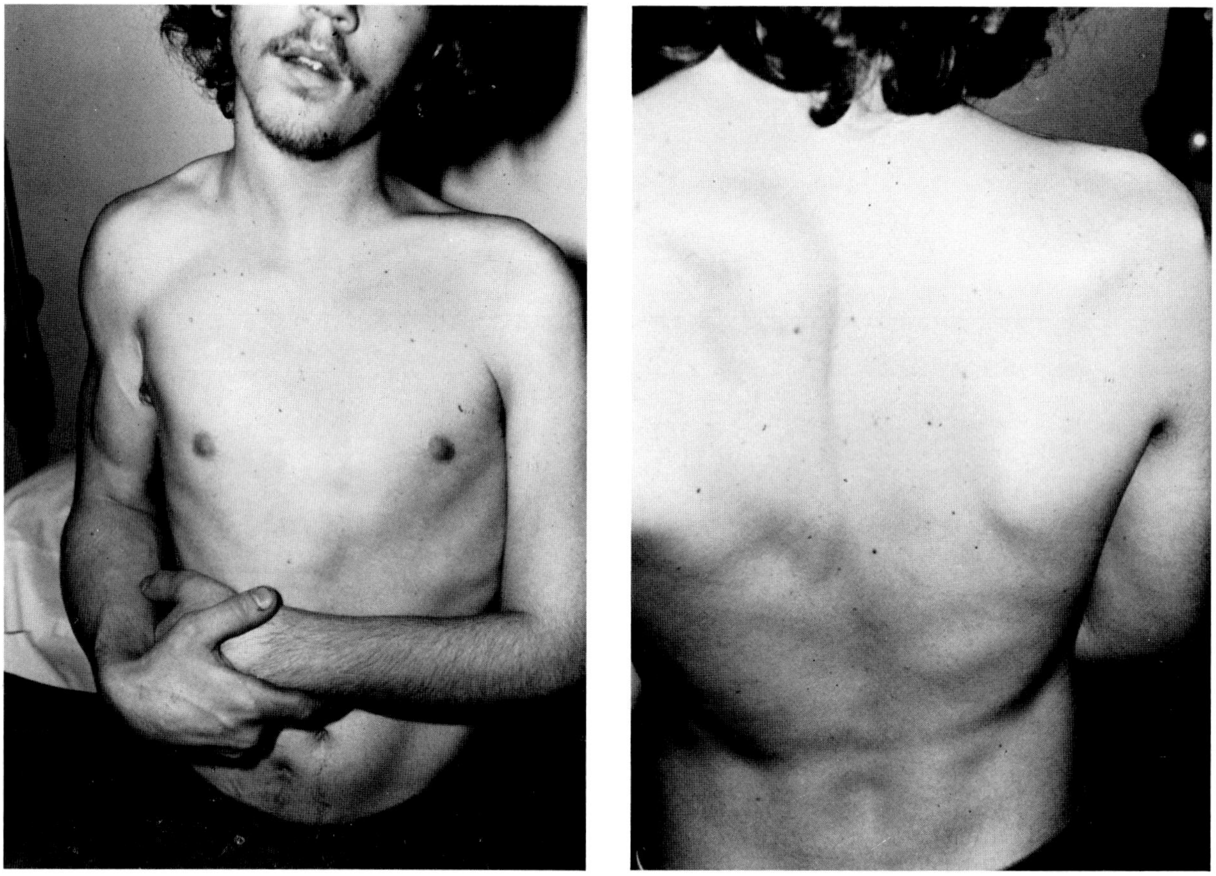

Fig. 1.24. Patient with complete avulsion of left brachial plexus and winging of scapula due to denervation of serratus anterior. There is also total paralysis of rhomboids.

may occasionally receive a branch from C4 and rarely may arise in C4. Usually, the nerve is a single trunk, although it may be composed of two branches and usually initially runs on the middle scalene, from which it descends in the interval between it and the posterior scalene. It then runs caudalward on the deep surface of the levator scapulae to the vertebral border of the scapula, where it ultimately supplies the major and minor rhomboids on their anterior surface.

The Long Thoracic Nerve

The nerve to the serratus anterior usually comes from two or three roots immediately after their emergence from the intervertebral foramina (Figs. 1.21, 1.23, 1.25). The C5 contribution may arise in common with the nerve to the rhomboids and levator scapulae before C4 joins C5. C6 usually contributes the largest branch according to Harris[13] and Hollinshead,[16] and that from C7 may be lacking. The first two roots, C5 and C6, usually join before they perforate the middle scalene, and C7, according to Cruveilhier,[5] joins the other two branches further distally. C5 may be the sole supply of the upper digitation of the muscle. The long thoracic nerve crosses the first rib, and then descends through the axilla behind the major branches of the plexus to gain the lateral aspect of the chest wall, where it supplies the fleshy digitations of the muscle. Because of its origin at the root level, denervation that results in scapular winging is a useful indicator of intraspinal injury or injury to any of its component roots. Harris[13] believed that atrophy of the serratus was often characteristic of a lesion involving C6.

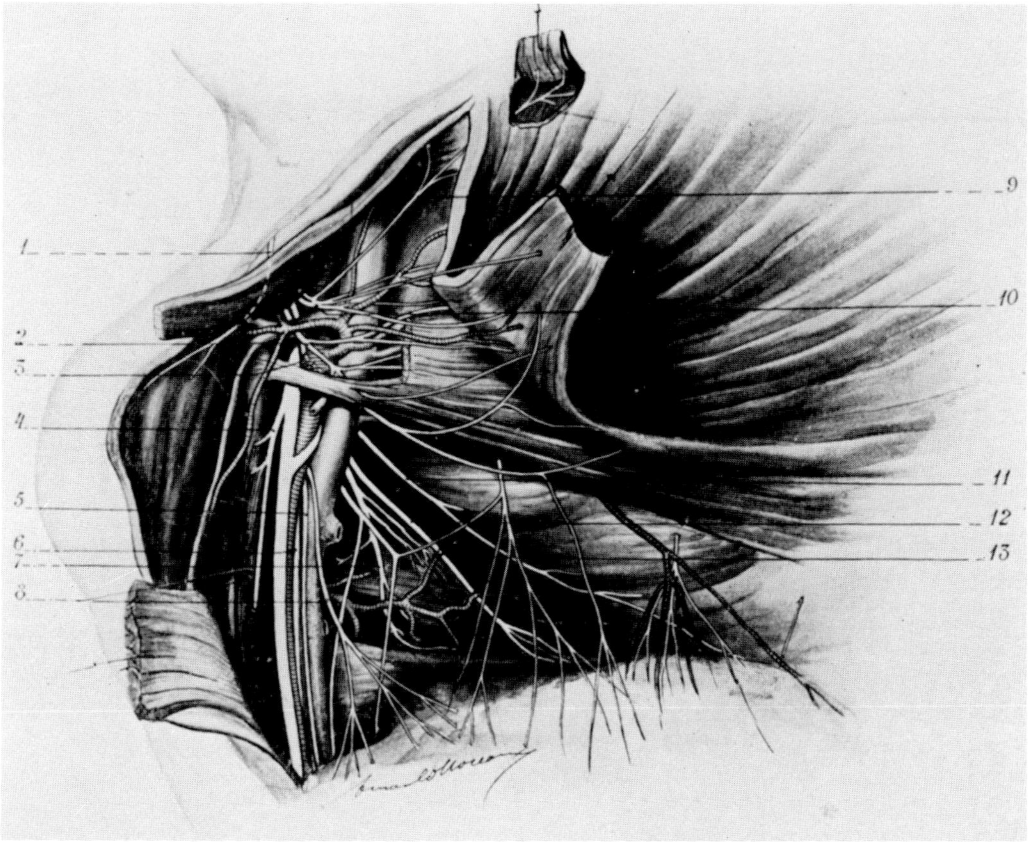

Fig. 1.25. The branches of the brachial plexus in the axilla. (Reproduced from Hovelacque A: Anatomie des nerfs craniens et rachidiens et du système grand sympathique. Doin, Paris, 1927.)

1. Subacromial branch of cervical plexus
2. Lateral pectoral nerve to pectoralis major passing anterior to axillary artery
3. Nerve to pectoralis minor
4. Musculocutaneous nerve
5. Medial brachial cutaneous nerve
6. Ulnar nerve
7. Nerve to latissimus dorsi
8. Branch of medial cutaneous nerve of arm to axillary skin
9. Branch to pectoralis major
10. Branch to pectoralis major
11. Long thoracic nerve
12. Nerve to latissimus dorsi
13. Intercostobrachial nerve

The Suprascapular Nerve

The suprascapular nerve (Figs. 1.22, 1.23, 1.26) usually arises from the superolateral aspect of the upper trunk shortly after its formation (Erb's point), but it may also be seen at the terminal part of C5, in which case it may receive a twig from behind C6, according to Hovelacque.[17] Kerr[20] found it to come from the cephalic trunk or its dorsal or ventral divisions in over 82%. C4 may also contribute to the nerve. The course of the nerve in the posterior triangle is from the superolateral border of the upper trunk down and posterior to the inferior belly of the omohyoid, between it and the anterior surface of the trapezius. It then passes into the notch of the scapula, under the superior transverse ligament and deep to the supraspinatus. From there it goes around the lateral border of the spine of the scapula into the infraspinous fossa, where it innervates the infraspinatus.

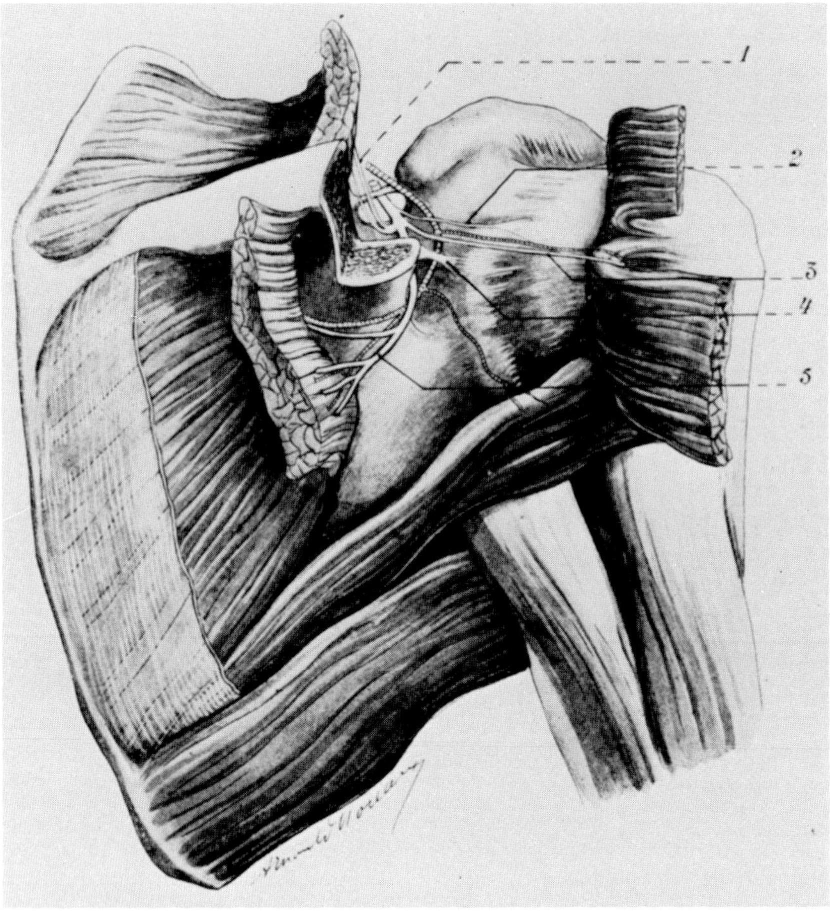

Fig. 1.26. The suprascapular nerve. (Reproduced from Hovelacque A: Anatomie des nerfs craniens et rachidiens et du système grand sympathique. Doin, Paris, 1927.)

1. Supraspinatus branches
2. Articular branch
3. Branch to the posterior aspect of infraspinatus
4. Spinoglenoidal ligament
5. Infraspinatus branches

The Phrenic Nerve

The phrenic nerve arises at the root level, chiefly from the fourth cervical nerve, with contribution from the third and fifth nerves as well. It crosses the anterior scalene from lateral to medial and extends into the thorax between the subclavian vein and artery. The accessory phrenic nerve is inconstant, and may come from either C5 or the nerve to the subclavius. It descends ventral to the subclavian vein and joins the phrenic nerve at the root of the neck or in the thorax.

The Nerve to the Subclavius

The clinically unimportant nerve to the subclavius arises from the upper trunk or the anterior division in 50% of the cases. In two thirds of these, the fourth, fifth, and sixth cervical nerves may send fibers to it. In over 26% it arises only from C5, and in

Table 1.3. Segmental Composition of Lateral Cords and Branches

Nerve	Usual Composition	Apparent Variations
Lateral cord	C4–7 or C5–7	C4–8
Lateral pectoral	C5–7	C5–6; C6–7, C7
Musculocutaneous	C5–7	C5–6; C5–8; C5–T1
Lateral root of median	C5–7	C5–6; C6–7
Median, both roots	C5–T1	C5–8; C6–T1

From Hollinshead WH: Anatomy for Surgeons. Vol 3: The Back and Limbs. 2nd Ed. Harper & Row, Hagerstown, MD, 1969, with permission.

over 21% it may receive fibers for both fourth and fifth cervical nerves, according to Kerr.[20]

COMPOSITION AND VARIATION OF THE CORDS OF THE BRACHIAL PLEXUS AND THEIR TERMINAL BRANCHES

The cords of the brachial plexus, even though often observed as depicted previously with relation to each other and the major vessels, may vary considerably in their derivation, interconnections, segmental composition, and in the manner in which they give off their terminal branches.

The descriptions of Hollinshead,[16] who relied heavily on Kerr, are particularly useful and will be paraphrased liberally in this section. Table 1.3 is reproduced from Hollinshead's *Anatomy for Surgeons.*

Several common variations in the lateral cord were noted. Kerr found that it gave a contribution to the ulnar nerve in 42.9% of his specimens.

The Lateral Root of the Median Nerve

The size of the lateral root of the median nerve varies considerably, according to Kerr; when it was small, he commonly found a communication from the musculocutaneous to the median in the arm. Kaplan and Spinner[19] quoted Vallois as indicating a 24% occurrence rate for this branch. They described that the lateral root may pass with the musculocutaneous nerve to join the medial root of the median nerve at varying levels in the arm. If these join sufficiently distally, there may be the appearance of a double median nerve. Finally, the lateral root of the median nerve can pass posterior to the axillary artery to join the medial root rather than anteriorly as normally seen.

The Musculocutaneous Nerve

The musculocutaneous nerve (Figs. 1.25, 1.27) usually arises as one of the two terminal branches of the lateral cord (88.6%, according to Kerr), but may be the only continuation of this cord with the lateral root to the median coming from the C7 only. Three of Kerr's cases had it arising from a single anterior cord formed by the union of lateral and medial cords. In 4.75% of the same series, it came from the anterior division of the upper trunk. It may arise late from the median nerve or combined median and ulnar trunk (5.1% of Kerr's cases). The actual incidence of representation of C7 and lower roots in the musculocutaneous nerve has been debated. Kerr stated that C7 is represented in about two thirds of the cases. Walsh[33] traced C7 to the musculocutaneous in about half that number. Kerr estimated that C8 and T1 are represented in 6 or 7%.

In the most common mode of origin, the musculocutaneous nerve arises from the lateral cord at the inferior border of the pectoralis major. The nerve then enters the coracobrachialis, which it innervates, and then crosses between brachialis and biceps brachii and on to the lateral side of the arm. Just above the elbow, it pierces the deep fascia lateral to the bicipital tendon and becomes the lateral cutaneous nerve of the forearm.

In summary, the usual branches are as follows:

1. Coracobrachialis
2. Biceps and brachialis
   a. Articular branch to elbow
   b. Osseous branch to humerus—into nutrient foramen
3. Lateral antebrachial cutaneous nerve
   a. Anterior and posterior divisions

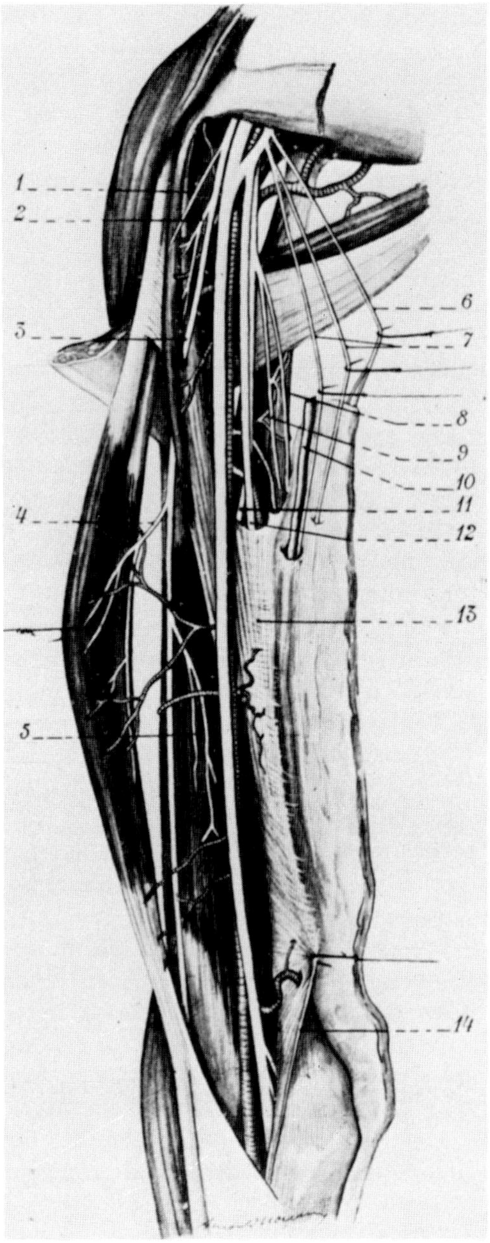

Fig. 1.27. The nerves in the anterior aspect of the upper arm. (Reproduced from Hovelacque A: Anatomie des nerfs craniens et rachidiens et du système grand sympathique. Doin, Paris, 1927.)

1. Superior branch of nerve to coracobrachialis
2. Inferior branch of nerve to coracobrachialis
3. Musculocutaneous nerve
4. Nerve to biceps
5. Nerve to brachialis
6. Accessory branch to medial brachial cutaneous nerve
7. Medial brachial cutaneous branches dissected
8. Medial cutaneous branch of radial nerve
9. Branch to long head of triceps—recurrent
10. Basilic vein
11. Radial nerve
12. Ulnar nerve
13. Medial intermuscular septum
14. Fibers of pronator teres originating from intermuscular septum

Kaplan and Spinner[19] have catalogued and illustrated a number of variations in the form of the musculocutaneous nerve. It can be seen to arise from a single structure that appears to give origin to median, musculocutaneous, and ulnar nerves, or it may divide soon after origin into its terminal branches before perforating the coracobrachialis muscle. It may appear as a "double musculocutaneous nerve" or, because of the combined median musculocutaneous nerve, may appear to be absent. Variations are therefore frequent. When C7 fibers are present, they may pass through a communication from the musculocutaneous nerve to the median, a branch found in approximately 24% of upper extremities, according to Kaplan and Spinner.[19] A median to musculocutaneous nerve communication is said to occur in approximately 2% of specimens.

The lateral pectoral nerve will be described in the next section.

BRANCHES OF THE MIDPORTION OF THE PLEXUS

Although the branches of the midportion of the plexus are usually thought to arise from the plexus at the level of the median, lateral and posterior cords, there may be significant variation in their origin that may bedevil the clinician in attempts to localize a lesion on the basis of physical examination. This is particularly true with reference to the innervation of pectoralis major and minor, as will be described. The other nerves to be considered in this section are the subscapular nerves, which include the thoracodorsal nerve.

The Pectoral Nerves

The innervation of the pectoralis major and minor is clearly described by Gray[12] as follows: The two pectoral nerves arise at the level of the clavicle on either side of the axillary artery and are thus termed lateral and medial pectoral nerves (Figs. 1.25, 1.28).

The lateral (lateral anterior thoracic) pectoral nerve, lateral to the artery, usually comes from the lateral cord but may come from the anterior division of the upper and middle trunks just before they unite into a cord. This anatomic variant is very important because it explains the riddle of the occasional patient with a severe traction injury to the plexus and a flail-anesthetic arm whose pectoralis major muscle is functioning while every other muscle in the limb is paralyzed. The lateral pectoral nerve then passes superficial to the first part of the axillary artery and vein, sends a branch to the medial pectoral nerve, and then reaches the deep surface of both portions of the pectoralis major by traversing the clavipectoral fascia.

The medial (medial anterior thoracic) pectoral nerve usually arises from the medial cord of the plexus, medial to the artery. Although it is designated as "medial," its origin is actually more lateral from the midline of the body than is the lateral or superior branch described above. It goes between the axillary artery and vein, branches to join the communication from the lateral pectoral nerve so that a loop is formed about the artery, and then enters the deep surface of the pectoralis minor. Two or three branches of this nerve pierce the muscle to supply the more caudal parts of the pectoralis major. The loop formed by the two nerves may supply both muscles.

Kerr described a single root for the lateral anterior thoracic nerve from the lateral cord in 43% of the cases. In over 78% of cases where there were two roots, one came from the anterior division of the upper trunk and one came from the anterior division of the middle trunk. In over 54% of the cases where there are three roots, one came from the anterior division of the upper trunk and the other two from the anterior division of the middle trunk. All of the nerves cephalic to C8 may send fibers to the lateral anterior thoracic in over 83% of the cases.

The medial pectoral nerve arose from the medial cord in 69% of Kerr's cases and from the lower trunk in 24%. It therefore can be said to receive fibers from C8 to T1 in most cases.

The Subscapular Nerves

Gray[12] described the subscapular nerves to be usually two in number, which arise from the posterior cord. The superior or upper subscapular, the smaller of the two, enters the superior part of the subscapularis. It is frequently double. The inferior subscapular supplies the distal part of the subscapularis and ends in the teres major.

By contrast, Kerr[20] found the origin of the subscapular nerves to be most commonly from the posterior division of the upper trunk, next in frequency from the posterior cord, and least often from the combined posterior divisions of the upper and middle trunks. He stated that the nerves usually contained fibers from C5, less commonly from C5 and C6. There was also significant variation in the origin of the lower subscapular nerve. In Kerr's series, it came from the posterior cord in about one third, from the axillary nerve in a slightly higher percentage, and from the proximal plexus in 25%.

The Thoracodorsal Nerve

The nerve to the latissimus dorsi is also known as the middle or long subscapular nerve and is described by Gray[12] as a branch of the posterior cord of the plexus arising between the two other subscapular nerves and following the course of the subscapular and thoracodorsal arteries along the posterior wall of

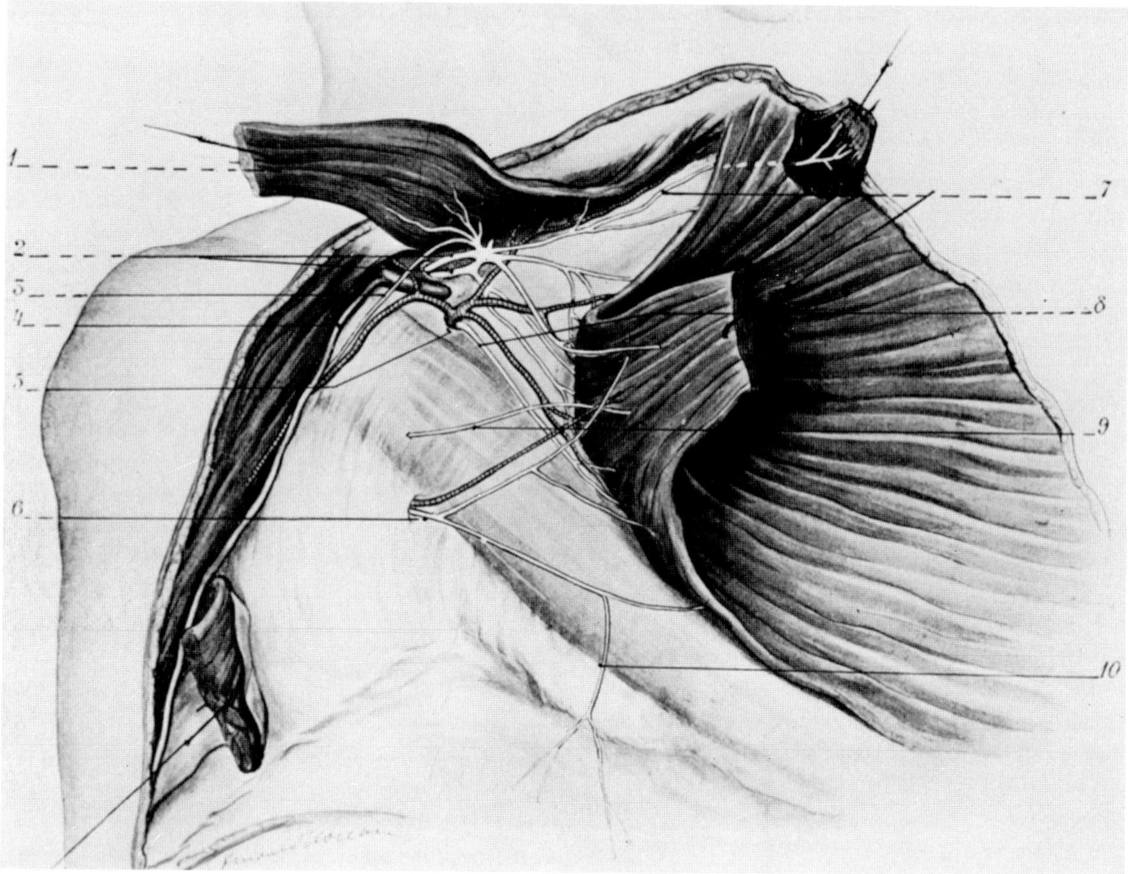

Fig. 1.28. The nerves to the pectoral muscles. (Reproduced from Hovelacque A: Anatomie des nerfs craniens et rachidiens et du système grand sympathique. Doin, Paris, 1927.)

1. Clavicular head of pectoralis major
2. Lateral anterior thoracic nerve to pectoralis major
3. An inconstant branch going to deltoid
4. Cephalic vein
5. Thoracoacromial artery
6. Medial anterior thoracic nerve to pectoralis major (medial pectoral nerve)
7. Lateral anterior thoracic nerve to pectoralis major (lateral pectoral nerve)
8. Medial anterior thoracic branch to pectoralis major (medial pectoral nerve) passing above pectoralis minor
9. Branch of medial anterior thoracic nerve traversing pectoralis minor
10. Branch of medial anterior thoracic going to axillary skin

the axilla under the ventral border of the latissimus dorsi, which it supplies. According to Kerr,[20] the posterior cord was the most common origin of the thoracodorsal nerve, and 70.2% came either from there or through the radial or axillary nerves. In others, it came off in a variable manner with or from the other subscapular nerves. Kerr cited C7 as the only root in 50% of cases, and in most of the other cases the nerve arose from C5-7.

COMPOSITION AND VARIATIONS IN THE FORMATION OF THE POSTERIOR CORD AND ITS TERMINAL BRANCHES

The posterior cord, as described by Hollinshead,[16] is most commonly formed by the posterior divisions of the upper and middle trunks, then joined at a lower level in the axilla by the smaller posterior division of the lower trunk. As has already been men-

Table 1.4. Segmental Composition of Posterior Cord and Plexus

Nerve	Usual Composition	Apparent Variations
Posterior cord	(C4?) C5–8	(C4?), C5–T1; C6–T1; C6–8
Upper subscapular	C5	C5–6; C7
Thoracodorsal	C7–8	C5–6; C5–7; C6–8; C8–T1
Lower subscapular	C5–6	C5; C5–7; C6; C6–7
Axillary	C5–6	C5; C5–7
Radial	C5–8	C5–7; C5–T1; C6–8; C6–T1; C7–8

From Hollinshead WH: Anatomy for Surgeons. Vol 3: The Back and Limbs. 2nd Ed. Harper & Row, Hagerstown, MD, 1969, with permission.

tioned, this last point, with reference to the contribution of T1, has been the subject of great debate. There are many variations described—Walsh[32] stated that there was no posterior cord proper but that the radial and axillary nerves arose independently from the plexus, and this situation was verified in 36 of 173 cases in Kerr's series. Other variations involved the level and manner in which the posterior divisions gathered together. Kerr stated that C5 does not send fibers to the posterior cord in about 20% of cases and that T1 does not in about 80%.

Hollinshead's summary of the segmental composition of the posterior cord and branches is reproduced in Table 1.4.

The subscapular nerves, including the middle subscapular or thoracodorsal, have been described in the previous section. It now remains to detail the manner of evolution of the two terminal branches, the circumflex or axillary and the radial.

The Axillary Nerve

The axillary (Figs. 1.29, 1.30) or circumflex nerve, according to Hovelacque,[17] should really be described as a collateral rather than a terminal branch of the plexus since it does not supply the free part of the limb. He describes it as arising from the posterior cord but at varying levels on the subscapularis, sometimes behind the pectoralis minor, rarely at the inferior border of that muscle, but always behind the axillary artery. It may come off in varying planes with reference to the radial nerve, but then descends on the subscapularis, bounded below by the superior border of the teres major, laterally by the long head of the triceps, and medially by the surgical neck of the humerus and the inferior capsule of the glenohumeral joint. The posterior circumflex humeral artery, which comes from the axillary artery, accompanies the nerve, usually medial and inferior to it. As the nerve exits the quadrilateral space, it gives off the branch to the teres minor, and other branches include articular branches and, according to Cruveilhier,[5] a constant branch to the subscapularis. A separate cutaneous branch to the skin over the deltoid often arises with the nerve to the teres minor, and the axillary nerve itself passes from posterior to anterior on the undersurface of the deltoid, and ultimately pierces the deltoid to provide additional branches to supply the skin overlying the muscle.

According to Kerr, the axillary nerve arose from the posterior cord in 79.7%, and in the remainder where there was no posterior cord per se, from the upper and middle divisions directly. He expressed doubt whether it ever received fibers from C8 or T1, and, although it usually did have C5 and C6 fibers, it could also have C5 fibers only and also include some fibers from C7.

The Radial Nerve

The radial nerve, the largest terminal branch of the brachial plexus, usually arises as one of the two branches of the division of the posterior cord (Figs. 1.1, 1.23, 1.29, 1.30). As has been described for the other branch, the axillary nerve, this division occurs on the inferior surface of the subscapularis muscle behind the pectoralis minor or just above its inferior border. In Kerr's series of 173 plexuses, 138 or 79% had the classical origin, while in the absence of a true posterior cord, which occurred in 35 or 20%, there was a variable manner of formation, most commonly (19 cases) with the posterior division of the upper and middle trunks forming a radiocircumflex trunk. In 10 cases, the posterior branches of the upper and middle trunks formed the circumflex, the posterior division of the upper trunk contributed the largest share of the radial. Sixteen others had a very variable origin. Kerr collected, in addition to his own figures, a com-

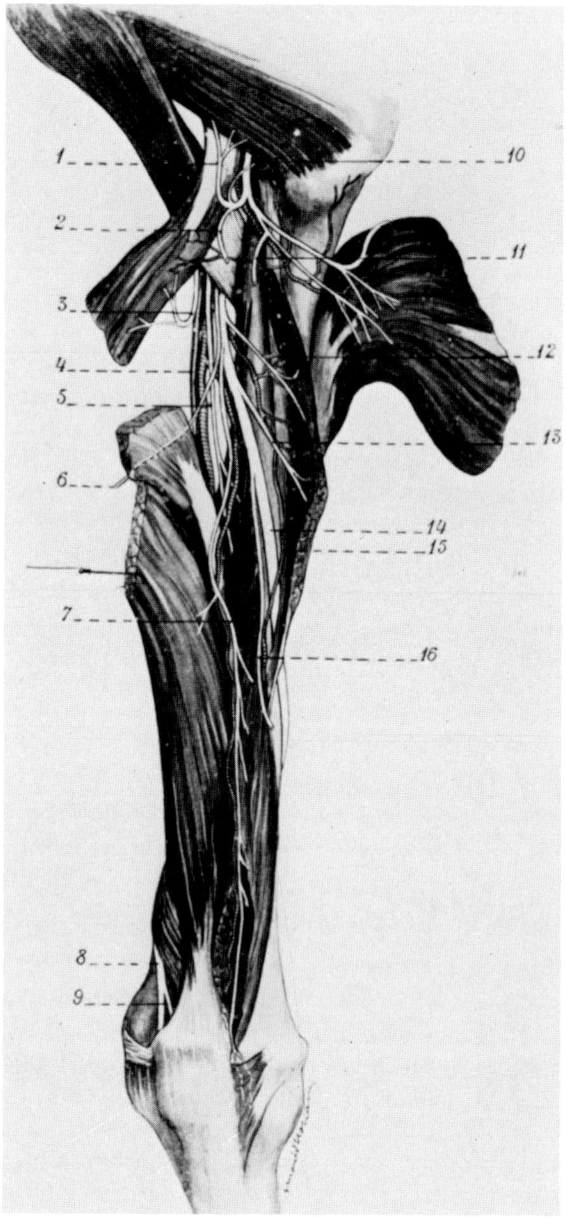

Fig. 1.29. The axillary nerve and the radial nerve on the posterior aspect of the arm. (Reproduced from Hovelacque A: Anatomie des nerfs craniens et rachidiens et du système grand sympathique. Doin, Paris, 1927.)

1. Nerve to teres minor
2. Posterior cutaneous branch to shoulder
3. Nerve to long head of triceps
4. Ulnar nerve
5. Superior branch to medial head of triceps
6. Radial cutaneous branch
7. Inferior branch to medial triceps and anconeus
8. Ulnar nerve
9. Branch of ulnar nerve to flexor carpi ulnaris
10. Articular branch of axillary nerve
11. Anterior cutaneous branch of the shoulder

12, 13. Nerves to lateral head of triceps

14. Radial nerve trunk
15. Profunda brachii artery
16. Lateral cutaneous branch of radial nerve

pendium of those from the literature as to the roots represented in the radial nerve. Walsh's[33] 67 cases had fibers from C5 to C8 in 67, and from T1 also only in 6, according to Hollinshead.[16]

The radial nerve is constantly located posterior to the axillary artery, which separates it from all other nerves of the plexus, except for the axillary. It crosses the latissimus and the teres major, then goes around the medial side of the humerus and descends between the medial and long head of the triceps.

The main branches of the radial nerve in the arm are, according to Gray, as follows:

1. Medial muscular branches arising in the axilla to the medial and long head of the triceps
2. Posterior brachial cutaneous nerve arising in the

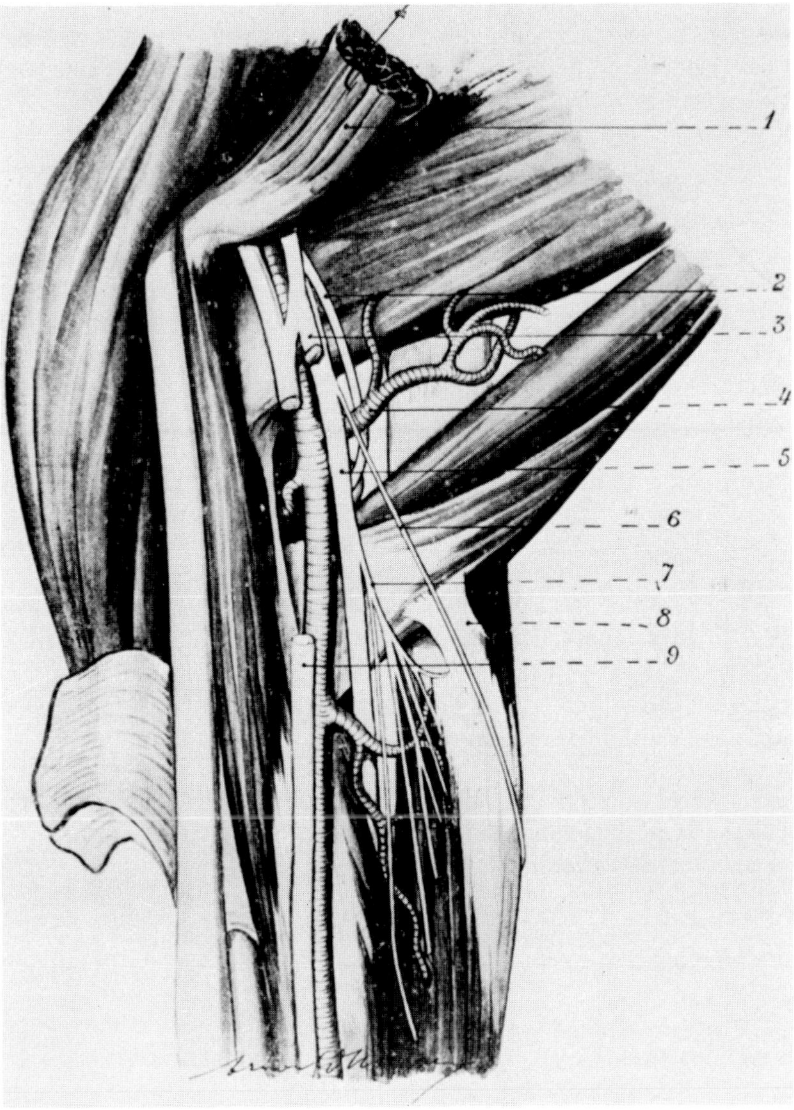

Fig. 1.30. The deep elements of the neurovascular bundle of the axilla. (From Hovelaque A: Anatomie des nerfs craniens et rachidiens et du système grand sympathique. Doin, Paris, 1927.)

1. Pectoralis minor sectioned and retracted
2. Axillary nerve
3. Ulnar nerve sectioned
4. Subscapular artery
5. Radial nerve
6. Medial cutaneous branch of radial nerve
7. Nerve to large head of triceps
8. Fibrous arcade stretched between latissimus dorsi and long head of triceps
9. Median nerve sectioned

axilla — to the dorsal skin of the arm as far as the olecranon

3. Posterior muscular branches arising in the spiral groove of the humerus to supply medial and lateral heads of the triceps and the anconeus
4. Posterior antebrachial cutaneous nerve
5. Lateral muscular branches to brachioradialis, extensor carpi radialis longus, and brachialis
6. Articular branches to elbow

The branches of the radial nerve in the forearm are as follows:

1. Superficial radial nerve
2. Deep branch of the radial nerve
   a. Muscular branches to extensor carpi radialis brevis and supinator, extensor digitorum, extensor digiti minimi, extensor carpi ulnaris, extensors to abductor pollicis longus, and extensor indicis
   b. Articular branches

COMPOSITION AND VARIATION OF THE MEDIAL CORD AND ITS BRANCHES

Because the medial cord usually represents the continuation of the anterior division of the lower trunk, it should contain fibers from C8 and T1, and Kerr[20] found this to be the usual situation in 94.58% of his specimens, despite some variation in their manner of distribution. In six cases, the medial cord received fibers from C7. Hollinshead's table of the variations in segmental composition is reproduced in Table 1.5.

The medial pectoral nerve has already been discussed in a previous section as has the lateral root of the median nerve, which ordinarily comes from the lateral cord. The latter is considerably more variable in size and composition than the medial root of the median nerve, which Hovelacque[17] considered to be relatively constant in size. The variations in the manner of formation of the median nerve proper have already been described. Kerr found the "classical description" to be the most commonly observed in 150 of 175 cases. Cruveilhier[5] stated that it was not rare to see the median receive a third medial root. According to Hovelacque,[17] Turner noted a case in which the medial root passed behind the artery, and Calori described one wherein the medial root passed medial to the axillary vein so that the "fork embraced both the artery and the vein."

The roots of the median nerve fix the axillary artery on both sides with the artery between them and the subscapularis. The median nerve is applied to the anterolateral aspect of the artery. It accompanies it down the arm, and gradually crosses to the medial side so that by the distal part of the arm, it actually is medial. At the antecubital fossa, it is superficial to the brachialis and passes between the two heads of the pronator teres, being separated from the ulnar artery by the deep head. Then it continues distally through the forearm between flexor digitorum superficialis and profundus into the carpal tunnel from which it supplies the hand.

The branches are as follows:

1. Above the elbow there is often a branch to the pronator teres.
2. Articular branches, usually one or two, are given off to the elbow joint.
3. Muscular branches are given off near the elbow to the flexor pronator muscles; pronator teres, flexor

Table 1.5. Segmental Composition of Medial Cord and Branches

Nerve	Usual Composition	Apparent Variations
Medial cord	C8–T1	C7–T1; C8–T2
Medial pectoral	C8–T1	C7–T1; C8
Medial brachial cutaneous	T1	C8–T1
Medial root of median	C8–T1	T1
Median, both nerves	C5–T1	C5–8; C6–T1
Ulnar	C7–T1	C5–T1; C6–T1; C7–T2; C8–T1

From Hollinshead WH: Anatomy for Surgeons. Vol 3: The Back and Limbs. 2nd ed. Harper & Row, Hagerstown, MD, 1969, with permission.

carpi radialis, palmaris longus, and flexor digitorum superficialis.
4. The anterior interosseous nerve accompanies the anterior interosseous artery along the interosseous membrane and supplies the radial half of the flexor digitorum profundus, the flexor pollicis longus, and the pronator quadratus.
5. The palmar cutaneous branch.
6. The muscular branches in the hand to abductor pollicis brevis, opponens pollicis, and the superficial head of the flexor pollicis brevis.
7. The common and proper digital nerves.

The Ulnar Nerve

The ulnar nerve (Figs. 1.27, 1.30) is usually seen as the termination of the continuation of the medial cord anterior to the lower border of the subscapularis, medial to the axillary artery, and between it and the vein. It arises below the origins of the medial root of the median nerve and the medial cutaneous nerves of the arm and forearm. As such, it is usually constant, although Kerr[20] did report 5 cases of 175 in which it came off a common trunk with the median and musculocutaneous below the fork of the median, and Hovelacque[17] quoted Sterzi's dissection of 50 cadavers and animals which led Sterzi to the conclusion that the ulnar was actually a collateral of the median. Nevertheless, most authors have designated it as the principal and constant terminal branch of the medial cord. It should, therefore, contain only fibers from C8 and T1. Very often, however, there is an additional branch, a "lateral root of the ulna," which is responsible for its receiving fibers from C7 (or higher), usually from the lateral cord or one of its branches. The fibers are usually destined for the flexor carpi ulnaris, although Harris[13] suggested that they may occasionally go to the muscles of the thumb. The actual incidence of this branch has varied from different authors. Kerr reported it in 75 of 175 cases and saw it crossing the medial head of the median. Linell[23] found it in 57% of 21 plexuses. Walsh[33] found it in 265 of 290 cases.

At its origin, the ulnar nerve is located deeply between the axillary artery and vein, at the inferior border of subscapularis, where it crosses anterior to the teres major and latissimus dorsi. It descends to the middle of the arm, where it goes posteriorly through the medial intermuscular septum and follows the medial head of the triceps to the region of the cubital tunnel. There are no branches of the ulnar nerve above the elbow, but those distally are as follows:

1. Articular branches
2. Muscular branches—to flexor carpi ulnaris and ulnar half of flexor digitorum profundus
3. Palmar cutaneous branch
4. Dorsal branch
5. Palmar branch
   a. Superficial branch
   b. Deep branch to hypothenar muscles, third and fourth lumbricals, interossei, adductor pollilcis, and deep head of flexor pollicis brevis

The Medial Cutaneous Nerve of the Arm

The medial cutaneous nerve of the arm is usually described as arising from the medial cord of the brachial plexus. Kerr studied this structure in 166 plexuses.[20] In 137 (83%), the nerve was represented by a single branch, in 28 there were two branches, and in one there were three separate filaments. In those cases in which the nerve was represented by a single branch, Kerr described it as originating in the following ways: It arose from the lower trunk or medial cord in 92 cases, and in two cases from the dorsal division of the lower trunk. In 11 cases it arose from the first thoracic nerve, from the ulnar nerve, or from C8 or T1. Numerous connections, especially with the intercostobrachial nerve, were demonstrated. The relations of the nerve to the basilic vein may be quite variable as the nerve descends to pierce the deep fascia in the middle of the arm, where it supplies the medial skin as far as the elbow.

The Medial Cutaneous Nerve of the Forearm

The origin of the medial cutaneous nerve of the forearm may be very variable, although Kerr[20] found it coming from the medial cord in 82% of the cases. It most often comes off immediately above the medial cutaneous branch to the arm, but may originate in common with it. It descends medial to the brachial artery, pierces the deep fascia at midarm with the basilic vein, and divides into anterior and posterior branches that supply the skin of the medial forearm as far as the wrist. There are numerous communications with adjacent cutaneous nerves.

VARIATIONS IN THE RELATIONSHIP BETWEEN THE AXILLARY ARTERY, ITS BRANCHES, AND THE BRACHIAL PLEXUS

The recent resurgence of interest in direct surgical intervention in the traumatized brachial plexus has brought well-deserved and vital focus on the work of Ruth Miller,[24] who in the 1930s studied the comparative anatomy of the brachial plexus of the vertebrates, especially the primates, in an attempt to understand some of the variations observed in the human plexus. A portion of her work, entitled "Observations upon the Arrangement of the Axillary Artery and Brachial Plexus" was published in 1939, and will be summarized and partially reproduced because of its direct applicability to the problems of contemporary brachial plexus surgery.

Miller studied the variations of the axillary structures among 480 human dissections and considered only those anomalies that showed aberrant arrangements of the brachial plexus with the axillary artery. Since the veins are so often variable, and in only 4% of the dissections studied could abnormalities be definitely associated with the veins, the veins were not documented. However, she found anomalous relationships between the brachial plexus and axillary artery in 42 out of 480 cases, or 8%. These were found to be of five general types, each including several specific kinds of variation. These will be described and illustrated.

The normal relationship of axillary structures, including the general sites of the artery-plexus variations in order of frequency, are seen in Figure 1.31, which indicates the sites of the five general types of variation in order of their frequency. Each general type includes several specific kinds of variation, listed below and illustrated in Fig. 1.32.

Type 1. The artery is superficial to the median nerve. This variant was found in 17 cases (40%), of which 15 were bilateral and two were unilateral.

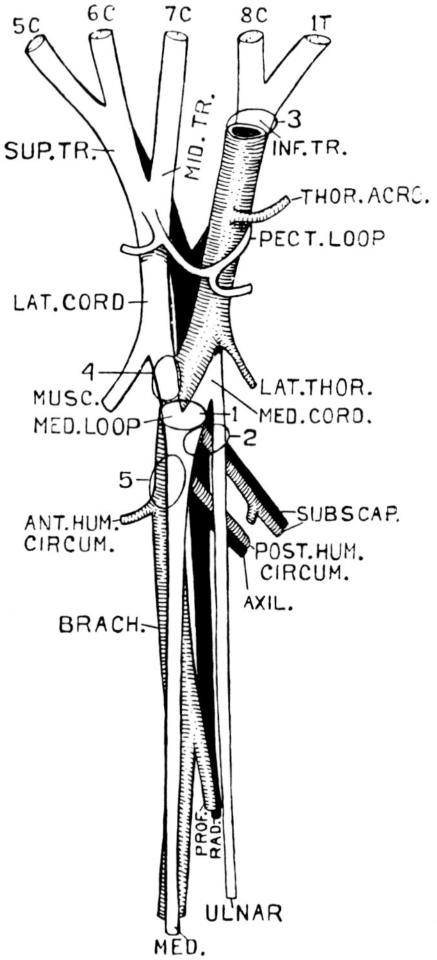

Fig. 1.31. Normal relationship of axillary structures, including general sites of artery-plexus variation in order of their frequency. (Reproduced from Miller RA: Observations upon the arrangement of the axillary and brachial plexus. Plate 1. Am J Anat 143:64, 1939.)

2. The most common variant of type 1 (15 cases) — a superficial radial superior artery, a branch of the axillary, is given off above the median loop.
3. One case. The superficial brachial superior artery arises from the axillary artery and passes over the median loop.
4. One case. An axillary brachial artery perforates the median loop.

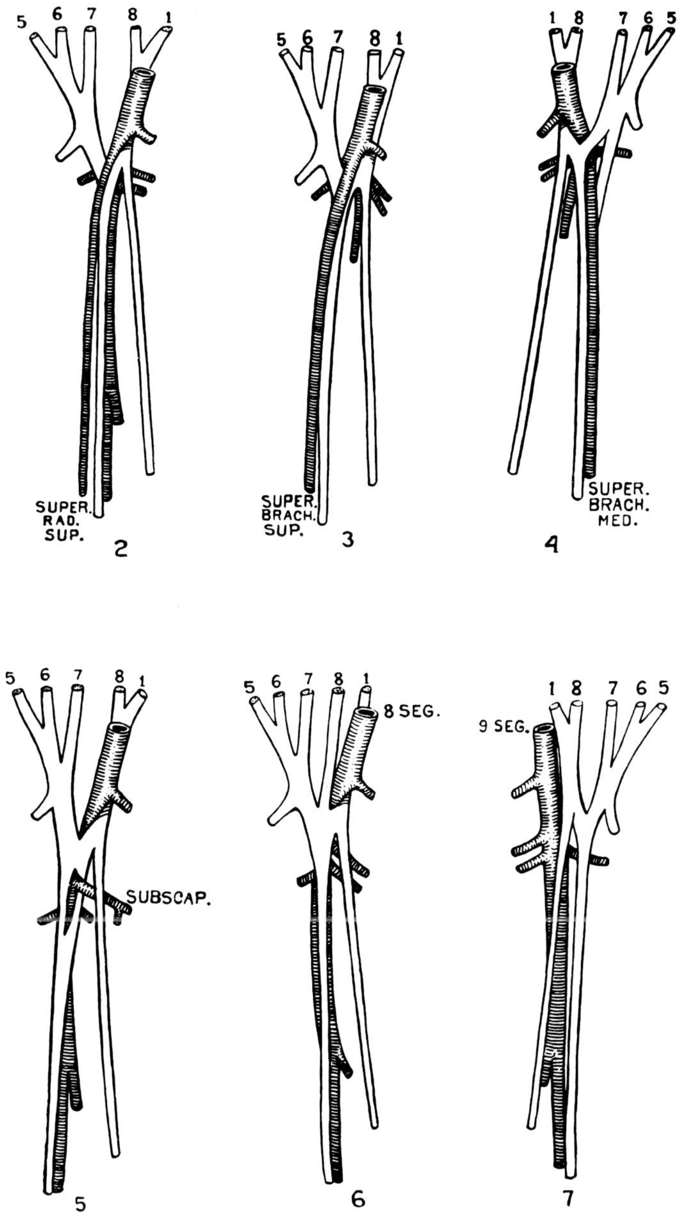

Fig. 1.32. Variants of relationship of axillary artery and plexus. See text. (Reproduced from Miller RA: Observations upon the arrangement of the axillary and brachial plexus. Am J Anat 143:64, 1939.)

(Figure continues on next page.)

Type 2. The median nerve is divided by a branch of the artery. There were eight cases (19%), of which seven were bilateral and one unilateral.

5. The subscapular artery perforates the nerve just below the median loop in five cases.

Type 3. The structure of the plexus is modified by an aberrant axillary artery. There were seven cases (17%), of which four were bilateral and three unilateral.

6. The eighth segmental artery passes through the median loop between the eighth cervical and first thoracic root of the medial cord in four cases.
7. One case. The ninth segmental artery lies caudad to the first thoracic nerve root and does not penetrate the plexus.

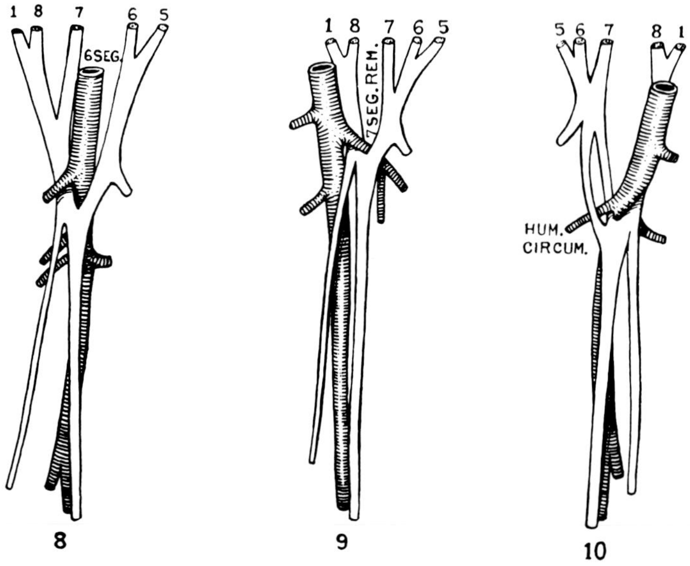

Fig. 1.32. *(continued)*

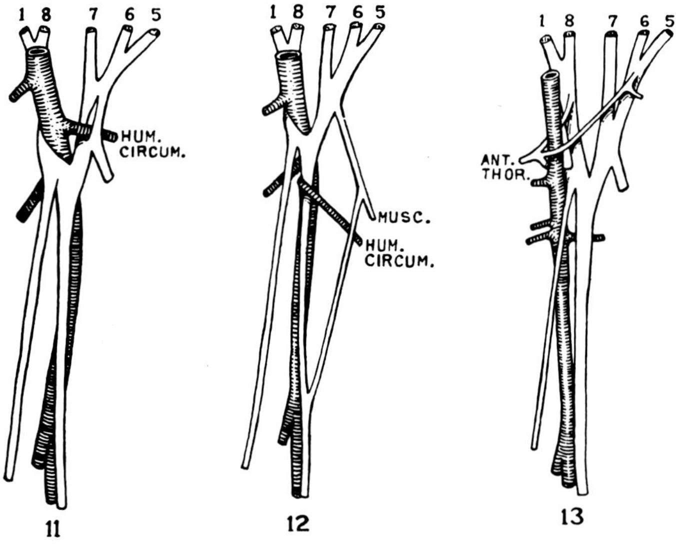

8. One case. The sixth segmental artery passes through the plexus between the superior and middle trunks. A branch of the artery perforates the lateral cord.
9. One case. The remnant of the seventh segmental artery is a branch of the ninth segmental vessel, which passes through the median loop and gives rise to the humeral circumflex and deep brachial branches.

Type 4. The cord of the plexus is divided by an arterial branch. Six cases were found (14%), two bilateral and four unilateral.

10. Three cases. The lateral cord below the origin of the musculocutaneous nerve is perforated by the common stem of the anterior and posterior humeral circumflex arteries.
11. One case. The lateral cord above the origin on

the musculocutaneous nerve is perforated by the common stem of the humeral circumflex artery.

Type 5. The nerves communicate around the axillary artery or its branches. This was found in four cases (10%), all unilateral.

12. Two cases. The musculocutaneous and median nerves communicate around the common stem of the humeral circumflex arteries.
13. One case. The anterior thoracic and ulnar nerves communicate around a ninth segmental artery. A remnant of the seventh segmental artery is also present.

Miller showed by her studies that more than one type of anomalous artery-plexus arrangement may occur in the same axillary region and that there may be numerous intrinsic variations of the nerves and blood vessels. In 41% of the anomalous cases, the plexus was normal, whereas the relationship with the artery was not. 14% of the cases showed a normal artery in an abnormal relationship with the plexus. In 45% of the anomalies, the artery and plexus were mutually aberrant. On the basis of these studies and those in other animals, Miller concluded that the problem of the relationship between the axillary artery and the brachial plexus is explained as a combination of embryologic and evolutionary processes.

The foregoing compendium of the variations in the anatomy of the brachial plexus is presented in the hope that rather than intimidating or stupefying the reader into a sense of hopelessness, it will stimulate thought and application in clinical situations. The pertinent surgical anatomy and operative approach will be found in Chapter 10.

REFERENCES

1. Abdullah S, Bowden REM: The blood supply of the brachial plexus. Proc R Soc Med 53:203, 1960
2. Alnot JY, Huten B: La systématisation du plexus brachiale. Rev Chir Orthop 63:27, 1977.
3. Bowden REM, Abdullah S, Gooding MR: Anatomy of the cervical spine, membranes, spinal cord, nerve roots and brachial plexus. In Lord Brain, Wilkinson M (eds): Cervical Spondylosis and Other Disorders of the Cervical Spine. Saunders, Philadelphia, 1967
4. Bufalini C, Pescatori G: Posterior cervical electromyography in the diagnosis and prognosis of brachial plexus injuries. J Bone Joint Surg 51B:4, 1969
5. Cruveilhier J: Traité d'anatomie descriptive. 2nd Ed. Labé, Paris, 1843
6. Cunningham DJ: Note on a connecting twig between the anterior divisions of the first and second dorsal nerves. J Anat Physiol 11:539, 1877
7. Engel J, et al: Choline acetyltransferase for differentiation between human motor and sensory nerve fibers. Ann Plast Surg 4(5):376, 1980
8. Ferrier D, Yeo GF: The function of the motor roots of the brachial plexus. Proc R Soc Lond 32:12, 1881
9. Frykholm R: The mechanism of cervical radicular lesions resulting from friction or forceful traction.
10. Frykholm R: Cervical epidural structures, periradicular and epineurial sheaths.
11. Gooding MR: The study of some aspects of the blood supply of the spinal cord. Thesis, MSC University of London, 1964
12. Goss CM (ed): Gray's Anatomy. 28th Ed. Lea and Febiger, Philadelphia, 1966
13. Harris W: The true form of the brachial plexus and its distribution. J Anat Physiol 38:399, 1903–1904
14. Haymaker W, Woodhall B: Peripheral Nerve Injuries. 2nd Ed. Saunders, Philadelphia, 1956
15. Herringham WP: Minute anatomy of the brachial plexus. Proc R Soc Lond 41:423, 1886
16. Hollinshead WH: Anatomy for Surgeons. Vol 3: The Back and Limbs. 2nd Ed. Harper & Row, Hagerstown, MD, 1969
17. Hovelacque A: Anatomie des nerfs craniens et rachidiens et du système grand sympathique. Doin, Paris, 1927
18. Kaplan EB: Functional and Surgical Anatomy of the Hand. 2nd Ed. Lippincott, Philadelphia and Montreal, 1965
19. Kaplan EB, Spinner M: Normal and anomalous innervation patterns in the upper extremity. In Omer GE, Spinner M (eds): Management of Peripheral Nerve Problems. Saunders, Philadelphia, 1980
20. Kerr AT: The brachial plexus of nerves in man, the variations in its formation and its branches. Am J Anat 23:285, 1918
21. Kline DG, Judice DJ: Operative management of selective brachial plexus lesions. J Neurosurg 58:631, 1983
22. Landi A, Copland SA, Wynn-Parry, CB, Jones SJ: The role of the somatosensory evoked potentials and nerve conduction studies in the surgical management of brachial plexus injuries. J Bone Joint Surg 62:492, 1980
23. Linell EA: The distribution of nerves in the upper limb with reference to variabilities and their clinical significance. J Anat 35:6, 1921
24. Miller RA: Observations upon the arrangement of the axillary and brachial plexus. Am J Anat 64:143, 1939
25. Narakas AO: Surgical treatment of traction injuries of the brachial plexus. Clin Orthop 133:71, 1978
26. Sherrington CS: Experiments in examination of the

peripheral distribution of the fibres of the posterior roots of some spinal nerves. Part II. Phil Trans R Soc Lond 190:45, 1898

27. Sunderland S, Bedbrook GM: The relative sympathetic contribution to individual roots of the brachial plexus in man. Brain 72:297, 1949
28. Sunderland S: Meningeal—neural relations in the intervertebral foramen. J Neurosurg 40:756, 1974
29. Sunderland S: Mechanisms of cervical root avulsion and injuries of the neck and shoulder. J Neurosurg 41:705, 1974
30. Sunderland S: Avulsion of nerve roots. In Braakman R (ed): Handbook of Clinical Neurology. Vol 25. Part 1. Chap. 16, p. 393. Injuries of the Spinal Cord and Column. North-Holland Publishing, Amsterdam, 1976
31. Sunderland S: Nerves and Nerve Injuries. 2nd Ed. Churchill Livingstone, Edinburgh, 1978.
32. Testut L: Mémoire su la portion brachiale du nerf musculocutane. Int Monatschr Anat Histol 1:305, 1884
33. Walsh JF; The anatomy of the brachial plexus. Am J Med Sci NS 74:387, 1877

2

Closed Injury to the Brachial Plexus

SUPRACLAVICULAR INJURY

Although patients with brachial plexus injury may present with a bewildering variety of patterns of neurological loss in the upper limb, there are useful generalizations that may be applied to clarify the approach to anatomic diagnosis and, ultimately, functional prognosis.

The mode of injury usually involves a high-velocity motor vehicle accident in a young patient. Motorcycles account for the great majority of closed injuries. Bonney[2] documented a series of 29 patients with complete supraclavicular traction injuries of the plexus. Twenty of them were in the age group 16 to 25. Of the 29 patients studied, 22 received their injuries from motorcycles, and four from bicycles, while one was run over by a car, and two had their arms caught in machines. A series of 103 patients with all types of plexus injuries reported by Wynn-Parry[15] included seven gunshot wounds. There were, however, 52 motorcycle accidents and 28 road traffic accidents, with the remaining 13 closed injuries resulting from a variety of "low-velocity" situations.

These statistics are meaningful if one considers the mechanism of injury responsible for most of the cases observed. Even though the occasional patient may, as stated above, incur his injury by other means, the typical patient falls from a speeding motorcycle, often striking the head and shoulder and stretching the neck. Without a safety helmet, the impact upon the cranial contents may cause a fatal head injury.[3] Then the plexus injury is of academic interest only, as observed at the autopsy table. With the protection afforded by the helmet, the chances of severe head injury are significantly lessened. Nevertheless, many patients with plexus injuries still are rendered unconscious by their fall. The details of the history of injury are lost and sometimes the lack of voluntary control of the limb is unappreciated because of the overriding effects of the central nervous system lesion.

It is the distracting force exerted between the head and shoulder that produces the common traction injury. The normal anatomic structures that surround the plexus have been already described. If, however, the tensile strength of the deep cervical fascia, the scalene muscles, the skeletal structures, and the meninges are exceeded, then the nerves have little protection against traction elongation. The cervical transverse processes may be avulsed, or the first rib may be fractured. If these bony lesions are seen on plain radiographs, one may infer that the corresponding nerve roots that are invested by the fascia have been similarly avulsed from the spinal cord. The scalene muscles may also be torn by the same force, producing further scarring around the neuromas that form.

Given the anatomic and biomechanical complexities of the brachial plexus, one could anticipate an almost infinite variety of possible sites and degrees of injury under these circumstances.

To understand the biomechanics of injury, let us consider the plexus as Stevens[12] did by means of a simple mechanical analogy. He pointed out that, in order to rupture a hypothetical cord by either longitudinal or transverse traction, the ends must be securely held. The brachial plexus may be so depicted with the deep fascia providing firm anchorage. Now, even though one could conceivably position the head, neck, and arm in any number of ways and then apply stress of varying magnitude to the system from different directions, the ultimate result would be that, if stress is reflected on the cords of the plexus, tension is developed. The relative position of the arm

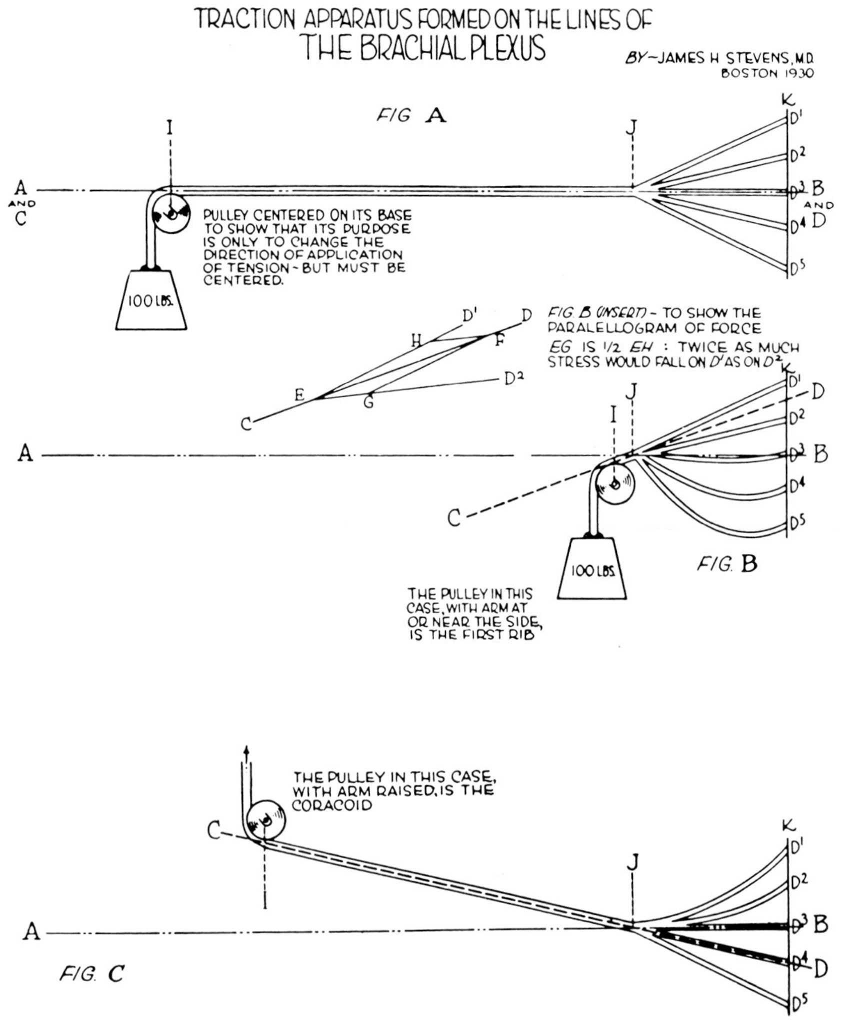

TRACTION APPARATUS FORMED ON THE LINES OF
THE BRACHIAL PLEXUS
BY—JAMES H STEVENS, M.D.
BOSTON 1930
FIG A
PULLEY CENTERED ON ITS BASE TO SHOW THAT ITS PURPOSE IS ONLY TO CHANGE THE DIRECTION OF APPLICATION OF TENSION—BUT MUST BE CENTERED.
100 LBS.
FIG. B (INSERT) — TO SHOW THE PARALELLOGRAM OF FORCE
EG IS 1/2 EH : TWICE AS MUCH STRESS WOULD FALL ON D' AS ON D²
THE PULLEY IN THIS CASE, WITH ARM AT OR NEAR THE SIDE, IS THE FIRST RIB
100 LBS.
FIG. B
THE PULLEY IN THIS CASE, WITH ARM RAISED, IS THE CORACOID
FIG. C

Fig. 2.1. Models of the forces causing different types of traction injury. (Reproduced from Stevens JH: Brachial plexus paralysis. In Codman EA (ed): The Shoulder. G. Miller, Brooklyn, NY, 1934.)

and head together with the velocity and magnitude of the stress applied then determine the nature and location of the lesion.

The cords of the plexus may be thought of as a traction apparatus with its normal axis passing through C7 (Fig. 2.1). With the arm horizontal, tension applied to this structure will fall equally on the five roots only if the force of the pull falls exactly through the neutral axis at its center. If, however, there is even a slight deviation from the neutral axis, the result is an offset pull to one side or the other. Transfer of the force to some of the roots would occur, while the others would be lax. A pulley introduced into this system would change the manner in which the force would fall to one side or the other of the neutral axis. If the pulley were elevated, the lines of tension would come below the neutral axis, and the acme of stress would be below. If the pulley were lowered, the acme of stress would be above. The movable scapula, with its coracoid process under which the integrated cord passes, acts like a movable pulley in the shoulder joint complex. One can then imagine various alternative positions of the shoulder and arm as the traction is applied, and the corresponding ways in which the resultant forces will differ in their ultimate pathways. With the arm at the side and pulled downward, the pulley is not the coracoid, but the superior surface of the first rib as the plexus passes over it. In this situation, the lower roots would bear the brunt of the stress. If, however, a weight falls on

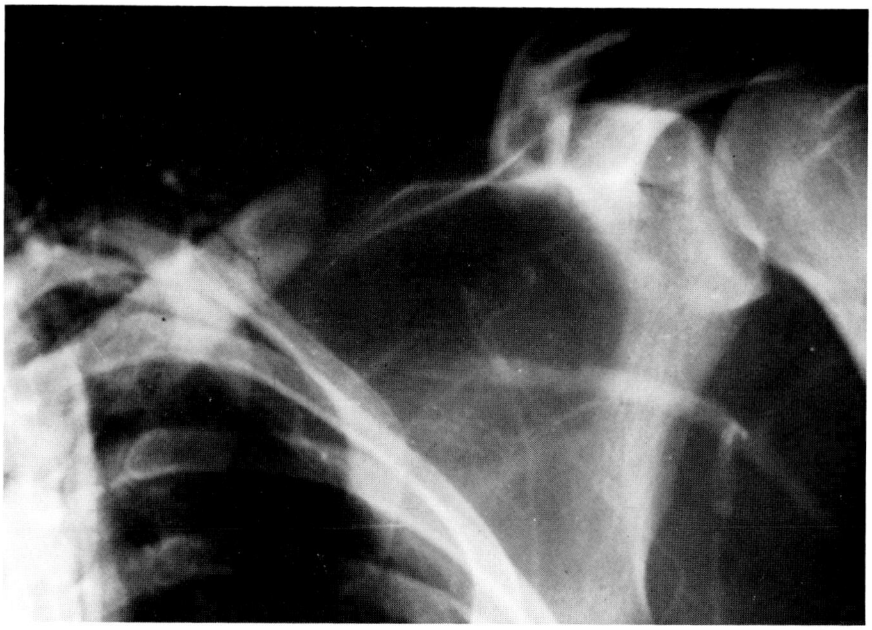

Fig. 2.2. Arteriogram of patient with flail, anesthetic arm due to traction injury of the brachial plexus incurred in a motorcycle accident. Not only was the clavicle fractured, but the entire brachial plexus was avulsed. No recovery or reconstruction is possible in this case.

the shoulder from above, the upper roots will suffer most. If the impact fractures the clavicle, abnormal excursion of the shoulder girdle will be possible, thus permitting greater stress to fall upon the nerves (Fig. 2.2). Since the plexus is firmly attached at both ends, the tension would build up rapidly and result in rupture of the nerves. If the arm were adducted and the head forced laterally to the other side, the upper roots would be affected (Fig. 2.3). A fall with the arm abducted would probably damage the lower roots primarily (Fig. 2.4). Not only can the neural elements be stressed, but the fascial investments and muscles can tear and also the bones fracture. Exudate and scar tissue can then solidify to further compromise nerve function.

It will be useful, although somewhat arbitrary, to divide the plexus into a supraclavicular and an infraclavicular portion (Fig. 2.5). This division is imprecise, of course, because the clavicle moves with movement of the arm in the scapular plane. Nevertheless, for the purposes of this discussion, we will assume that the patient has the arm at the side. Therefore, the supraclavicular portion will include the plexus from the intradural spinal roots to the divisions, and the infraclavicular, the cords, and the terminal branches as individual peripheral nerves.

It is the supraclavicular plexus that is most consistently and severely damaged by the type of traction injury described above. As with traction lesions in other parts of the peripheral nervous system, the damage to the individual neural components may vary from trivial and reversible to catastrophic and irreparable (Fig. 2.6). Although Sunderland's[14] classification of nerve injury is more precise in some situations, that of Seddon[10] simplifies designation of the severity of a particular lesion and will be used in this discussion (Table 2.1).

In general, a neurapraxia is not as common in the supraclavicular plexus as other types of injury, although it occurs more often here than in other parts of the plexus. It results from a moderate degree of stretch, which produces a physiological block to conduction rather than an identifiable anatomic lesion. Motor fibers tend to be affected more than sensory, and electrophysiological responses are normal. Usually, spontaneous recovery is largely complete within six weeks of injury.

Axonotmesis, which results from a greater degree of stretch, involves interruption of axonal continuity, and therefore total loss of distal neurological function. However, because the neural tubes are intact and capable of conducting the regenerating axons, spontaneous recovery is possible. Since Wallerian degeneration does occur distal to the site of

(Text continues on p. 44)

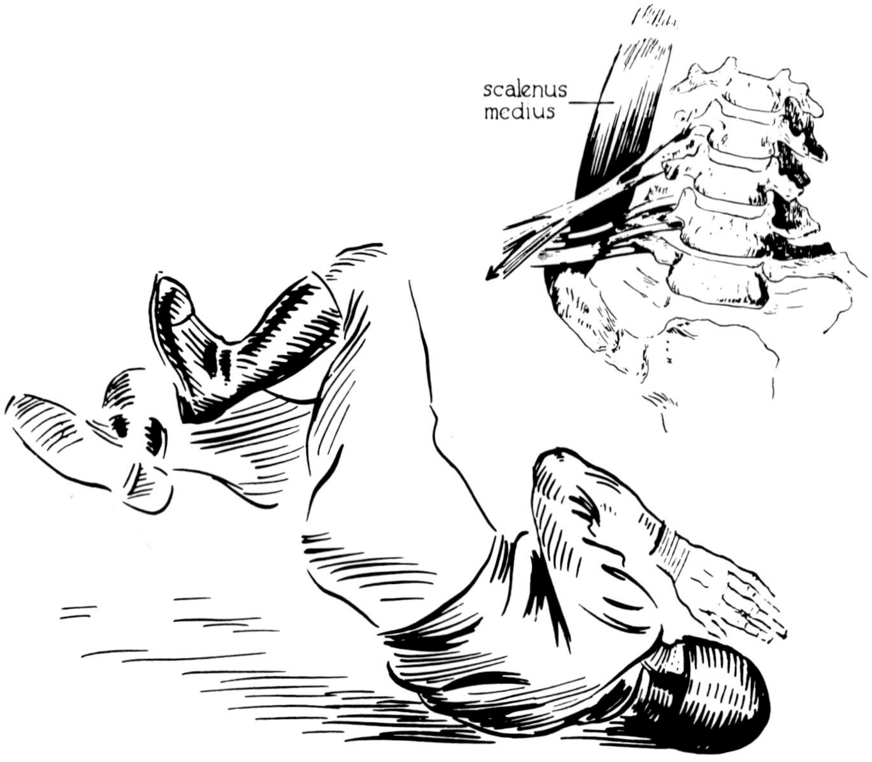

Fig. 2.3. Type of fall producing upper root injury. (Reproduced from Barnes R: Traction injuries of the brachial plexus in adults. J Bone Joint Surg 31B:10, 1949.)

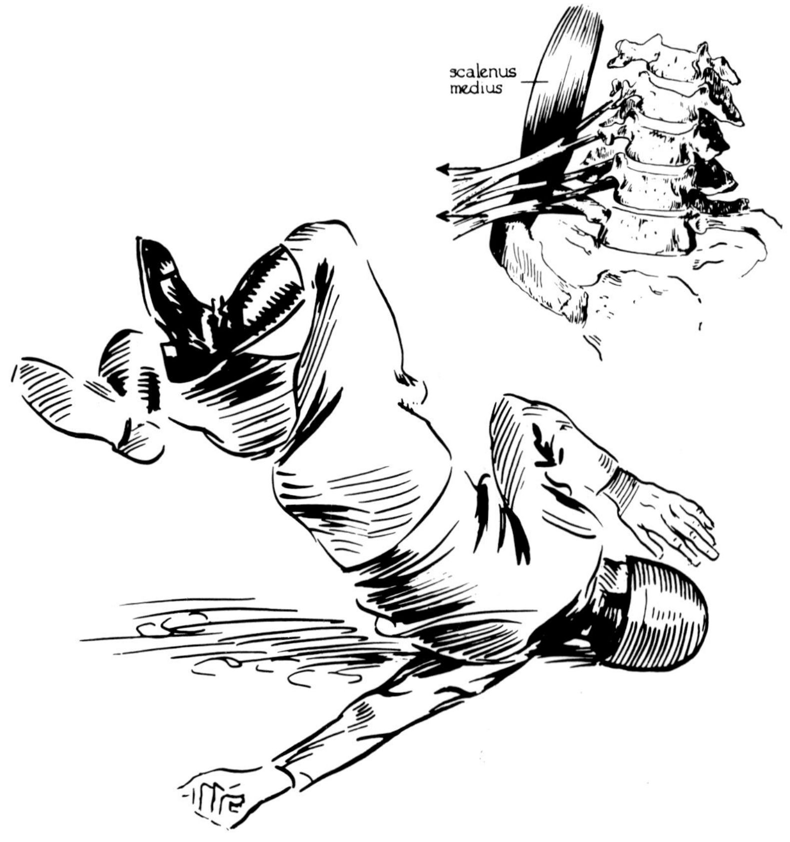

Fig. 2.4. Type of fall producing lower root injury. (Reproduced from Barnes R: Traction injuries of the brachial plexus in adults. J Bone Joint Surg 31B:10, 1949.)

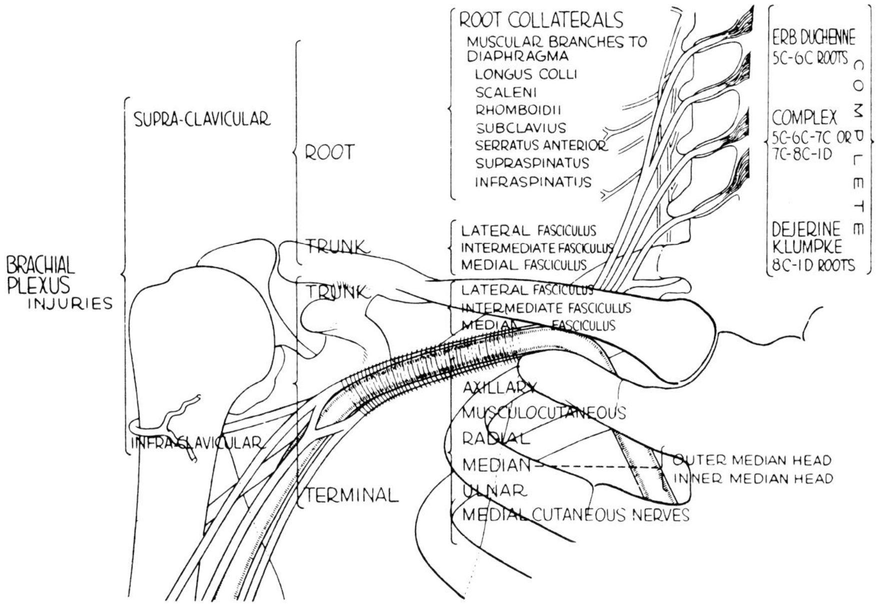

Fig. 2.5. The brachial plexus, according to Stevens. (Reproduced from Stevens JH: Brachial plexus paralysis. In Codman EA (ed): The Shoulder. G. Miller, Brooklyn, NY, 1934.)

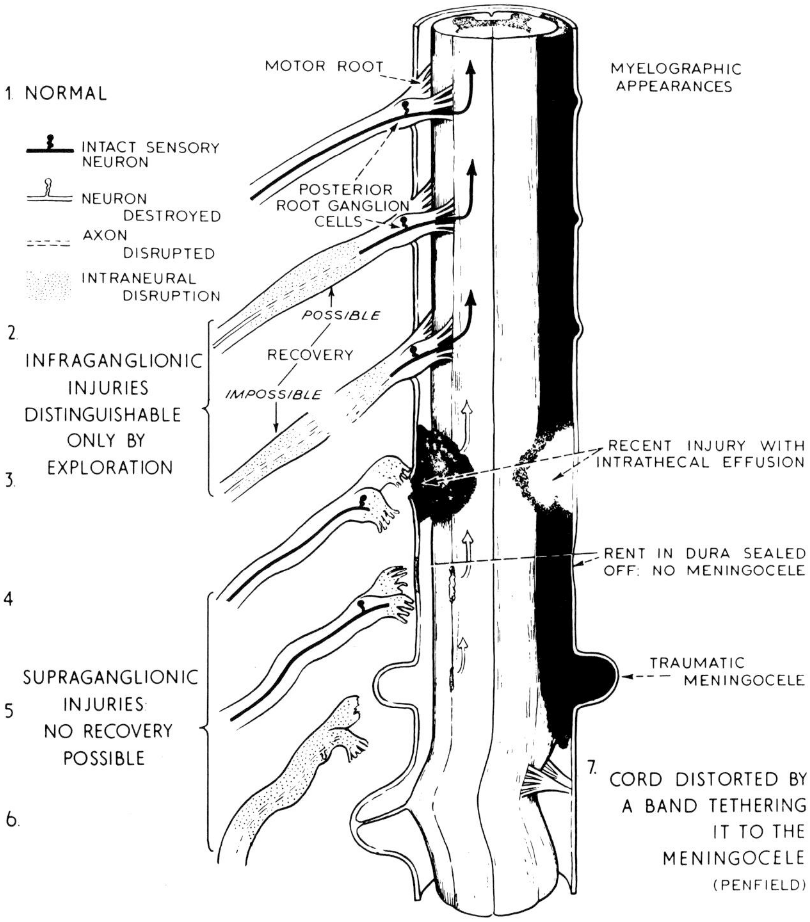

Fig. 2.6. Types of injury suffered by the roots of the brachial plexus. (Reproduced from Seddon HJ: Surgical Disorders of the Peripheral Nerves. Copyright 1972 The Williams & Wilkins Co., Baltimore.)

Table 2.1. Classification of Nerve Injuries

	Neurapraxia	Axonotmesis	Neurotmesis
Common causes	Compression Traction Freezing Ischemia Missiles	Compression Traction Missiles Ischemia Freezing Friction	Lacerations Missiles Traction Injections Ischemia
Pathology (involving all or part of nerve circumference)	Local demyelination; axons intact	Axons interrupted; supporting stroma (Schwann sheaths) intact	Axons and sheaths both interrupted
Clinical findings	Complete motor paralysis; partial sensory loss	Complete motor and sensory loss	Complete motor and sensory loss
Electromyographic findings	Rare fibrillations; no voluntary action potentials	Fibrillations seen after 3 wks; no voluntary action potentials	Fibrillations seen after 3 wks; no voluntary action potentials
Operative findings	Nerve continuity preserved	Nerve continuity preserved; occasional neuromatous swelling	Anatomic gap in nerve; continuity may be apparent because of scar
Spontaneous recovery	Usually within 4–6 wks; no regular order of recovery	Recovery at rate of 1 mm/day in order of innervation	None without surgical repair
Quality of recovery	Complete	Complete or nearly complete	Never complete, even after surgical repair

Adapted from Seddon HJ: Three types of nerve injury. Brain 66:237, 1943.

injury, the electrical responses are those of denervation, and therefore indistinguishable except by serial examination from neurotmesis.

Neurotmesis, the most severe degree of nerve injury (literally, "a cutting of nerve"), results from complete disruption of all elements of the nerve so that spontaneous recovery is impossible. To apply this term to traction injuries of the brachial plexus, however, it is necessary to further define the site of the lesion as either within the spinal canal (supraganglionic or preganglionic) or distal to the dorsal root ganglion and intervertebral foramen (infraganglionic or postganglionic). Supraganglionic injury involves avulsion of the root from the spinal cord, while infraganglionic involves distal rupture of the nerves. While both situations result in total loss of motor and sensory function mediated by the particular root involved, there are important differences in both pathophysiology and potential for surgical reconstruction (Fig. 2.7).

The mechanism of traction and avulsion injuries of the brachial plexus has been studied by many authors, a number of whom came to widely divergent conclusions.

Fieux[7] experimentally ruptured the trunks of the brachial plexus in stillborn infants and found that they were regularly torn at a distance of 5–6 mm lateral to the transverse processes. Others, such as Duval and Guillain[5,6] claimed that rupture occurred more centrally. Stevens[12] and Barnes[1] found a more peripheral site to be most common.

The experiments of Frykholm[8] are of interest in elucidating the mechanism of intradural rupture. He performed cervical laminectomy in eight adult cadavers and then observed the intraspinal structures while the head was turned in different directions. The visible movements of the dural sac, cord, nerve roots, and radicular nerves were recorded, and the influence of the position of the shoulder girdle and arm on these structures were studied. Frykholm concluded that the trunks of the plexus are protected from direct strain by their epineurial sheaths, which are firmly attached to the cervical transverse processes. If these attachments give way, the strain is transmitted to the periradicular sheaths. If the periradicular and epineurial sheaths both rupture, the strain falls directly on the nerve trunk. Since the weakest point of the nerve trunk is at the duroradicu-

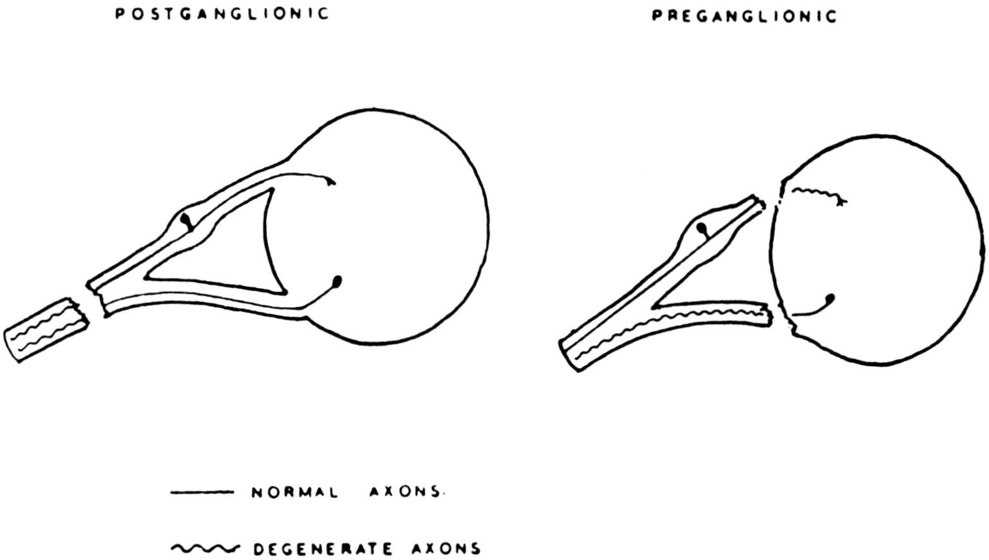

Fig. 2.7. Postganglionic (infraganglionic) lesion produces motor and sensory loss and Wallerian degeneration of all axons distal to the rupture of the nerve because they have been separated from their neurons, both in the dorsal root ganglion (sensory) and the anterior horn cell within the spinal cord (motor). Neither motor nor sensory nerve conduction can be demonstrated. Nevertheless, surgical repair of the lesion may be possible. The preganglionic (supraganglionic) avulsion of the roots from the spinal cord also produces total sensory and motor loss. In this case, because the dorsal root ganglion has been avulsed in continuity with its axon (the central connection is lost), there is no Wallerian degeneration in the sensory axon, and even though there is peripheral anesthesia, there is preservation of normal conduction velocity in the sensory components of the nerve. Motor conduction is lost. Such root avulsions cannot be repaired surgically.

lar junction, the root stems are torn off from the dural sac, and the roots are avulsed from the cord.

The type of injury to the plexus and its roots is determined both by the magnitude of the force and by where along the neural pathway it is applied. The roots may be avulsed wholly or partially, and differential avulsion of the sensory and motor components can occur. When a root is avulsed, the dura usually ruptures as well, and leakage of cerebrospinal fluid occurs. There may also be significant intrathecal bleeding. The cord may rarely be injured directly, with disruption of adjacent spinal pathways and demonstrable distant spasticity in the lower extremity.

The meningeal tear may sometimes be sealed off when the local effusion organizes. Usually, however, a pouch lined by the stretched and scarred meninges develops. These pseudomeningoceles are demonstrable by laminectomy, but since root avulsions are not surgically reparable, indirect means of diagnosis are usually employed. They will be described in detail in a chapter devoted to the evaluation of plexus injuries.

CLINICAL CLASSIFICATIONS OF CLOSED SUPRACLAVICULAR TRACTION INJURIES

Despite the variety of possible injuries to the plexus, most patients have neurological deficits that fall within relatively few, well-recognized groups. They may be classified as follows: (1) C5–6 or upper trunk lesions, (2) C5, C6, C7 lesions, (3) diffuse lesions of the plexus, and (4) C8, T1 lesions. Each group will be discussed separately along with factors of prognostic significance. Overall expected rates for spontaneous recovery in adults will be given.

The C5–6 or Upper Trunk Lesion

Shoulder control and elbow flexion are lost in the C5–6 or upper trunk lesion (Fig. 2.8). Typically there is atrophy of the supraspinatus and infraspinatus muscles beneath the trapezius, and of the deltoid as well. The result is an adducted and medially rotated shoulder which lacks abduction, lateral rotation, and forward flexion.

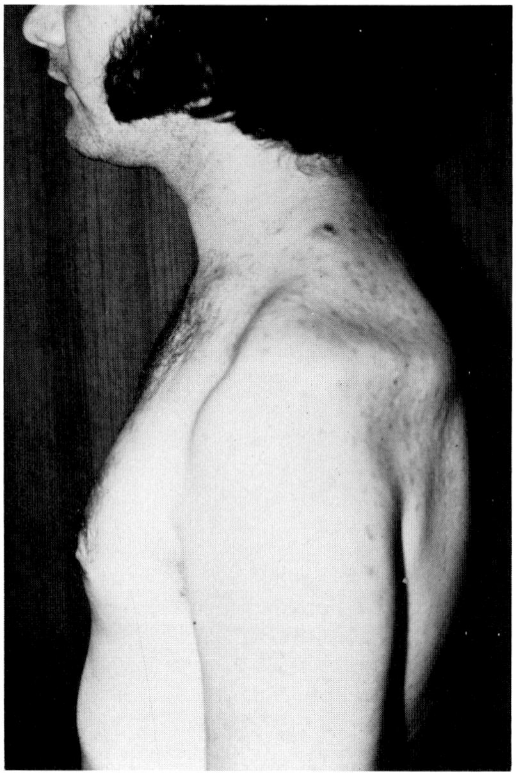
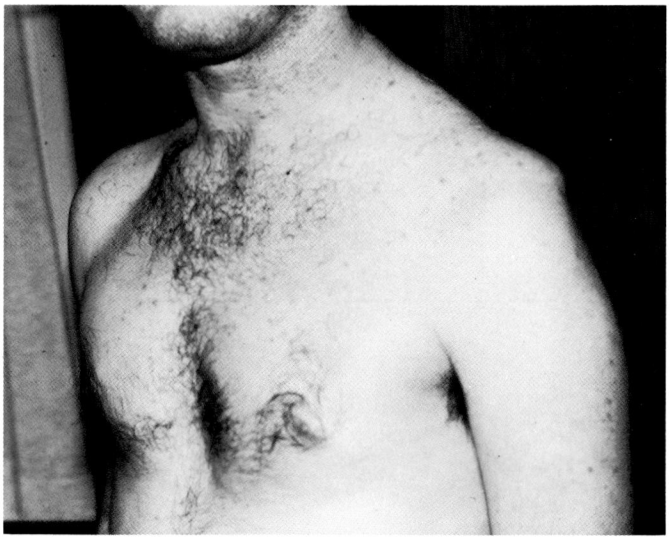
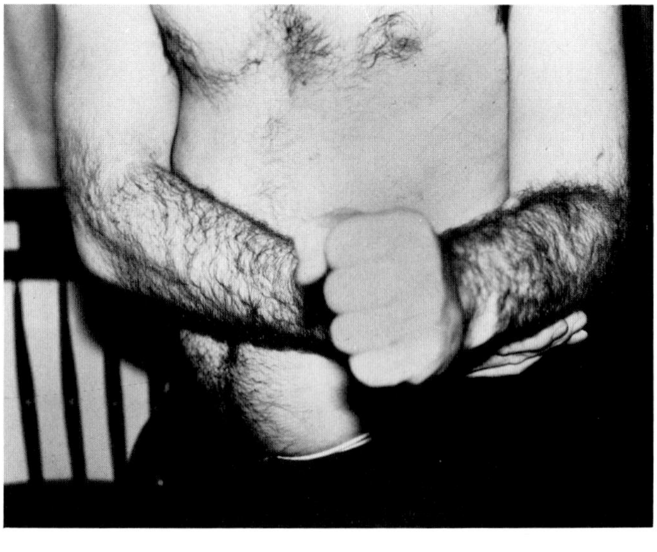

Fig. 2.8. A patient with an upper trunk C5, C6 lesion. Note the profound atrophy of the rotator cuff musculature as well as the inferior subluxation of the shoulder. Hand motor function is preserved.

Scapular control is usually preserved because of an intact trapezius and serratus anterior, which allow some shrugging motion, but little purposeful positioning of the limb. Although the clavicular pectoralis major is paralyzed, the more massive sternal portion is usually spared. All of the primary elbow flexors, including biceps and brachialis, are paralyzed, as is the brachioradialis. There may be a variable amount of wrist extension weakness, which can be disguised by supplementary extension through intact finger extensors.

If there has been a supraganglionic avulsion of C5, there may, in addition, be paralysis of the rhomboids and weakness of the serratus anterior, the latter resulting in winging of the scapula. These muscles are innervated by root collaterals coming off the roots themselves (the serratus by C6 and C7 in addition to C5). It is important for anatomic localization of the injury to recognize weakness in these muscles. Occasionally, with a large contribution of C5 to the innervation of the diaphragm, root avulsion will cause paralysis of the ipsilateral hemidiaphragm that can be demonstrated by fluoroscopy or inspiration–expiration chest x-ray. All of these simple, noninvasive examinations can provide valuable insight into the state of the intradural C5.

If, however, the serratus and rhomboids are intact and the muscles innervated by the suprascapular nerve are weak, the lesion can be placed between the origins of the root collaterals and the confluence of C5 and C6 into the upper trunk, from which the suprascapular nerve arises. This is the most common situation—root avulsion at C5 or C6 is uncommon.[15,16]

Sensory loss in the C5, C6 group usually involves the lateral brachium 2 cm below the acromion and the radial forearm extending to the thumb and index finger. Complete anesthesia in this area is unusual.

Because atrophy of the rotator cuff and deltoid progresses with time, the unsupported weight of the limb causes an inferior subluxation of the glenohumeral joint. This can be an annoying cause of shoulder pain due to stretching of the joint capsule and ligaments. In addition, a secondary chronic traction lesion of the remainder of the plexus can result in significant discomfort unless it is recognized and prevented. Although a sling will unweight the shoulder and prevent or correct the downward subluxation, constant use can produce an adduction–medial rotation contracture which can be very difficult to treat.

The prognosis for spontaneous recovery of function is generally felt to be better for patients with these injuries than with any of the supraclavicular traction injuries of the brachial plexus. Barnes[1] reported 14 patients whose major deficit was of the upper trunk: 11 regained flexion of the elbow and abduction and external rotation of the shoulder against gravity and resistance, although not all were capable of sustained effort. He stated that in all cases rated as satisfactory, weak contraction was noted in the paralyzed muscles within nine months of injury. In his patients there was an unspecified number of nondegenerative lesions, which would help to explain why four of the 10 patients with pure C5, C6 lesions achieved satisfactory functional recovery within six months, and one case considered to be a C4, C5 lesion also recovered within that time. Certainly, if the time required for recovery is calculated using an overall rate of 1 mm of nerve growth per month, most adult patients with degenerative lesions of the upper trunk will require longer than six months to achieve that degree of recovery. Outcome was less favorable in a similar group of upper trunk lesions in our clinic, many of whom were not seen until 3 or 4 months had elapsed. Failure to detect significant motor activity in these muscles by 9 months, and certainly by 12 (even in the presence of some low-level voluntary EMG activity), almost always indicates permanent paralysis. For the anatomical purist, it might seem desirable to attempt to separate the C5 lesion from the C6, but on the basis of clinical examination, it is impossible to so do. In all probability, C5 is the major motor root, and C6 may be the sensory, but no clinical advantage is gained from these considerations, and the two are best thought of as one unit, the upper trunk, even though the component parts may be used as individual sources of axons in reconstruction of the plexus.

Even if no neurological recovery at all occurs in these patients, as long as the joints have been maintained mobile and no contractures exist, the extremity can still be salvaged and reconstructed to provide useful function. Motor impairment of the the hand is minimal, although sensory loss on the radial side of the hand is significant.

The C5, C6, C7 Lesion

Patients with a C5, C6, C7 lesion (Fig. 2.9) have, in addition to deficits found in the C5, C6 lesion, a functional loss of active extension of the elbow, wrist and fingers—as though a radial nerve palsy were added to the usual results of C5–C6 injury. Not only is the C7 root the central one of the plexus, but it is the major root mediating extension. A deficit of C7 alone is rare, but in combination with an upper trunk palsy it is quite common. Such lesions are usually severe, because they reflect extensive damage to the plexus, and the prognosis for spontaneous recovery is worse than for C5–C6 injury.

Barnes[1] studied a series of 19 patients with C5, C6, C7 injury. Eleven patients regained extension of the wrist and fingers, flexion of the elbow, and abduction of the shoulder against gravity and some resistance. Six patients had incomplete recovery of function of the paralyzed muscles, and two had no recovery.

Two of the 19 patients had evidence of concomitant injury to the cervical plexus. Of the remaining 17, four achieved what was described as satisfactory functional recovery within six months. This again points to a mixed lesion, with a significant nondegenerative element present. Barnes reported a propensity for the flexors of the elbow to recover within

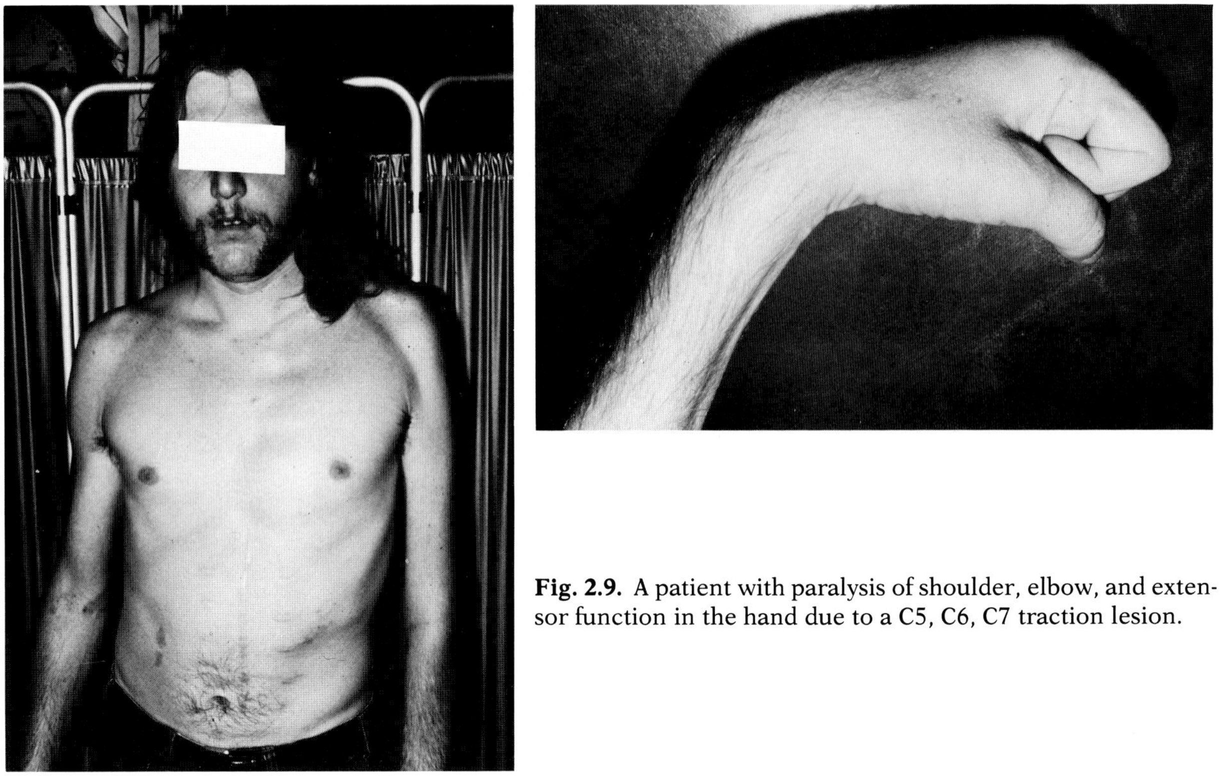

Fig. 2.9. A patient with paralysis of shoulder, elbow, and extensor function in the hand due to a C5, C6, C7 traction lesion.

two months of injury, and satisfactory recovery could occur in the deltoid even when voluntary contraction was first noted at 13 months. This result has not been duplicated in our patients. However, the lesions are most often infraganglionic when confined to these levels. Again, despite the increased resultant deficit in both motor and sensory function in those patients who do not experience spontaneous recovery, the outlook for a useful extremity following reconstruction is good. Of particular importance is the danger of contractures of the unopposed wrist and finger flexors if they are not properly splinted. It must be noted, however, that inappropriate constant splinting of wrist and fingers in extension can produce contractures that are even more disabling to the patient than if he had been left unattended.

In general, we have proceeded with surgical reconstruction in those patients who do not experience spontaneous recovery by 12 months, and for reasons to be explained later, have almost always begun distally in the limb and left the more proximal parts until later.

The C8, T1 Palsy

The C8, T1 palsy is the least common of the supraclavicular traction injuries to the adult brachial plexus. Seddon[11] quotes Yeoman as saying that these lesions are less likely to result from motorcycle accidents than the other types of traction injuries, and are more often the result of home accidents such as falls. The mechanism is presumed to be either a fall with the arm abducted or traction on the abducted arm itself, resulting in damage to the C8 and T1 or lower trunk.

Typically, the patient has Horner's syndrome and what would appear to be a combined median and ulnar palsy affecting the hand. Although this is an uncommon injury in adults, it is the well-recognized Klumpke paralysis seen with congenital palsies.

If C7 is also involved, finger and thumb extension is lost as well (Fig. 2.10). The prognosis for spontaneous recovery of the lost function in these patients is poorer, and the incidence of supraganglionic root avulsion higher than in the more cephalad portions of the plexus. Even so, since sensibility is usually

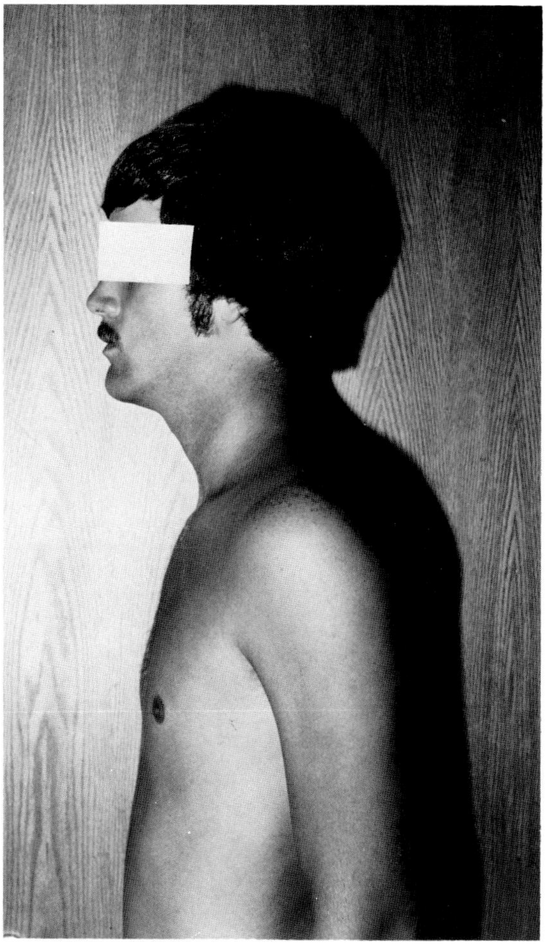

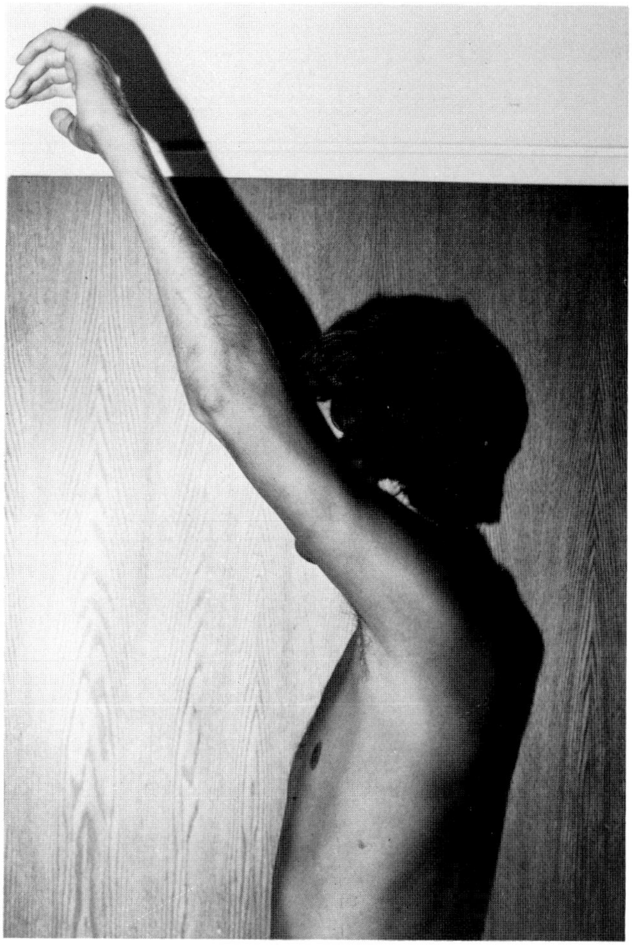

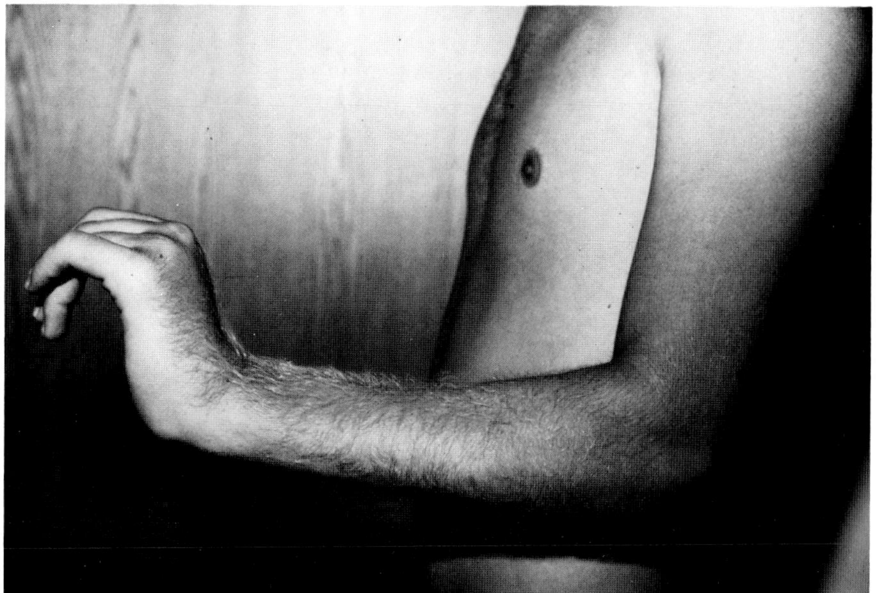

Fig. 2.10. This patient with a C7, C8, T1 lesion had Horner's syndrome. The C7 injury in this case caused paralysis of elbow, finger, and thumb extension. C5 and C6 function was preserved.

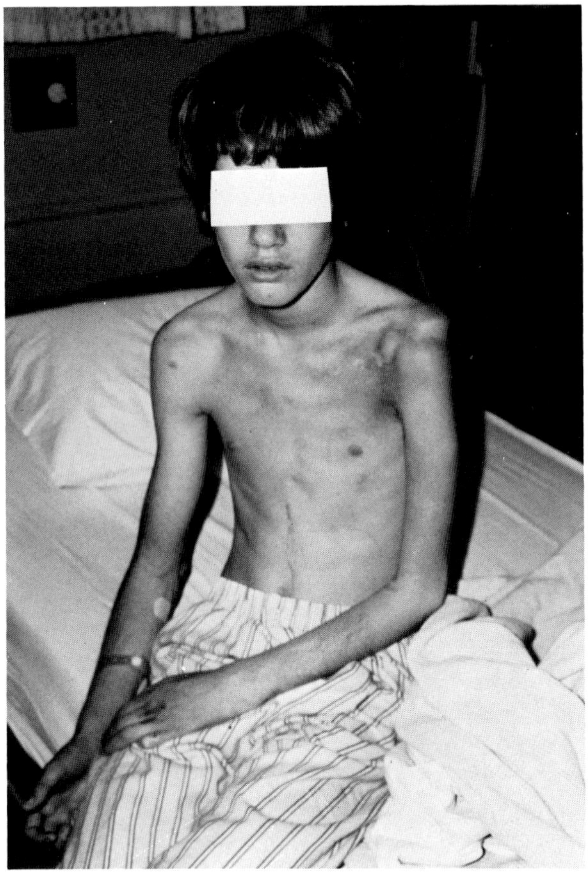

Fig. 2.11. A 12-year-old victim of a dirt-bike accident. He has a flail anesthetic arm and Horner's syndrome.

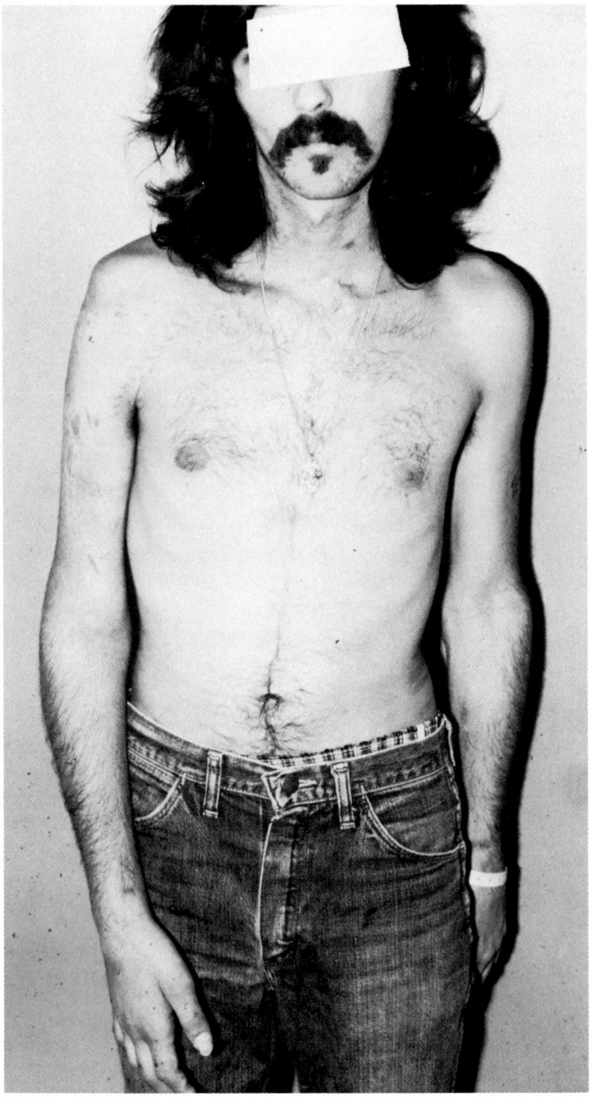

Fig. 2.12. This patient with a complete brachial plexus injury had Horner's syndrome and sensory loss on the lateral aspect of his neck, the latter indicating injury to the cervical plexus. C8 and T1 had been avulsed, and C5, C6, and C7 were ruptured distally in the posterior triangle of the neck.

preserved in the thumb and index fingers, and often in the middle finger as well, there is great potential for salvage of a useful hand by means of peripheral operative procedures involving tendon transfers and selected arthrodeses, particularly of the wrist.

The Whole-Plexus Injury

Patients with a whole-plexus injury (Figs. 2.11, 2.12) present the most difficult problem of all. Not only are the nerve lesions the most extensive, but they are also the most severe, and they usually result from major trauma. Often there are associated injuries to the head, chest, abdomen, or extremities that can be life-threatening. In the presence of a severe head injury, even if the patient is not in coma, one can fail to appreciate major paralysis of one arm. The possibility of brachial plexus injury should always be kept in mind, to avoid misdiagnosing a central nervous system lesion. The neurological loss is always greatest at the time of injury, rather than occurring hours later, after the beleaguered intern in the emergency ward has recorded "normal extremity function." The possibility of worsening of the neurological deficit by scar, as advanced by Davis et al.,[4] is debated, but certainly is not a consideration in the immediate hours or days following injury.

Some of these patients may be diagnosed from across the room by the observation of a unilateral Horner's syndrome of ptosis, myosis, and enophthalmos. This sign is an indication of a supraganglionic lesion of the first thoracic nerve root, assuming there is no local lesion of the eye or a central nervous system lesion. There may be a tender mass or ecchymosis in the supraclavicular fossa on the affected side, with Tinel's sign on percussion over the brachial plexus. The dermal distribution of the cervical plexus, which includes the lateral neck, cap of the shoulder, and tip of the ear, may by hypesthetic, and, if so, one can infer injury to the cervical plexus as well. Sometimes the ipsilateral trapezius may be weak or paralyzed, the result of an extensive traction lesion that also involves the spinal accessory nerve.

Manual muscle testing in a cooperative patient may be accomplished very quickly. One should specifically test the strength of the rhomboid. In the absence of trapezius weakness, a winged scapula is indicative of serratus weakness, and presumptive evidence of supraganglionic damage to C5, C6, and/or C7. In a patient with involvement of the entire plexus, the remainder of the musculature of the limb will be flail. Sensory examination will demonstrate anesthesia, certainly below the elbow, and to a variable degree above, except for the medial brachium and axilla, which is innervated by the intercostobrachial nerve. Rarely, T2 is involved to the point where this area loses sensation as well.

The general picture of spontaneous recovery in patients with lesions of the whole plexus has been well documented by Barnes[1] and Bonney.[2] Although the former described four patients with nondegenerative lesions of the entire plexus who recovered completely within six months, this favorable lesion has been rare in our experience. Bonney's series of 19 patients whose period of observation was 24 months or longer should be considered in detail for a representative picture of expected recovery. Muscle grading was according to the Medical Research Council system (Table 2.2).

All patients preserved or recovered normal or useful (Grade 3) power in trapezius, rhomboids, and serratus anterior. Undoubtedly, many of these patients had minimal loss in these muscles at the time of injury. The pectoralis major recovered to grade 3 in 12 cases. Only two patients got useful recovery of the deltoid, and two recovered to the same level in the lateral rotators of the humerus. The biceps recovered useful function in six cases, of whom two experienced confused reinnervation. In these patients, the triceps contracted simultaneously with the biceps to lock the elbow. Six patients recovered triceps function. In only five did one or more wrist flexors recover to grade 3 or better. Four patients achieved useful recovery in one or more finger flexors. No useful recovery was achieved in the extensor muscles of wrist or fingers, or in the intrinsic muscles of the hand. The overall picture is summarized in Figure 2.13. The quality of both motor and sensory recovery was extremely poor; more than half of the patients had motor recovery of grade M3 or lower and insignificant sensory recovery. The three patients who had the best sensory recovery also had motor recovery of grade M5 or better, according to Bonney.[2]

The pattern of timing of recovery is shown for Bonney's overall series of 28 patients from whose records this information could be obtained. The chart shows the time in months when contraction was first noted in a muscle that subsequently regained useful function (Fig. 2.14).

Although much of the initial contraction of these muscles was observed in the period between 6 and 18 months, it should be noted that in the wrist and finger flexors, recovery was first appreciated after two years post injury. Undoubtedly, this is a manifestation of the long distance necessary for the regenerating axon to grow before reaching the denervated muscles. Considering the extensive atrophy that intrinsic muscles of the hand would have by the time required for their reinnervation, it is not sur-

Table 2.2. Medical Research Council Motor Grading

Grade 1	Trace of contraction
Grade 2	Active movement of unloaded joint
Grade 3	Contraction against gravity
Grade 4	Contraction against gravity and mild resistance
Grade 5	Contraction against gravity and strong resistance (normal)

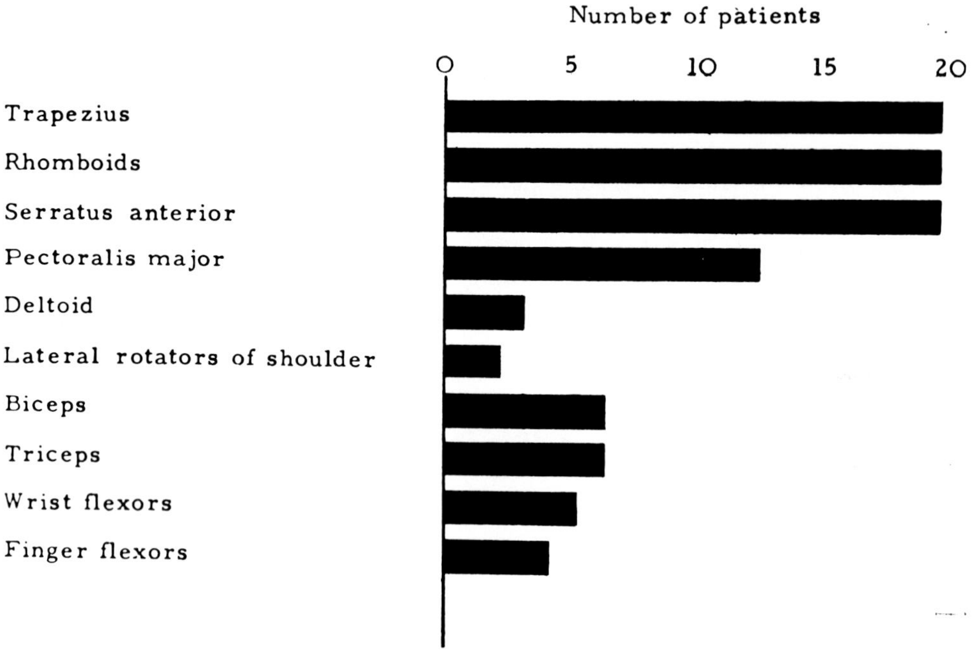

Fig. 2.13. Analysis of motor recovery to Medical Research Council grade 3 or better. Nineteen patients with traction injuries of the brachial plexus. Period of observation 24 months or longer. (Reproduced from Bonney G: Prognosis in traction lesions of the brachial plexus. J Bone Joint Surg 41B:4, 1959.)

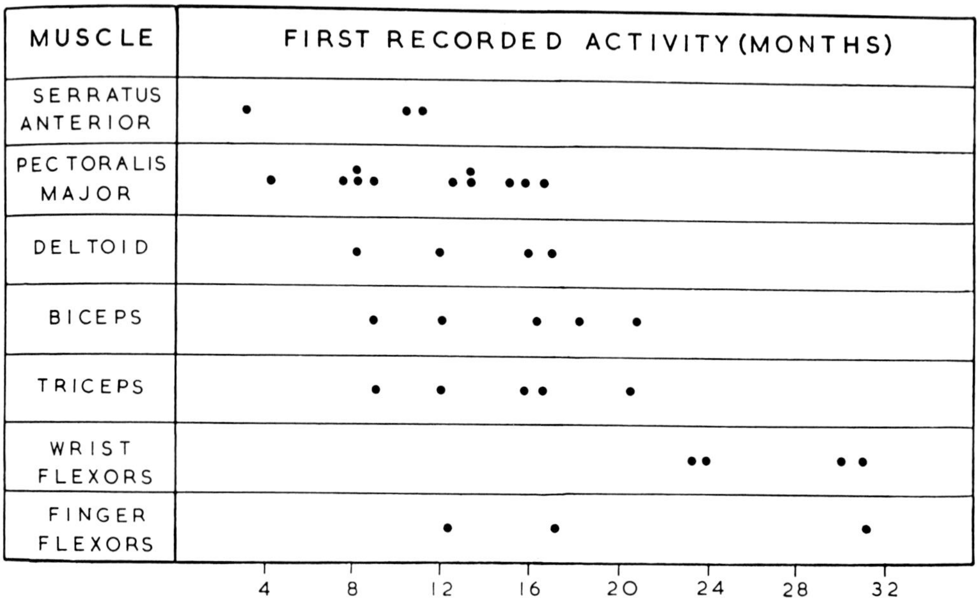

Fig. 2.14. Motor recovery in traction injuries of the brachial plexus. Time of first recorded activity of muscles which later went on to recovery of Medical Research Council grade 3 or better. (Reproduced from Bonney G: Prognosis in traction lesions of the brachial plexus. J Bone Joint Surg 41B:4, 1959.)

prising that they did not recover. Whether it is failure of the end organ or the axons themselves is a question, since sensibility in the distribution of the lower trunk rarely recovers either.

General sensory recovery in these patients was poor. Bonney commented that "not only was the extent of sensory recovery poor, but its quality was extremely defective." Nevertheless, his patients experienced very few problems as a result of defective sensibility, with only one patient developing a small ulcer, and another a blister from a burn.

The sensibility of the "anesthetic" limb is of interest, in that a variety of types of sensation may be reported by patients who are reliable reporters. The causalgia-like discomfort or paresthesias of which many patients complain should really be considered as "pain," and are of prognostic significance. The sensations perceived in response to external stimuli are poorly localized on the skin, and are sometimes felt as vibrations. Although most patients have no proprioceptive feedback from the muscles or joints of the hand, a surprisingly large percentage will have some awareness of the spatial position of the elbow. It is important to be able to test this sensation, since it may well make a difference in the usefulness of a prosthesis, even with anesthetic skin over the stump.

Although the lack of voluntary control of the flail-anesthetic arm makes it unlikely that the skin will be damaged by functional use, cutaneous vulnerability can be a significant problem. Common and seemingly unavoidable household objects such as steam pipes, stoves, and doors or lids can inflict serious damage on the hand and arm before the patient has any awareness of what has happened (Fig. 2.15). Long, brittle fingernails accompanying long-standing denervation can catch on clothing and be avulsed or cause finger fractures. Finally, one occasionally sees emotionally disturbed patients who will pick at the anesthetic fingers until ulcerations develop and amputation is the only available treatment.

There are a number of factors that can be considered of prognostic significance in the patient with whole plexus lesion. Since it is obvious that one must be careful to specify whether neurological or "functional" recovery is under consideration, the following factors relate only to the former, or that which can be defined as "impairment" rather than "disability."

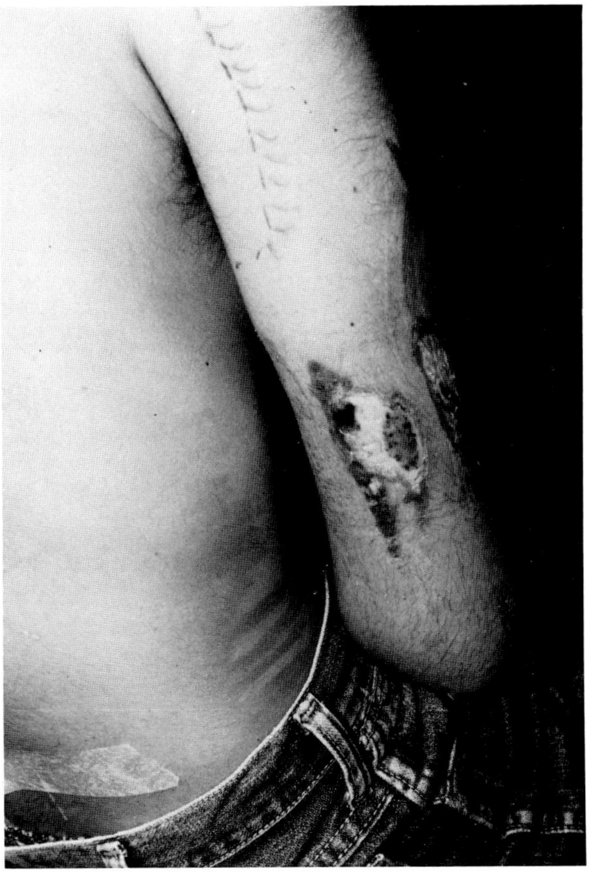

Fig. 2.15. This patient with a complete brachial palsy and an insensate limb sustained third-degree burns of the arm on a radiator and never felt them. Note intact sensibility in the distribution of T2 on the medial aspect of the arm and axilla.

Prognosis for Spontaneous Recovery of Traction Injuries

Mode of Injury. As has been stated previously, supraclavicular traction injuries to the brachial plexus caused by major violence, such as a fall from a speeding motorcycle or a high-velocity car crash, tend to be more extensive and severe than those caused by lesser trauma. The prognosis for recovery generally matches the severity of injury.

Associated Injuries. Bonney[2] studied patients with flail anesthetic arms with and without an associated fracture in the ipsilateral limb. He found that there was no difference in motor or sensory recovery in the two groups.

However, some bony injuries can be related to prognosis because they represent significant factors in the injury itself. The avulsion fracture of a cervical transverse process or of the first rib is good presumptive evidence that the nerve root at that level has been avulsed as well, although I have seen several cases where this proved to be false. Roaf[9] has called attention to the lateral tilt of the cervical spine that can be seen in the frontal radiograph of patients with root avulsion. In patients who have sustained a fracture of the clavicle along with their plexus injury, the extra mobility of the shoulder as it is distracted can produce more traction damage than might otherwise occur with an intact shoulder girdle. All of these bone injuries are associated with poor prognosis.

However, it should be noted that there is a much smaller group of traction injuries to the plexus associated with bony injury in the region of the shoulder girdle. These infraclavicular injuries in which the skeletal injury actually causes the nerve injury have a significantly better prognosis for recovery. They are discussed in Chapter 3.

Horner's Syndrome. Barnes[1] noted the association of ipsilateral Horner's syndrome with poor prognosis for recovery of the total brachial plexus palsy. Of 13 such patients, seven had no recovery and six regained only shoulder abduction and elbow flexion. Bonney's series of 29 patients with complete supraclavicular traction lesions included four who had no disturbance of the cervical sympathetics. Three of these went on to excellent recovery. In Yeoman's series of 99 patients with total paralysis, Horner's syndrome was present in 91% of the patients who failed to recover and in 80% of patients with total paralysis in whom there was no recovery in C8 and T1. These last statistics were quoted by Seddon[11] who considered Horner's syndrome a most unfavorable sign.

The pathogenesis of Horner's syndrome is as follows. The cervical portion of the sympathetic division of the autonomic nervous system originates in the intermediolateral cells of the spinal cord, extending from the eighth cervical or first thoracic segment through the upper four, five, or six thoracic segments. The fibers controlling oculopupillary action probably come from the eighth cervical and first and second thoracic segments. Preganglionic fibers extend from these roots to the inferior sympathetic ganglion and travel through middle and superior ganglia, where postganglionic fibers then travel with the internal carotid artery to the cavernous sympathetic plexus. From here they accompany the fifth cranial nerve to the orbit. The ciliary nerves then supply the dilator of the pupil, the tarsal muscles, and the orbital muscles of Müller. Interruption of this system by avulsion of the first thoracic nerve root causes the clinically observed syndrome. The myotic pupil results from paralysis of pupillary dilation. Ptosis is caused by paralysis of the tarsal muscles, and enophthalmos is due to paralysis of Müller's muscle. Sudomotor function is lost ipsilaterally on the face and neck, where sensation is normal, as well as in the anesthetic upper limb.

Horner's syndrome is difficult to detect in a patient who is unconscious due to a head injury. Sometimes the other, normal, pupil may be mistakenly thought to be dilated, which may lead to diagnostic confusion. However, there is no excuse for missing the presence of this important sign because of failure to remove the patient's eyeglasses.

Pain. In most cases of severe traction injury of the brachial plexus, the patient experiences severe pain in the limb, even though the limb may be essentially anesthetic to external stimuli. The pain is often described as constant, deep and boring, or burning, and it may be intermittently exacerbated. The onset is almost always immediate, and it may persist unremittingly for years. Fortunately, in many patients the pain tends to diminish to tolerable levels with time. Persistance of severe pain, however, has been correlated with a poor prognosis for recovery.[1] In Bonney's series of 25 patients followed for two years, 12 patients had persistent pain and 13 patients did not have severe pain. Of the patients with pain, 11 had motor recovery of grade M3 or less. More than half the patients with less severe or no pain, experienced motor recovery of grade M4 or better. Seddon[11] quoted Yeoman's series as follows: pain was severe in 32 of the 46 patients who suffered permanent paralysis of the whole plexus. Pain was also severe in 22 of the 40 patients who had total paralysis initially but who later showed some recovery proximal to the elbow.

In addition to the unfavorable prognosis for recovery, the problem of achieving relief of intractable pain has been thus far largely unsolved.

REFERENCES

1. Barnes R: Traction injuries of the brachial plexus in adults. J Bone Joint Surg 31B:10, 1949
2. Bonney G: Prognosis in traction lesions of the brachial plexus. J Bone Joint Surg 41B:4, 1959
3. Cairns H, Holbourn H: Head injuries in motor-cyclists with special reference to crash helmets. Br Med J May, 1943
4. Davis L, Martin J, Perret G: The treatment of injuries of the brachial plexus. Ann Surg 125:647, 1947
5. Duval P, Guillain G: Sur le mécanisme de production des paralysies radiculaires traumatiques du plexus brachial. Gaz Hebd Sci Med Bordeaux 5:649, 1900
6. Duval P, Guillain G: Les paralysies radiculaires du plexus brachial. G. Steinheil, Paris, 1901
7. Fieux: De la pathogenie des paralysies brachials chez le nouveau-né; paralysies obstetricales. Ann Gynecol Obstet 47:52, 1897
8. Frykholm R: The mechanism of cervical radicular lesions resulting from friction and forceful traction. Acta Chir Scand 102:93, 1951
9. Roaf R: Lateral flexion injuries of the cervical spine. J Bone Joint Surg 45B:36, 1936
10. Seddon HJ: Three types of nerve injury. Brain 66:237, 1943
11. Seddon HJ: Surgical Disorders of the Peripheral Nerves. Williams & Wilkins, Baltimore, 1972
12. Stevens JH: Brachial Plexus Paralysis. In Codman EA (ed): The shoulder. G. Miller, Brooklyn, NY, 1934
13. Sunderland SA: A classification of peripheral nerve injuries producing loss of function. Brain 74:491, 1951
14. Sunderland S: Nerves and Nerve Injuries. 2nd Ed. p. 69. Churchill Livingstone, Edinburgh, London, and New York, 1978
15. Wynn-Parry CB: The management of injuries of the brachial plexus. Proc R Soc Med 67:488, 1974
16. Yeoman PM: Brachial plexus injuries. J Bone Joint Surg 47B:187, 1965
17. Yeoman PM: Cervical myelography in traction injuries of the brachial plexus. J Bone Joint Surg 50B:253, 1968

3

Infraclavicular Brachial Plexus Injuries

Although traction injuries to the brachial plexus may occur anywhere from within the spinal canal to below the axilla, those that primarily involve the infraclavicular segments merit separate consideration. Not only is their mechanism of injury distinct from the more common supraclavicular injuries, but, because of this difference, their prognosis for spontaneous recovery is considerably better. The pathomechanics of supraclavicular injury have already been described. Let us now consider how skeletal injury in the region of the shoulder joint produces injury to the adjacent neurovascular structures.

The anatomical site of lesions of the brachial plexus caused by traction was the subject of lively debate in the late nineteenth and early twentieth centuries. In 1910 Delbet and Cauchoix[3] published a classic study in which they pointed out that the plexus lesions accompanied by shoulder dislocations were caused by them and involved the infraclavicular plexus and its terminal branches rather than the more proximal parts. They stated that the prognosis for recovery of these lesions was favorable. However, the paper received little attention in the English-speaking world, and were it not for Stevens'[9] comprehensive work published in 1934, which reiterated this concept and its importance, it would never have been appreciated. Although Delbet and Cauchoix[3] reported three surgical cases of their own and studied 36 cases of dislocations with nerve injuries from other sources, verification was still lacking.

In 1953 G. W. Milton[7] published an anatomical study of the possible mechanisms by which axillary nerve palsy could be produced during dislocation and reduction of the shoulder. The tensions produced on the other branches of the brachial plexus during the same maneuvers were studied. Fifteen recent cadavers were used to make the observations, which will be described in some detail since they are important to the understanding of this distinctive variety of nerve injury.

With the arm in the anatomical position, all the terminal branches were lax. Strong downward traction was applied to the adducted arm, which was then rotated internally and externally to the fullest extent while maintaining traction. The tension of the nerves was then recorded with the arm abducted 90 degrees in the extremes of rotation while exerting lateral traction. Finally the arm was hyperabducted with traction. The results of these experiments were as follows: Downward traction on the arm held at the side produced pull on the plexus, and internal rotation increased tension on the axillary and radial nerves. External rotation with traction caused a slight increase in radial nerve tension. With the arm at 90 degrees of abduction there was little traction on the posterior cord or its branches. Full external rotation increased the pull on the musculocutaneous nerve. In the hyperabducted position, there was no significant pull on the plexus.

In the second part of the study the shoulders were dislocated by lateral rotation and hyperabduction. The findings from this experiment are most important.

During the hyperabduction stage of dislocation the axillary nerve was rendered taut as it was stretched across the humeral head. With the arm by the side and the shoulder dislocated, the nerves in the axilla were more relaxed than normal. Then, if the arm was pulled downward and internally rotated, the axillary nerve was tightly stretched, especially if it

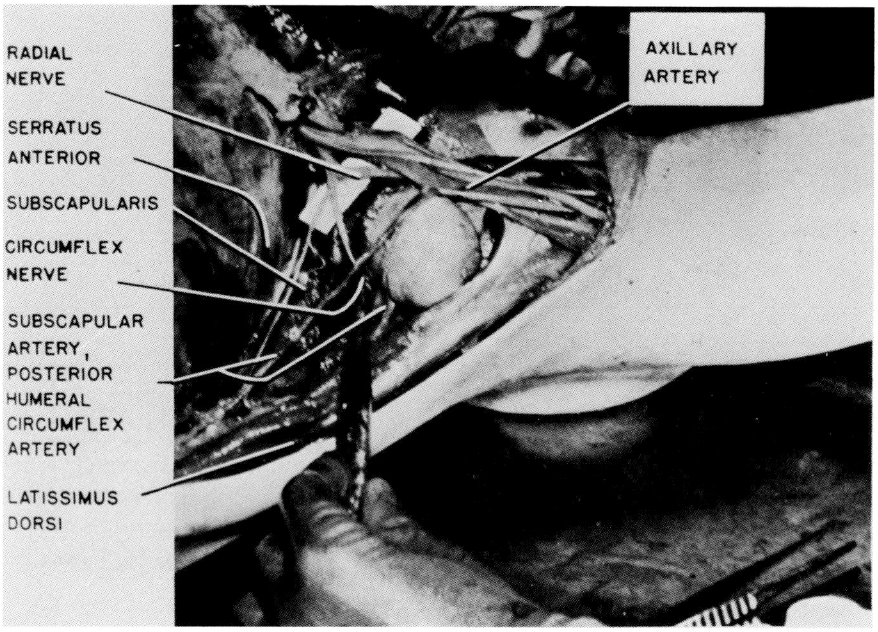

Fig. 3.1. The axillary (circumflex) nerve stretched over the humeral head during experimental dislocation of the shoulder in a cadaver dissection. (Reproduced from Milton GW: The mechanism of circumflex and other nerve injuries in dislocation of the shoulder and the possible mechanism of nerve injury during reduction of dislocation. Aust NZ J Surg 23:4, 1953.)

remained hooked over the head, rather than sliding down to its more normal position at the humeral neck (Fig. 3.1).

Downward traction on the arm produced tension on the axillary nerve, and the tension on the nerve was proportional to the traction on the arm. However, if the arm was first laterally rotated, the nerve could slip down off the head which relieved the tension. Internal rotation of the arm under these conditions increased the tension on the radial nerve and posterior cord as well as the axillary nerve. In the 90-degree abducted position, traction on the arm increased the tension of all the main branches of the brachial plexus except for the axillary nerve. The tension on the radial nerve was greatest in full internal rotation, and the musculocutaneous nerve in full external rotation. In the hyperabducted arm the tension of the nerves was lessened, although the axillary artery was severely stretched.

The implications of these findings with reference to reduction of dislocated shoulders are as follows: In using the Hippocratic method of longitudinal traction with the arm at the side, the humerus should be first laterally rotated to allow the axillary nerve to slip down off the head to avoid injury. In using the Kocher maneuver, for the same reason, strong downward traction and full internal rotation at the same time should be avoided.

In 1962 Gariepy, Derome, and Laurin[4] published a report on six patients who dislocated their shoulders and sustained severe brachial plexus injury. All had anterior dislocations, and two first noted their paralysis after reduction. A fifth patient, with a recurrent dislocating shoulder left unreduced for 24 hours, experienced the gradual onset of paralysis during that time. All patients experienced complete recovery from their neurological deficits; only one was operated upon. In this case the postoperative recovery was not attributed to the operation. From these cases and several cadaver dissections following experimental dislocation, the authors concluded that the most common mechanism of nerve injury is local traction because of the local excursion of the dislocated humeral head. Less commonly, direct pressure on the nerves by the humeral head was felt to be the cause. In those patients who experienced delayed onset of paralysis with unreduced dislocations it was postulated that the development of edema rendered the plexus more susceptible to the effects of compression. Gariepy, Derome, and Laurin concluded that the plexus lesions with shoulder dislocations are infraganglionic and always in continuity. They stated that the prognosis is excellent, and that no surgical exploration of the plexus is indicated.

In 1963 Sir Herbert Seddon proposed the study of a large series of patients seen at the Wingfield-Morris Orthopaedic Hospital, Oxford, and the Royal National Orthopaedic Hospital, London, to verify Steven's statement that "Lesions of the plexus caused by, or at the time of, dislocation soon get well." In 1965 Leffert and Seddon[6] described the results of that study. Of the available records of 230 cases of closed injury to the brachial plexus, 31 were considered infraclavicular, according to the following criteria:

> Injury to the brachial plexus and its terminal branches accompanying closed injury in the region of the shoulder except where there was
>
> 1. Fractured clavicle or cervical transverse processes
> 2. Evidence of injury to known supraclavicular branches of the plexus, i.e., dorsal scapular, suprascapular, and long thoracic nerves
> 3. Horner's syndrome
> 4. Swelling, induration, or tenderness in the supraclavicular fossa

All of these findings indicate supraclavicular injury, which would primarily determine the prognosis. Those cases of plexus injury with fractured clavicle are usually supraclavicular and were, therefore, excluded.

Table 3.1 Distribution of Skeletal Injuries: 31 Patients

Type of Skeletal Injury	No. of Patients
Dislocated shoulder and fractured greater tuberosity	12
Dislocated shoulder and fractured scapula	1
Dislocated shoulder	4
Fractured humerus—surgical neck	5
Fractured humerus—surgical neck and fractured scapula	1
Fractured humerus—surgical neck and greater tuberosity	1
Fractured greater tuberosity	2
Fractured shaft of the humerus	2
Fracture of glenoid neck	2
Fractured scapula—axillary border	1

From Leffert RD, Seddon HJ: Infraclavicular brachial plexus injuries. J Bone Joint Surg 47B:9, 1965.

The mode of injury of the 31 patients involved lesser degrees of violence occurring at lower velocity than in supraclavicular injuries. Although 12 cases resulted from falls from moving vehicles, seven patients fell while walking, a mechanism virtually never seen in the supraclavicular group. The distribution of skeletal injuries is given in Table 3.1.

RECOVERY OF THE INFRACLAVICULAR BRACHIAL PLEXUS INJURY

In order to document the recovery of the 31 patients with infraclavicular brachial plexus injury, the various patterns of neurological involvement had to be grouped according to the predominant nerve or nerves affected. In 14 the entire limb was involved; these were designated as having "diffuse infraclavicular injuries." The remaining patients had lesions of one or two cords or their terminal branches, and for analysis the combined lesions were examined separately. This resulted in eight patients appearing under two headings. The major categories to be considered, then, in addition to "diffuse," were "posterior cord or part thereof," the "lateral cord," or the "medial cord."

The "diffuse" group documented in Table 3.2 contrasts sharply with supraclavicular injuries involving the entire limb, for all patients with diffuse infraclavicular injury regained at least good and often normal power proximal to the hand. Intrinsic hand muscles of median innervation returned to grade IV in 11 of the 14 patients studied. The interossei did only slightly less well, with eight having near-normal or normal power and three more having a useful grade of recovery after more than two years (Fig. 3.2). It should be noted, however, that if the joints are allowed to stiffen, then neurological recovery will not result in return of function. This point will be further emphasized in the section on treatment in Chapter 9.

In the posterior cord group (Table 3.3) it was seen that recovery of the deltoid was poorest in the six isolated axillary nerve lesions. Recovery of the deltoid in the seven patients in the combined posterior cord group was considerably better (Fig. 3.3). Although this result could be anticipated, since the force producing the injury might be dissipated by its distribution over several nerves rather than the sin-

Table 3.2 Diffuse Infraclavicular Lesion—Motor Recovery

A. Initial Examination

Case No.	Electrical Reactions	Deltoid	Elbow Extension	Wrist Extension	Extension of Digits	Elbow Flexion	Wrist Flexion Median	Wrist Flexion Ulnar	Flexion of Digits Median	Flexion of Digits Ulnar	Median Intrinsic	Ulnar Intrinsic
1	Yes	—	0	0	0	0	0	0	0*	0*	0*	0*
2	Yes	0	0	0*	0	0	0	0	0*	0	0	0
3	Yes	3*	0*	0*	0	1+*	0	0*	3	3	2+	0*
4	No	2	1	0	0	0	0	0	0	3	0	0
5	Yes	0	0*	0*	0*	0	0	0*	0	0*	0	0*
6	Yes	—	—	0	0	0	0	0*	0	0*	0	0*
7	Yes	0	0	0	0	0	0	0	0	0	0	0*
8	Yes	0	0	0	0	0	0	0	0	0	0	0
9	No	2	0	0	0	0	1	2	3	2	3	1
10	Yes	5	0*	0	0*	0	0	0	0	0	0	0
11	No	0	0	0	0	3	3	—	4	4	3	0
12	Yes	2*	0*	1*	0*	0*	0*	0*	0*	0*	0*	0*
13	Yes	0	0*	0	0*	0*	0	0	0	0	0	0
14	Yes	0	0	0	0	0	0	0	0	0	0	0*

B. Final Examination

Case No.	Period of Observation from Time of Injury (months)	Deltoid	Elbow Extension	Wrist Extension	Extension of Digits	Elbow Flexion	Wrist Flexion Median	Wrist Flexion Ulnar	Flexion of Digits Median	Flexion of Digits Ulnar	Median Intrinsic	Ulnar Intrinsic (Interossei)
1	37	5	5	5	5	5	5	5	5	5	5	5
2	48	5	4	5	5	4	5	5	5	5	0	0
3	25	4+	4+	4+	4+	4+	4+	4+	4+	4+	4+	3+
4	23	5	5	5	5	5	5	5	5	5	5	0
5	24	5	5	5	5	5	5	5	5	5	5	4+
6	36	5	5	5	5	5	5	4+	5	4+	5	4+
7	29	5	5	5	5	5	5	5	5	5	5	3+
8	25	5	5	5	5	5	5	5	5	5	5	3+
9	14	5	5	5	5	5	5	5	5	5	5	5
10	12	5	5	5	5.3+	4+	5	5	4	—	3	5
11	19	3+	4+	4+	4+	4+	4	4	4+	4	4+	4
12	49	5	5	4	4	5	4	4	4	4	4	4
13	42	5	5	5	5	5	5	5	5	5	5	5
14	17	5	5	5	5	5	5	5	5	5	3	2

* Reaction of degeneration.

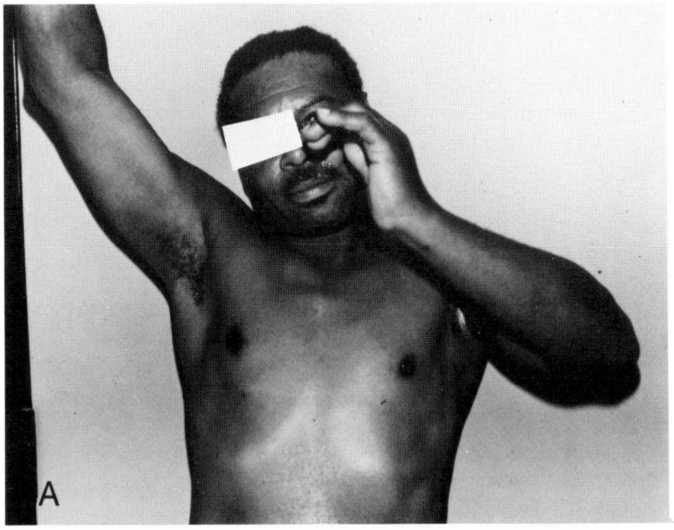

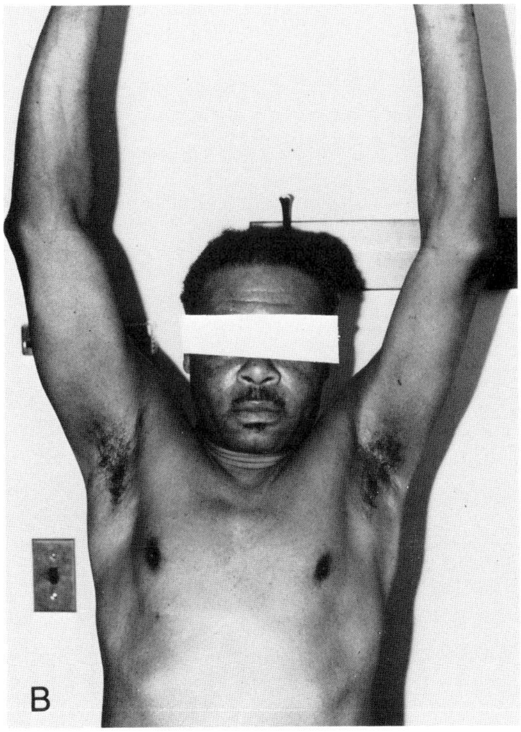

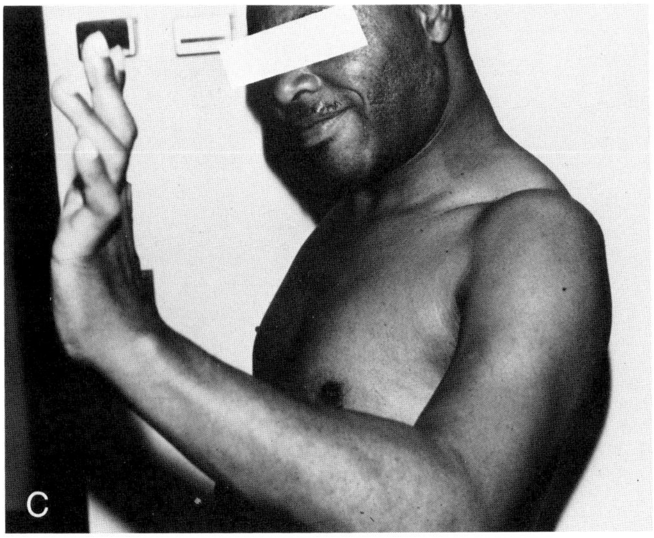

Fig. 3.2. A: Patient with beginning recovery four months following diffuse infraclavicular brachial plexus injury caused by shoulder dislocation. **B** and **C**: Same patient one year later. Note recovery of all musculature proximal to the hand in absence of intrinsic function causing clawing of fingers.

gle short length of nerve, there may be a different explanation for this observation: the axillary nerve is the nerve most predisposed to injury by anterior dislocation of the shoulder. In a fresh dislocation, where nerve injury is suspected, supporting evidence can be gained by demonstrating the appropriate sensory loss, even though motor power of the deltoid cannot be accurately assessed because of the pain of recent injury. Yet it is rare to observe permanent deltoid paralysis in most of the patients seen in the general practice of orthopedics (Fig. 3.4). It is therefore possible that the bias in this series results from selection of patients from a Nerve Injury Center. It may well be that many patients with shoulder dislocations and axillary nerve lesions either never have their nerve injuries recognized, or simply are not referred to a Nerve Injury Center. Hence, only the severe ones were there to be counted.

Sunderland[10] noted that most such lesions recover spontaneously because they are first- or second-degree injuries, but cautioned that, in the latter case, spontaneous recovery occurs more slowly than would be expected. Signs of recovery may be delayed for 3–6 months or even longer. Sunderland quoted from the 1929 work of Foerster, who gave a range of 4–9 months for the onset of recovery. Finally, in

(Text continues on p. 64)

Table 3.3 The Posterior Cord—Shoulder Abduction

Case No.	Nerve Injury	Electrical Reaction	Period of Observation from Time of Injury (months)	Deltoid Power (Initial) Posterior	Deltoid Power (Initial) Middle	Deltoid Power (Initial) Anterior	Deltoid Power (Final) Posterior	Deltoid Power (Final) Middle	Deltoid Power (Final) Anterior	Functional Result	Remarks
15	Isolated circum-flex	No	34	0	0	0	4	4	4	Poor because of pain and stiffness	Stiff shoulder persisted
16	Isolated circum-flex	Yes	26	0	0	0*	2	3	1	Full abduction — no disability	Slight feeling of weakness in shoulder
17	Isolated circum-flex	Yes	14	0	0	0*	0	0	0	Active abduction to 160 degreess	Air Force pilot — slight weakness pushing throttle forward
18	Isolated circum-flex	No	41	0	0	0	4	2	1	Full abduction — no disability	
19	Isolated circum-flex	Yes	28	0	0	0*	0	0	0	Combined active abduction to 100 degrees	No disability as a truck driver
20	Isolated circum-flex	Yes	96	0	0	0*	4	2	1	Poor because of pain and stiffness	Arthrodesis of shoulder 8 years after injury

21	Circumflex combined	Yes	9	—	0*	—	—	3	—	Active abduction to 140 degrees	
22	Circumflex combined	Yes	23	0	0	0	5	5	5	Normal shoulder	
23	Circumflex combined	Yes	11	—	4*	—	—	5	—	Normal shoulder	
24	Posterior cord	Yes	36	0	0	0*	4	4	0	Abduction 60 degrees	Suprascapular nerve probably cut by fractured scapula — paralysis of spinati
25	Posterior cord	Yes	31	0	0	0*	0	0	0	Abduction 60 degrees "very useful"	Patient 69 years old
26	Posterior cord	Yes	44	—	0*	—	—	5	—	Normal shoulder	
27	Posterior cord	Yes	21	4	2	2*	—	4+	—	Normal shoulder	Tendon transplantation for residual radial paralysis below triceps

* Reaction of degeneration.
From Leffert RD, Seddon HJ: Infraclavicular brachial plexus injuries. J Bone Joint Surg 47B:9, 1965.

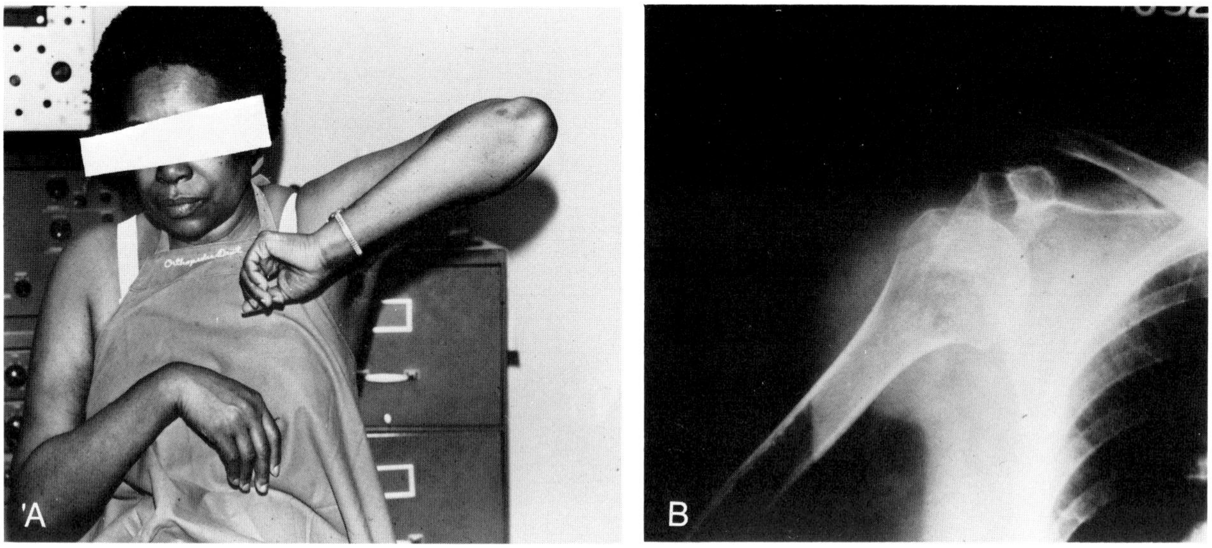

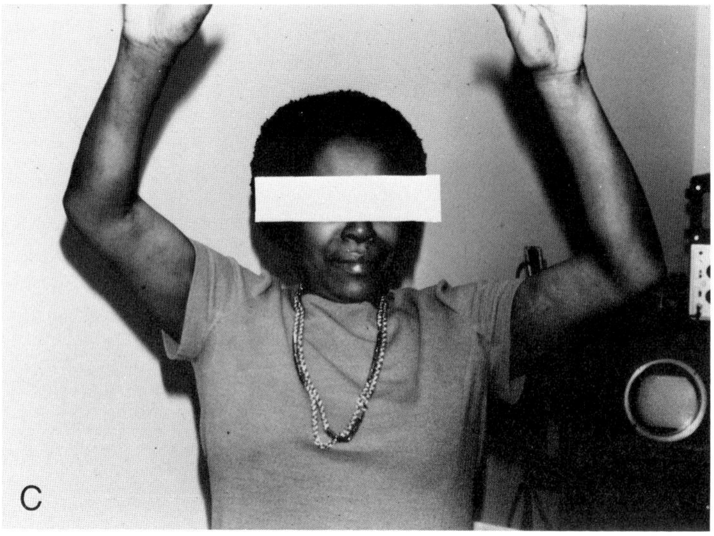

Fig. 3.3. A: Patient with posterior cord paralysis following anterior shoulder dislocation. **B**: Radiograph of dislocated shoulder. **C**: Recovery at four months.

1952 Watson-Jones[11] reported 15 cases of axillary palsy with shoulder dislocations. Ten patients recovered spontaneously within 6 months, and three recovered between 6 and 12 months. In two patients the deltoid remained permanently paralyzed.

As shown in Table 3.4, the spontaneous recovery of lesions of the posterior cord or radial nerve was quite good. A similar situation prevails for the lateral cord or musculocutaneous nerve (Table 3.5). For patients who do not recover function of the biceps and brachialis, powerful elbow flexion may still be possible if the brachioradialis is intact, although some may complain of weakness of supination (Fig. 3.5).

The medial cord recovery is shown in Table 3.6.

In order to document the progress of motor recovery of the various functional-anatomical groups, all records were analyzed in terms of when the first evidence of muscular contraction was noted and when a useful degree of strength was attained. These are illustrated in Figures 3.6, 3.7, 3.8, and 3.9. These analyses show that in the posterior cord group, all patients but one had recovered finger extension to grade III by 18 months.

The recovery of elbow flexion occurred in nine of 16 patients by 6 months, and all but one attained grade IV by 18 months.

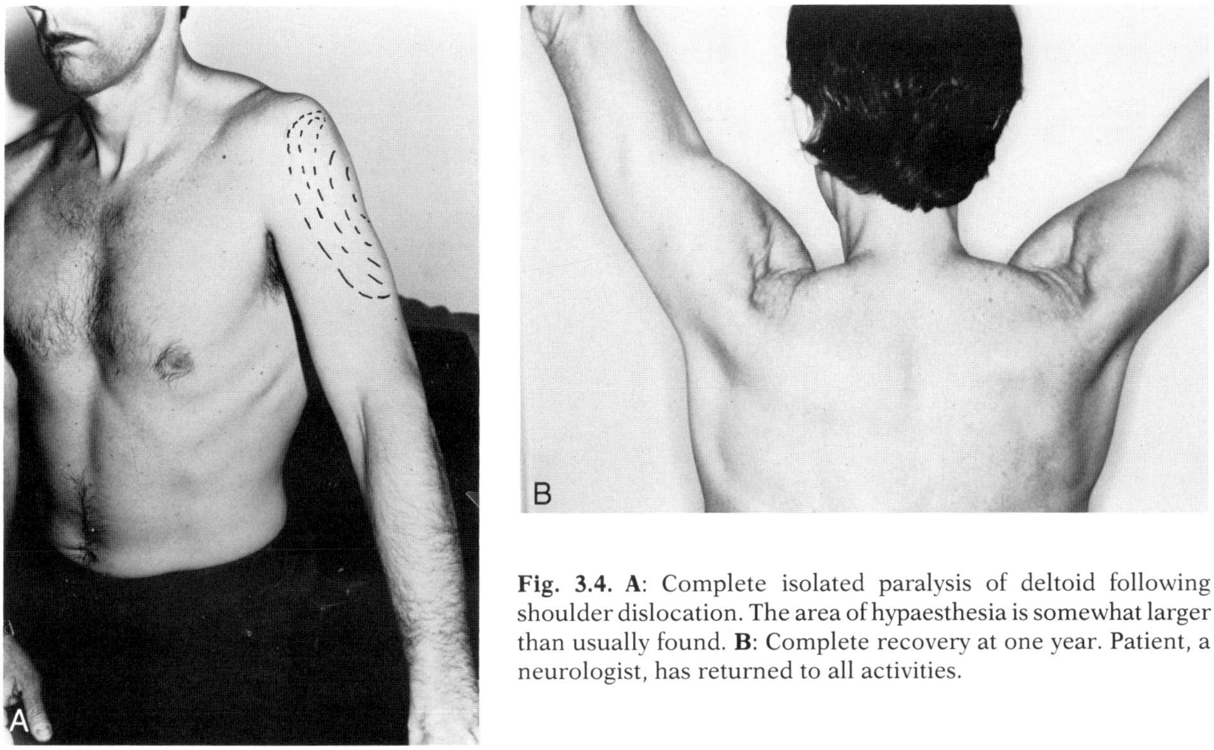

Fig. 3.4. A: Complete isolated paralysis of deltoid following shoulder dislocation. The area of hypaesthesia is somewhat larger than usually found. **B**: Complete recovery at one year. Patient, a neurologist, has returned to all activities.

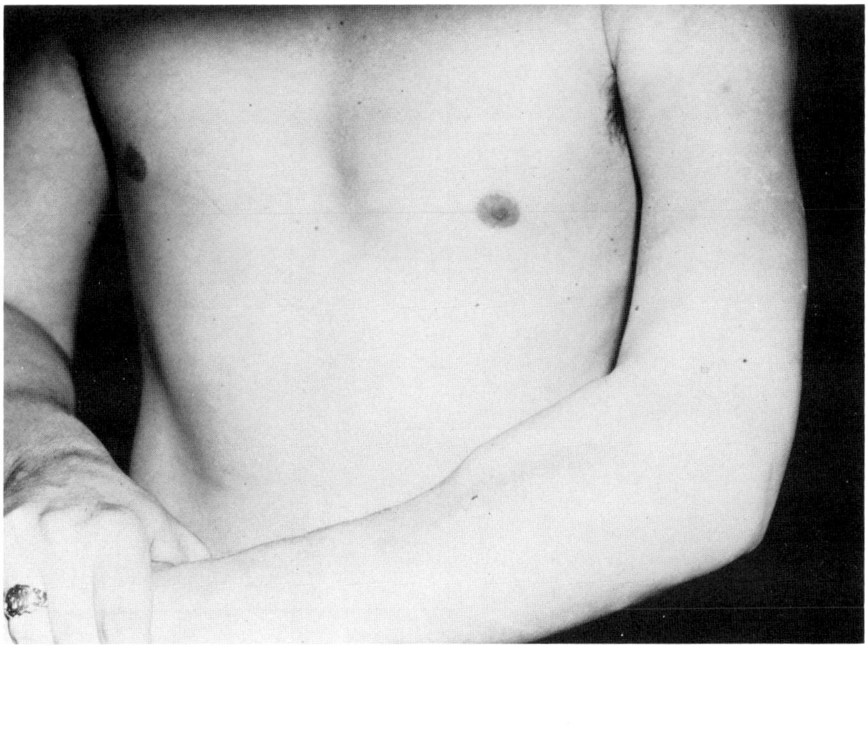

Fig. 3.5. Complete paralysis of muscles innervated by musculocutaneous nerve. Note the bulging brachioradialis.

Table 3.4. Posterior Cord—Recovery of Extensor Muscles

	Initial Examination					Final Examination			
Case No.	Electrical Reactions	Period of Observation from Time of Injury (months)	Elbow Extension	Wrist Extension	Extension of Digits	Elbow Extension	Wrist Extension	Extension of Digits	Remarks
24	No	36	0	5	5	5	5	5	Drives truck
25	Yes	31	4*	0*	0*	5	5	5	When seen 5 months after injury triceps largely recovered
26	Yes	44	5	0*	0*	5	5	5	Fit for military duty
27	Yes	37	0*	0*	0*	4	0	0	Tendon transplantation
28	No	15	2+	0	0	5	5	5	—

* Reaction of degeneration.

From Leffert RD, Seddon HJ: Infraclavicular brachial plexus injuries. J Bone Joint Surg 47B:9, 1965.

Table 3.5. Recovery of Flexion of the Elbow After Lateral Cord or Musculocutaneous Nerve Injury

Initial Examination					Final Examination	
Case No.	Period of Observation from Time of Injury (months)	Electrical Reactions	Associated Nerve Lesion	Biceps and Brachialis	Biceps and Brachialis	Remarks
22	23	Yes	Circumflex	0*	5	Normal elbow flexion
23	11	Yes	Circumflex	0*	5	Normal elbow flexion
24	36	No	Posterior cord	1	5	Normal elbow flexion
27	21	Yes	Posterior cord	2	4	Normal elbow flexion
29	34	No	Medial cord	0	0	Powerful elbow flexion due to intact brachioradialis

* Reaction of degeneration.
From Leffert RD, Seddon HJ: Infraclavicular brachial plexus injuries. J Bone Joint Surg 47B:9, 1965.

Intrinsic function of the hand, as expected, took longer to recover than other groups. Opposition of the thumb continued to improve for up to 3 years. Five of 11 patients showed significant improvement in the interossei between 18 and 36 months post injury.

The recovery of sensibility in the hand was considered in the distribution of the median and ulnar nerves, since only these are of functional importance. Table 3.7 illustrates the grade of recovery in 15 of 21 patients with corresponding motor loss. Of 11 patients with median sensory loss, eight were followed for at least 2 years, and six regained normal sensation.

Of the 14 patients with ulnar sensory loss, six were followed for more than 3 years, and four of

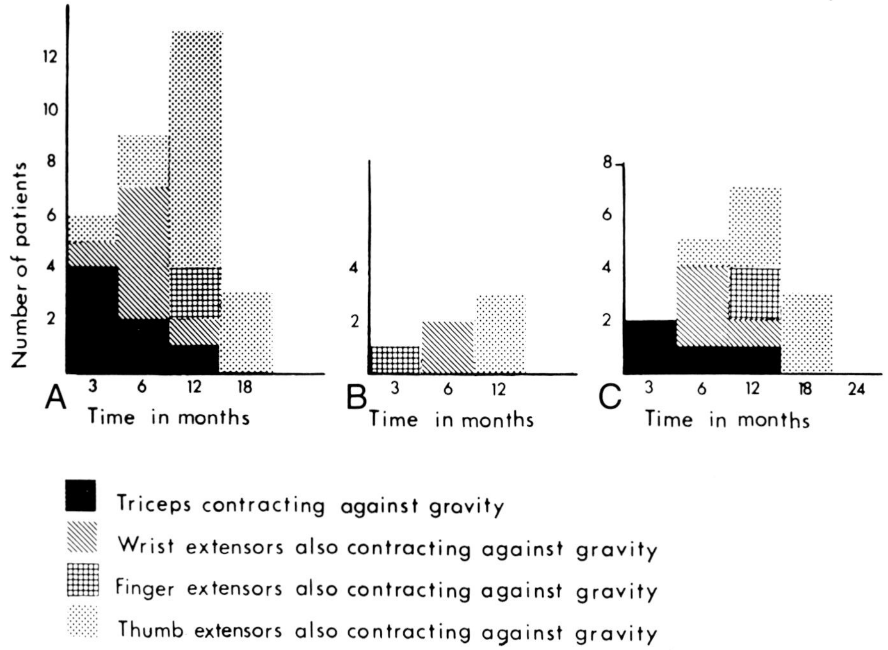

Fig. 3.6. Progress of motor recovery after injury to the posterior cord. **A**: Sixteen degenerative and nondegenerative lesions. **B**: Three nondegenerative lesions. **C**: Eight degenerative lesions. (Reproduced from Leffert RD, Seddon HJ: Infraclavicular brachial plexus injuries. J Bone Joint Surg 47B:9, 1965.)

Table 3.6. Medial Cord Injury—Motor Recovery

			Initial Examination					Final Examination			
Case No.	Period of Observation from Time of Injury (months)	Electrical Reactions	Associated Nerve Injury	Flexor Carpi Ulnaris	Flexor Digitorum Profundus (medial)	Median Intrinsic	Ulnar Intrinsic	Flexor Carpi Ulnaris	Flexor Digitorum Profundus	Median Intrinsic	Ulnar Intrinsic
26	44	Yes	Posterior cord	0*	0*	0*	0*	4+	4+	4+	4+
28	15	No	Posterior cord	4	3	5	3	5	5	5	5
29	34	Yes	Musculocutaneous	0	0	0*	0	5	5	5	5
30	51	No	Radial nerve	±	0	2	0	5	3	4	3+

* Reaction of degeneration.

From Leffert RD, Seddon HJ: Infraclavicular brachial plexus injuries. J Bone Joint Surg 47B:9, 1965.

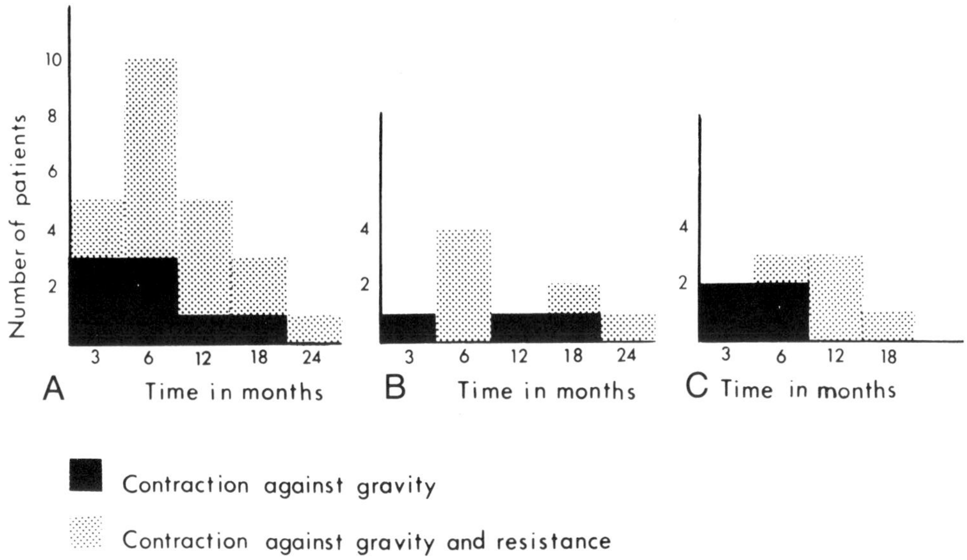

Fig. 3.7. Progress of recovery of the flexors of the elbow after injury to the lateral cord. **A**: Sixteen degenerative and nondegenerative lesions. **B**: Six nondegenerative lesions. **C**: Five degenerative lesions. (From Leffert RD, Seddon HJ: Infraclavicular brachial plexus injuries. J Bone Joint Surg 47B:9, 1965.)

these recovered completely. Eight were followed for less than 3 years, and five had a useful grade of sensibility when seen.

Of the 31 patients, only four underwent exploratory operations. Two operations were for posttraumatic aneurysms of the axillary artery, which were treated by ligation. Of the remaining two patients, one had an irreparable axillary nerve lesion, and the other a lesion of axillary, radial, and musculocutaneous nerves.

In 1971 Allende[1] reported his experience with infraclavicular plexus injuries, among which were

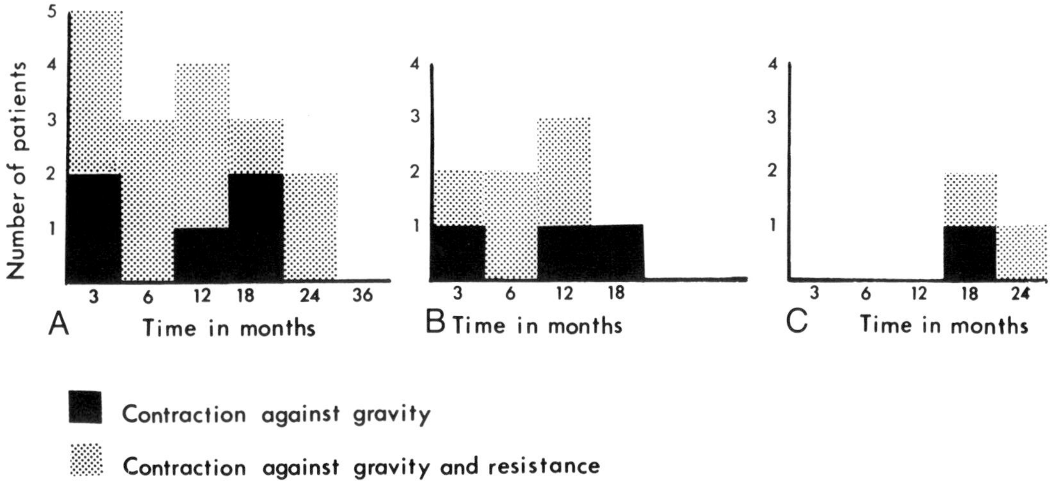

Fig. 3.8. Progress of recovery of the thenar muscles after injury to the medial cord. **A**: Fourteen degenerative and nondegenerative lesions. **B**: Seven nondegenerative lesions. **C**: Two degenerative lesions. (From Leffert RD, Seddon HJ: Infraclavicular brachial plexus injuries. J Bone Joint Surg 47B:9, 1965.)

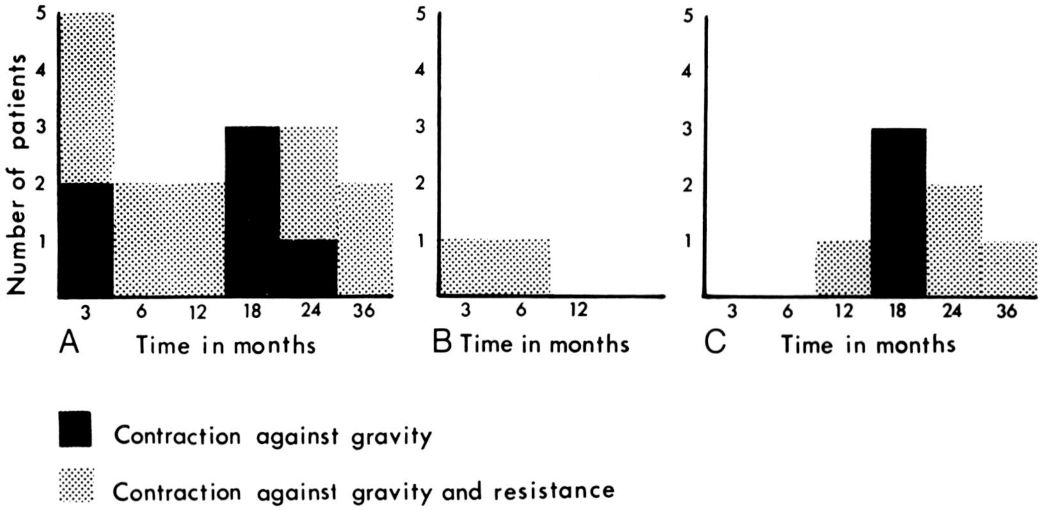

Fig. 3.9. Progress of recovery of interossei in injury to the medial cord. **A**: Eleven degenerative and nondegenerative lesions. **B**: Two nondegenerative lesions. **C**: Four degenerative lesions. (From Leffert RD, Seddon HJ: Infraclavicular brachial plexus injuries. J Bone Joint Surg 47B:9, 1965.)

nine complete closed injuries accompanying fracture or fracture-dislocation of the proximal humerus and scapula. Two had complete motor and sensory recovery while three failed to recover intrinsic hand function. One patient was found to have a concomitant distal radial nerve lesion that did not recover. One patient, who was an elderly diabetic with a spastic hemiparesis preceding the plexus injury, failed to recover function below the elbow in the already impaired upper limb. One patient who had a fracture of the vertebral border of the scapula as well as the clavicle and humerus only recovered the posterior

Table 3.7. Sensory Recovery in the Hand

	Initial Examination			Final Examination	
Case No.	Period of Observation from Time of Injury (months)	Median	Ulnar	Median	Ulnar
1	37	S:0	S:1	S:4	S:4
2	48	S:0	S:0	S:2	S:2
3	25	S:1	S:1	S:4	S:4
4	23	S:0	S:0	S:3	S:3
5	24	S:0	S:0	S:4	S:4
6	36	S:0	S:0	S:4	S:4
8	25	*	S:0	*	S:2
10	12	S:0	*	S:2	*
11	17	*	S:1	*	S:3
12	49	S:0	S:0	S:4	S:4
13	42	S:0	S:0	S:4	S:4
14	17	S:1	S:0	S:2	S:2
28	15	*	S:0	*	S:2+
29	34	S:0	S:0	S:0	S:4
30	51	*	S:1	*	S:2

* Indicates no loss initially.

From Leffert RD, Seddon HJ: Infraclavicular brachial plexus injuries. J Bone Joint Surg 47B:9, 1965.

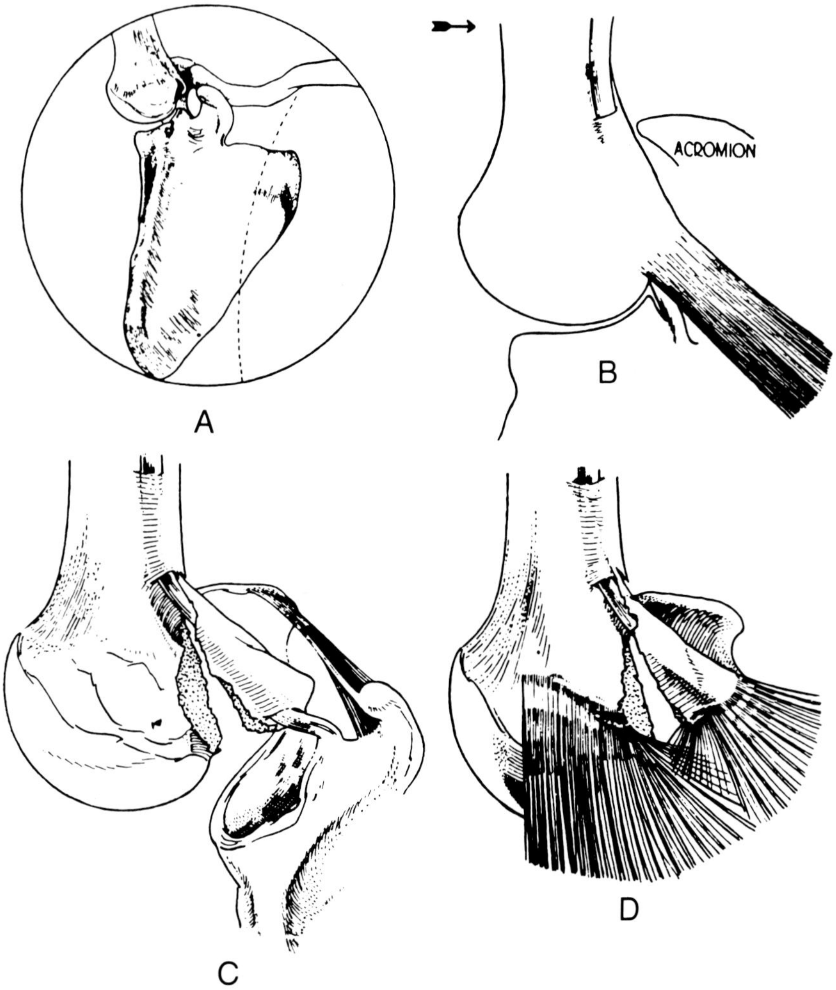

Fig. 3.10. The mechanism of fracture of the greater tuberosity of the humerus as sustained during dislocation, which may be momentary. (Reproduced from Codman EA: The Shoulder. G. Miller Medical Publishers, Brooklyn, NY, 1934.)

deltoid, the remaining nerves being transected by the fracture fragments. This lesion is identical with one reported in 1965 by Leffert and Seddon,[6] and emphasizes the important point that, although the mechanism in infraclavicular brachial plexus injury is often simple lateral traction on the nerves, or, less commonly, compression, more sinister lesions involving actual nerve laceration by fracture fragments may occur. Furthermore, in Allende's series there were two axillary artery lesions, one with a fractured scapula and one resulting from a dislocated shoulder that had been unreduced for 48 hours and caused a thrombosis. A case of axillary artery aneurysm, reported by Leffert and Seddon, had as its only skeletal lesion a fracture of the greater tuberosity of the humerus, the result of a momentary dislocation and relocation of the proximal humerus (Fig. 3.10). An arterial rupture complicating shoulder dislocation had previously been reported by Kirker[5] in 1952. It is therefore quite clear that one must be alert to the possibility of arterial injury in such cases.

In 1975 Seddon[8] reported an updated series of infraclavicular plexus injuries due to shoulder injury. There were 45 cases, with spontaneous recovery given as 33 "near-normal," 10 "impaired," 1 "poor," and 1 "bad." The distribution of nerve injury was not given. Figure 3.11 illustrates the generally favorable prognosis for this type of injury.

The generalizations accruing from the above experience can be summarized as follows: The infraclavicular portions of the plexus may be injured by fractures and dislocations in the region of the shoulder

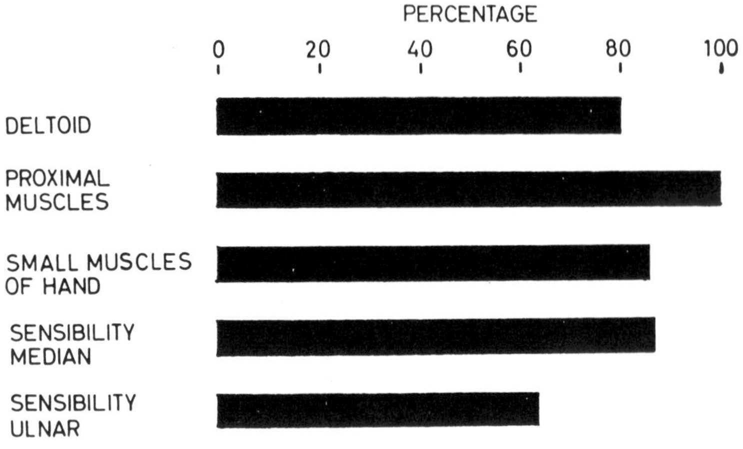

Fig. 3.11. Recovery after closed injuries in the region of the shoulder that damaged one or more nerves in the upper limb. In all cases the treatment was conservative. (Reproduced from Seddon HJ: Surgical Disorders of the Peripheral Nerves. 2nd Ed. Churchill Livingstone, Edinburgh, 1975, with permission.)

joint, and because of the mechanism of injury, the prognosis for neurological recovery is usually considerably more favorable than for the supraclavicular injuries. The milder nature of the nerve injuries is due to the restricted excursion of which the fractured or dislocated humerus is capable as well as the level at which the nerve injury occurs. Since the traction on nerves is usually exerted laterally at a point relatively far removed from an anatomical point of anchorage (spinal cord or muscle), the normal elasticity of the nerve roots protects them from more severe damage. The branch of this part of the plexus that is nearest its anchorage is the axillary nerve, which explains its increased liability to injury.

Although it is not generally possible to define a direct relationship between a particular skeletal injury and the type of nerve injury it may produce, those fractures that involve large, sharp bone fragments are much more likely to produce neurotmesis by direct laceration. The axillary border of the scapula is particularly apt to do this, and vascular injury at the same level is a hazard, which may force surgical exploration as soon as the nature of the lesion is recognized. Allende[1] documented that an arterial lesion can cause a significant lesion of the adjacent nerves. His patient developed a false aneurysm of the axillary artery following puncture for cardiac catheterization, resulting in progressive loss of median nerve function and development of intense causalgic pain.

Whether an infraclavicular lesion of the brachial plexus unaccompanied by vascular injury should be explored depends on the injury. Obviously, open injuries caused by knives or other sharp objects usually produce their nerve lesions by laceration, so that delay in exploration would serve no function. Projectiles that cause no vascular injury can produce neurapractic or axonotmetic lesions by their concussive effect and the shockwaves generated within the tissues. These lesions do not require surgical manipulation to achieve spontaneous recovery. However, a finite waiting period based on expected regeneration rates should not be exceeded nor surgery delayed lest excessive atrophy occur in the paralyzed muscles. Unless the closed skeletal injury, because of its fracture-fragment configuration, is likely to have caused direct nerve laceration, the recovery of these patients is not enhanced by operation on their nerves.

It must be emphasized that this discussion of the prognosis for spontaneous recovery of the patients with infraclavicular brachial plexus injuries pertains only to injuries resulting from skeletal injury as described, and not to more generalized nerve injury involving the supraclavicular plexus as well. The mechanism in the latter is usually traction, and the damage may reach below the level of the clavicle. The prognosis for spontaneous recovery and the indications for operative intervention are then determined by the state of the supraclavicular plexus.

Although the prognosis for neurological recovery is generally good, functional recovery may be prevented by a number of factors. The most significant of these is joint stiffness, which is most likely to occur in the older age groups. The unremitting use of a sling to support the shoulder and to prevent edema in the limb will, if not accompanied by regular daily range-of-motion exercises, produce a stiff shoulder with limited abduction and lateral rotation as well as a flexion contracture at the elbow. The inadvisable splinting of the "dropped fingers" in extension at all joints can produce contracture of the metacarpal phalangeal joints or extensor tendons that may be difficult to overcome. Edema of the hand is a constant danger in patients with a weak shoulder or elbow, and if it occurs, it must be vigorously combated. The atrophy of the larger muscles in the limb is usually not sufficient to cause serious functional deficits. Their size and proximity to their neurons are favorable factors in regeneration and ultimate recovery. The intrinsic muscles of the hand, because of their small size, complex function, and long distance from the site of injury, are likely to undergo serious and sometimes irrevocable atrophy before reinnervation can take place. Whether regular galvanic stimulation of the paralyzed muscles can retard atrophy has been long debated. In my opinion, it is not worthwhile, and I do not employ it in the treatment of my patients.

REFERENCES

1. Allende BT: Lesions traumatique du plexus brachial dans la region infraclavicular. Rev Chir Orthop 57(2):131, 1971
2. Codman EA: The Shoulder. G. Miller, Medical Publishers, Brooklyn, NY, 1934
3. Delbet P, Cauchoix A: Les paralysies dans les luxations de l'epaule. Rev Chir 41:327, 1910
4. Gariepy R, Derome A, Laurin CA: Brachial plexus paralysis following shoulder dislocation. Can J Surg 5:418, 1962
5. Kirker JR: Dislocation of the shoulder complicated by rupture of the axillary vessels. J Bone Joint Surg 34B(1):72, 1952
6. Leffert RD, Seddon HJ: Infraclavicular brachial plexus injuries. J Bone Joint Surg 47B:9, 1965
7. Milton GW: The mechanism of circumflex and other nerve injuries in dislocation of the shoulder and the possible mechanism of nerve injury during reduction of dislocation Aust NZ J Surg 23:4, 1953
8. Seddon HJ: Surgical Disorders of the Peripheral Nerves. 2nd Ed. Churchill Livingstone, Edinburgh, 1975
9. Stevens JH: Brachial plexus injuries. In Codman EA (ed): The Shoulder. G. Miller Medical Publishers, Brooklyn, NY, 1934
10. Sunderland S: Nerves and Nerve Injuries. 2nd Ed. Churchill Livingstone, Edinburgh, London, and New York, 1978
11. Watson-Jones R: Fractures and Joint Injuries. 4th Ed. Vol 1. Churchill Livingstone, Edinburgh, 1952

4

Clinical Assessment of Closed Traction Injury to the Brachial Plexus

The superposition of an infinitely varied spectrum of trauma on the anatomical complexity of the brachial plexus can create a seemingly impossible puzzle for the treating physician or surgeon. Nevertheless, by application of an orderly diagnostic approach, it is possible in most cases to formulate a rational treatment program. This chapter will be concerned with those nonoperative and indirect methods of assessment used in evaluation of closed traction injuries to the brachial plexus.

Depending on the circumstances of medical practice, or the chain of referral, the patients will be seen either acutely, or, as is often the case, some time after the accident. The multiply injured patient may have had a life- or limb-threatening trauma that diverts attention away from, or prevents recognition of, a brachial plexus injury. A head injury may render the patient unconscious, or a concurrent spinal cord injury may becloud the issue. Sometimes a severed or avulsed arm may be replanted in vain because the possibility of injury to the brachial plexus is not considered. Fractures or soft-tissue injuries in the limb may contribute greatly to the difficulty of precise neurological diagnosis. The object in all cases, whether acute or chronic, is to accurately assess the nerve lesion and document it in a way that facilitates the formulation of a prognosis and treatment program.

PHYSICAL DIAGNOSIS

History Taking

Demographic data should include occupation and handedness, since these factors can have an effect not only on the assessment of motor responses, but also on ultimate functional requirements. The circumstances and mode of injury may be vividly etched in the patient's memory, or he may be amnesic for all events surrounding the episode. Sometimes family members, friends, or fellow-workers may fill in the details, from which certain inferences may be made. In general, assuming a fall from a motorcycle or a car crash, the greater the speed, the more grave the injury is likely to be. Where direct traction of the arm has caused the paralysis, its orientation with respect to the axis of the body will generally indicate where in the plexus the damage may be expected. Obviously, these historical details are of inferential value only, since more specific methods are available in physical examination and other diagnostic maneuvers. Nevertheless, all potentially useful data should be collected. The question as to when in relation to the trauma the neurological deficit was first noted should always be asked, since the possibility of a previously existing deficit or injury should not be overlooked. Furthermore, it is not at all rare for the brachial plexus palsy to be noted only after several observers have attended the patient in the emergency situation. This can make it difficult to establish the magnitude and extent of the initial neurological deficit as well as its course with time. For the patient whose palsy and sensory loss can be documented to be increasing under careful observation, there may well be a remediable etiological factor, such as an expanding false aneurysm or compressing bone fragment. These situations are rare, but when they occur prompt surgical action may have a decisive effect. The majority of patients will have their maximal loss initially, to be followed either by a variable amount of improvement, or none at all. It is of crucial impor-

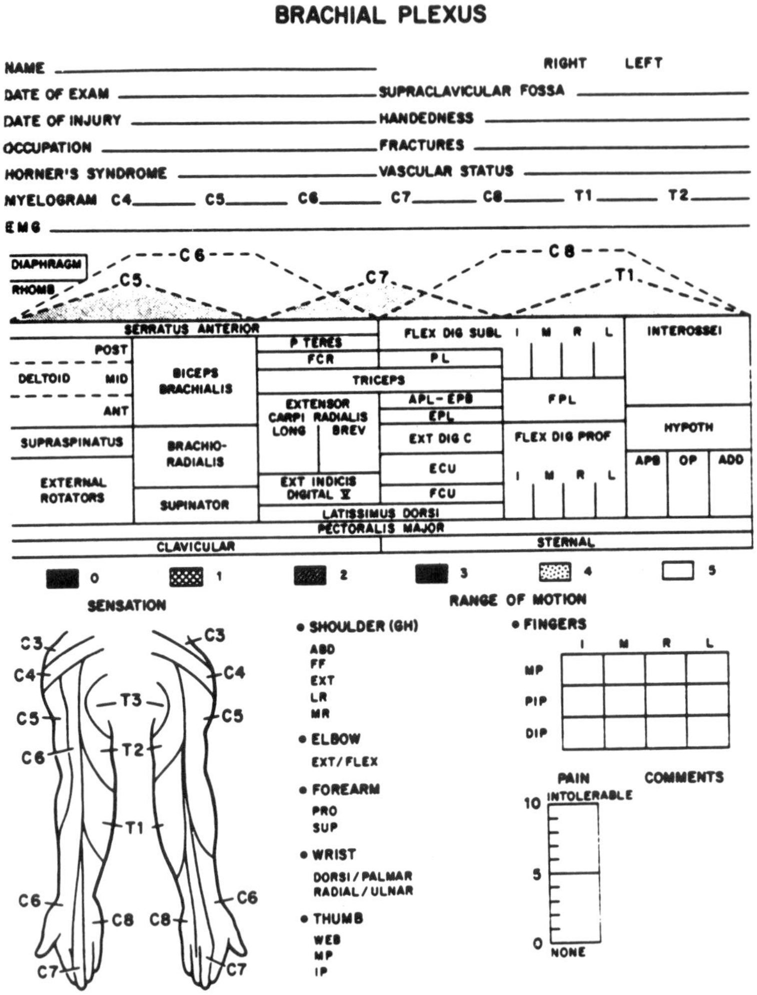

Fig. 4.1. The recording form, modified from d'Aubigne.

tance to have an accurate record of improvement or lack thereof, so that well-reasoned treatment plans can be made. Recording should be in a standard manner, using conventional terms and either a careful narrative format or one of a number of preprinted forms that can facilitate neurological deduction (Fig. 4.1).

The presence, localization, and quality of pain as well as any factors noted to intensify or alleviate it should be recorded. Particulars of analgesic requirements, including dosage, frequency, and effectiveness, are noted. The effect of the pain on activities of daily living is useful historical detail. Finally, direct inquiry regarding the patient's past or habitual use of drugs, prescribed or otherwise, completes the assessment.

Physical Examination

The physical examination should be conducted in a compulsive manner and adhered to without significant deviation so that the information derived will be uniform and inclusive in format. General affect, station, and gait, where applicable, are noted. Observation of the manner in which the patient disrobes for the examination can be quite enlightening regarding the degree of dependence or initiative that may be expected during the course of treatment.

Before the patient is touched, a number of specific things should be noted. The presence or absence of Horner's syndrome cannot be ascertained in poor light while the patient is wearing eyeglasses, and if anisocoria is noted, it should be established that it did not exist prior to the injury. Sometimes the lid lag will have diminished with the passage of time. As has been previously indicated, a winged scapula will be obvious on inspection, and is presumptive evidence of a supraganglionic lesion of the plexus, assuming the trapezius muscle is intact.

The examiner should note the position of the limb as well as abnormalities of the joints (for example shoulder subluxation) or long bone deformities, and the presence of wounds, either from the initial trauma or sustained because the limb is insensate. Evidences of trophic changes, sympathetic dysfunction, or changes resulting from vascular insufficiency are recorded.

In patients who have recently sustained traction injuries to the brachial plexus, the supraclavicular fossa may demonstrate swelling or ecchymosis. With the passage of time, the soft and doughy swelling will be gradually replaced by induration that may be confined to the specific path of the brachial plexus. Or, when there has been diffuse muscle damage and extensive hemorrhage, the entire posterior triangle of the neck will be involved in an indurated and tender mass. A neuroma or Tinel's sign may be present.

Tinel's Sign

The distal tingling that can be produced by percussing the injured plexus in the neck is a useful diagnostic maneuver. In order to elicit it from the supraclavicular fossa of a patient with a flail, anesthetic arm, some central connection of the plexus must be preserved, even if it is ruptured in its infraganglionic portion. In cases of distal rupture of a trunk, a positive sign gives strong evidence of the availability of proximal axons from which to graft for central reconstruction. For the patient with an incontinuity axonotmesis, repeated examinations over time will demonstrate distal migration along the nerves of the point from which tingling can be obtained. In the early stages of recovery, before any testable muscle has been reinnervated, Tinel's sign[6,9] may be the only means of monitoring progress or lack thereof. However, the intensity of subjective sensation cannot be quantitated or translated into expected levels of recovery. Some inferences may be made as to which roots are being stimulated according to where in the arm or hand the patient perceives the paresthesias.

Prior to formal manual muscle testing, it is essential to assess the passive range of motion of the cervical spine and all joints of the shoulder girdle and upper extremity. Failure to do this first, or to determine if any of the joints are unstable or painful, will result in spurious results of muscle testing. Joint range of motion is recorded with a goniometer, designating neural position as 0 degrees. Articular contractures may or may not be accompanied by shortening of musculotendinous units, which can directly affect the range of the joints they cross. Contractures are common in parts of the limb where there has been preservation of some function as well as total paralysis, and in patients seen late, these contractures may be a result of injudicious splinting. The shortening of finger extensor tendons seen after constant splinting in extension is common and is a preventable cause of ineffective grasp following tendon transfers for finger flexion.

Since the virtual elimination of paralytic poliomyelitis from everyday practice in the western hemisphere, the development of proficiency in manual muscle testing techniques has become considerably harder. A useful text is by Kendall, Kendall, and Wadsworth,[17] which also has tables of variations of motor and sensory innervation. It also considers so-called "trick and supplementary" motions that are sources of confusion and error in motor assessment. The method of recording of motor power employed by an individual examiner should be standard and reproducible.

Sensory Examination

Although sensory examination[11,27] can be performed to a high degree of sophistication, and many modalities tested, those pertinent to the examination of the patient with injury to the brachial plexus are considerably simpler:

1. Touch
2. Pain
3. Two-point discrimination
4. Joint position sense (proprioception)

Touch can be tested by stroking the surface of the skin with a fine brush, wisp of cotton, or even the examiner's fingertip, and pain sense by the use of a pin. Two-point discrimination and "moving two point" represent a higher level of sensibility, and will not be applicable to patients with profound defects. Having the patient differentiate between the milled and smooth edges of coins by blind touch indicates preservation of virtually normal sensibility in the fingers used, and may screen those in which it is defective, assuming the skin is not heavily calloused.

Since joint-position sense is of great importance in the function of the extremity, and especially one with major sensory loss, it is important to evaluate it. A useful method of accomplishing that is to blindfold the patient and then have the examiner position the joint of the injured limb in various ways to be duplicated by the patient with his sound limb. Even if there is cutaneous anesthesia of the forearm and elbow region and complete paralysis, the joint may have useful position sense. Preservation of this feedback can significantly enhance the limb's worth if, for example, a forearm amputation is elected rather than one above the elbow.

Vascular Status

Because of the intimate relationship of the brachial plexus to the subclavian artery and its branches, traction that is severe enough to rupture the nerves may also tear the vessels, resulting in a life-threatening emergency necessitating surgery to arrest the hemorrhage. Even though the limb will usually survive following ligation of the artery, repair should be done to give the compromised limb every potential benefit. Unfortunately, those cases in which arterial rupture accompanies rupture of the plexus have a generally poor prognosis for neurological recovery because of the magnitude and extent of the avulsion injury.

For patients seen after the acute injury, the status of the peripheral circulation and pulses must be noted. Patients in whom there is a history of significant vascular injury and in whom operative intervention for the nerves is contemplated should have the exact nature of the local circulation determined by whatever means necessary, including arteriography and venography.

Even in the absence of significant arterial insufficiency, the denervated limb will be cold-sensitive to the patient and feel cool and often appear cyanotic to the examiner. In limbs where sympathectomy has been accomplished by the injury, the skin will be dry.

ELECTRODIAGNOSTIC STUDIES

Electrodiagnostic studies, properly employed, are of considerable assistance in augmenting the clinical evaluation of the extent and severity of a brachial plexus injury.[38] If the physician performing these tests is not directly involved in the care of the patient, then good communication must avoid unnecessary delays or, worse, spurious conclusions. The techniques that can be employed with benefit are (1) electromyography of limb and shoulder girdle musculature, (2) electromyography of paravertebral musculature, (3) motor and sensory nerve conduction velocity determinations, and (4) somatosensory evoked potentials.

Electromyography

A thorough consideration of basic electromyography is neither possible nor desirable in a monograph of this nature. Fortunately, there are numerous references available.[1,21,34]

Following axonal interruption, whether accompanied by loss of continuity of the Schwann sheaths or not (the former having the potential for spontaneous regeneration and recovery of nerve function), the process of Wallerian degeneration of the distal segment occurs over an approximately three-week period. The electrophysiological counterpart of this neuropathological series of events is the alteration of the electrical characteristics of the denervated muscle. Whereas normal muscle is "silent" at rest, the denervated or even partially denervated muscle spontaneously generates minute electrical potentials that can be sampled by needle electrodes, displayed, measured, and recorded from the cathode ray tube of the electromyograph. The totally denervated muscle has no "voluntary" potentials on attempted contraction, and a partially denervated one has fewer or abnormal mixtures of potentials. By examination of the limb muscles on the side of the injury it is possible to map those parts of the plexus that are totally or partially affected by the injury. Repetition of the process at monthly or bimonthly intervals can often indicate recovery well before it is clinically evident, or simply confirm the impression that recovery is not occurring.

The anatomic configuration of the spinal nerves provides a method whereby extension of this technique to the cervical paravertebral musculature can help to differentiate supraganglionic from infraganglionic lesions. Since the posterior primary rami that innervate these muscles are given off immediately after the exit of the roots from the intervertebral foramina, a supraganglionic lesion will also denervate the outflow of the posterior rami. Electromyographic examination of these muscles for this purpose was described in 1969 by Bufalini and Pescatori[5] and is an extremely useful test. The posterior cervical muscles are found in four distinct layers. The first, and most superficial, is the trapezius, innervated by the spinal accessory nerve. The second level, consisting of the splenius and levator scapulae muscles is innervated by the cervical plexus. Both these layers are usually spared denervation even in severe injuries to the brachial plexus. The next, third, layer, has a longitudinal innervation with the medial parts supplied by C3 and C4, and the more lateral part by C7 and C8. The deepest layer, level 4, which is composed of tranversus spinosus and interspinosus intertransversalis, is horizontally innervated and gets nerve fibers from the corresponding spinal nerves at each level. Although the spinal nerves, after innervating the muscular layers, become sensory and innervate the back of the neck, the distribution of the sensory branches is inconstant and not useful in diagnosis.

These anatomic facts are employed in interpretation of the electromyogram of the patient with brachial plexus injuries as follows: The involved limb and shoulder girdle musculature are examined with needle electrodes for the presence of spontaneous electrical activity and voluntary potentials. The cervical paravertebral muscles are also examined at each spinal level. During the test, the patient's head must be supported by a chin rest to eliminate voluntary potentials, and the needles are introduced down to bone and then slightly withdrawn to insure sampling of the deepest muscle layer (Fig. 4.2). If the paravertebral muscles are normally innervated, and the plexus muscles denervated, then the strong implication is that the lesion is infraganglionic (Fig. 4.3). The finding of a single level of denervation of both paravertebral and limb girdle muscles would point to a supraganglionic or intraforaminal lesion. The method is as reliable as any indirect method can be, but is subject, as are all, to the inaccuracy of one level because of pre- or postfixation of the plexus. A practical consideration in doing the test is the cooperation of the patient, who obviously will feel no discomfort from the needles in areas of total denervation. It is therefore prudent to examine the neck muscles at the beginning, lest the patient become disturbed and terminate the test before the paravertebrals can be sampled.

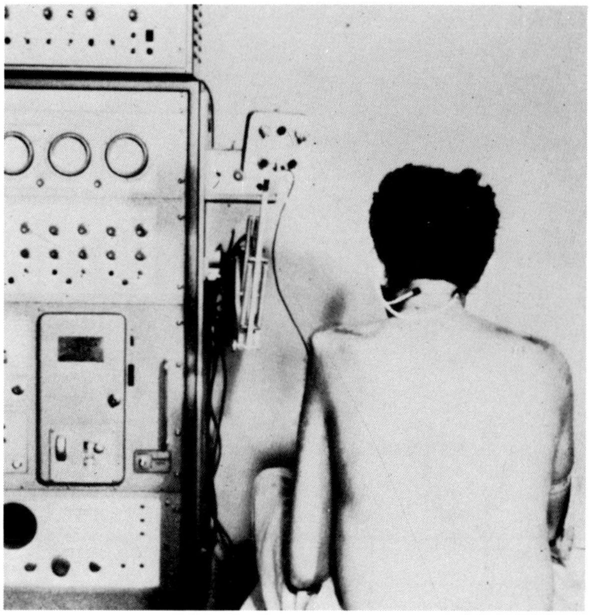

Fig. 4.2. Needle electromyographic examination of the posterior cervical musculature. (Reproduced from Bufalini C, Pescatori G: Posterior cervical electromyography in the diagnosis and prognosis of brachial plexus injuries. J Bone Joint Surg 51B:627, 1969, with permission.)

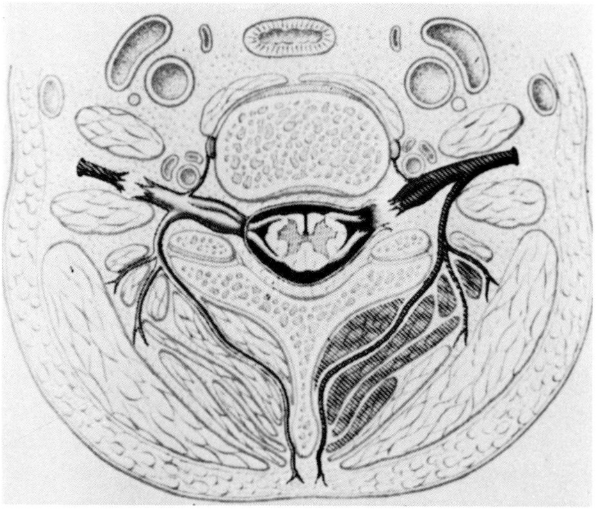

Fig. 4.3. The left side of the illustration shows a rupture distal to the dorsal root ganglion. The erector spinae musculature is not denervated. On the right, the root is avulsed (supraganglionic) and the erector spinae are denervated. (Reproduced from Bufalini C, Pescatori G: Posterior cervical electromyography in the diagnosis and prognosis of brachial plexus injuries. J Bone Joint Surg 51B:627, 1969, with permission.)

Nerve Conduction Velocity Determination

Understanding the application of the technique of nerve conduction velocity determination to the evaluation of a brachial plexus injury requires a review of the sequence of events following transection or avulsion of the nerve roots.[31] Immediately following trauma there will be cessation of voluntary activity and anesthesia in the limb. Assuming that root avulsion has occurred, the process of Wallerian degeneration will begin in the motor nerves, since these axons have been separated from their parent neurons, the anterior horn cells, within the spinal cord. The sensory nerves will not degenerate; although the central connections between the dorsal root ganglion outside the cord will be lost, causing anesthesia, the continuity of the axon and its cell body will be maintained, unless in addition to the supraganglionic avulsion there is an infraganglionic rupture.

Measurement of nerve conduction velocity immediately following root avulsion will be essentially normal, both motor and sensory. Within the succeeding 7 to 11 days, according to Warren and colleagues,[35] the normal motor action potentials will disappear as Wallerian degeneration occurs. Still, the sensory potentials and nerve conduction will remain unchanged for up to six months, as shown in two patients that these authors described in 1969. In my experience the sensory nerves can sometimes continue to conduct for a year or more where the root avulsion has resulted in centripetal, but not centrifugal, degeneration, unless there has been concomitant infraganglionic damage. The finding of absent motor conduction and intact sensory conduction in a peripheral nerve of a flail, anesthetic limb is therefore a poor prognostic sign in terms of the pathology and the possibility of surgical reconstruction of the plexus. If both motor and sensory action potentials are absent, one cannot infer that an underlying supraganglionic lesion is not present, unless paravertebral electromyography and myelography indicate otherwise.

Somatosensory Evoked Potentials

In 1970 Zalis and coworkers[38] reported on the diagnosis of cervical root avulsion with examination of somatosensory evoked potentials.[15,16] By stimulation of the median and/or ulnar nerves at the wrist and elbow, if the afferent pathways are intact, using scalp electrodes over the contralateral centroparietal region of the brain, an evoked potential may be recorded. In patients in whom root avulsion has occurred, even though sensory peripheral nerve conduction is normal, an evoked potential will not be obtainable from the cortex. To verify the integrity of the pathway between the cord and brain, an evoked potential can be obtained by stimulating the ipsilateral and contralateral peroneal nerves. In this way, the weight of objective evidence can be strengthened, even though it remains indirect.

PLAIN RADIOGRAPHY

Plain radiographs of the cervical spine and shoulder girdle should be obtained in every case of brachial plexus injury because valuable diagnostic and prognostic inferences may be made from them. Most often, the patient with a traction injury will have sustained a fall from a motorcycle. If he was wearing a helmet, much of the force that might have caused a fatal head injury will be expended in forcing the head and shoulder apart. Certainly, the possibility of injury to the cervical spine and cord exists, and in a patient who is unconscious, a plain radiograph may help to clarify the situation. In severe traction injuries of the brachial plexus, a lateral tilt of the cervical spine due to separation of the vertebral bodies may be seen in the anteroposterior view[28] (Fig. 4.4).

The frontal view radiograph should also be examined for the presence of fractures of the cervical transverse processes. Since the deep cervical fascia is tightly adherent to the nerve roots as well as the adjacent bone, an avulsed transverse process usually tears the root at that level (Fig. 4.5). Although for many years I believed that the bony injury was incontrovertible evidence of root avulsion, I have seen several patients in whom myelography and the subsequent course of recovery proved this to be untrue. It should be remembered, however, that variation in organization of the plexus may alter the expected neurological deficit based on the radiograph.

The first rib, in particular, should be seen in its entirety to establish that its anatomic relationships are normal and comparable to the other side, since the lower trunk of the brachial plexus is intimately associated with it. Downward displacement of the rib due to avulsion, or fracture of it or its transverse

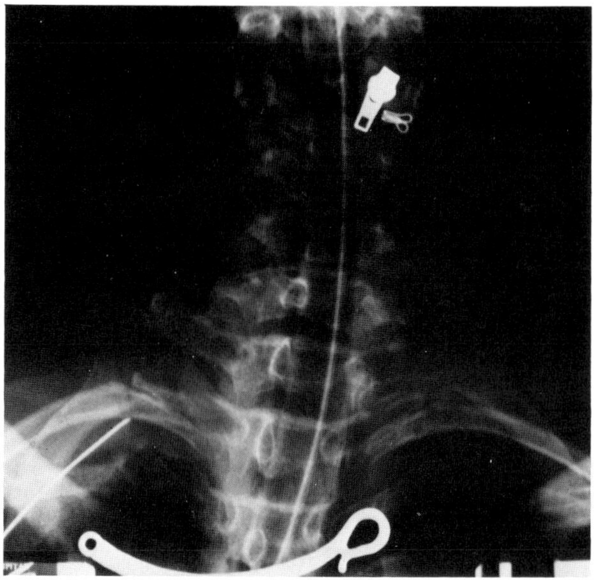

Fig. 4.4. Anteroposterior radiograph of patient with a severe traction injury of the brachial plexus. Note curve of the cervical spine outlined by endotracheal tube.

process, is a poor prognostic sign for that trunk and potentially for the accompanying artery[29] (Fig. 4.6).

Although fractures and dislocations of the shoulder girdle are usually associated with infraclavicular injuries, they do not exclude the possibility of supraclavicular nerve damage. Although fractures of the clavicle have the potential for causing acute injuries to the plexus, this usually does not occur. More commonly, the same force that distracts the head and shoulder fractures the clavicle, which then allows even greater excursion between these structures and increased traction on the nerves (Fig. 4.7). The neurological damage accompanying such clavicular fractures is usually severe and indicative of supraclavicular plexus injury.

In addition to these radiographic findings, some patients may even develop a high thoracocervical scoliosis due to muscle imbalance and unequal forces on the spine.

Additional information regarding the condition of the C5 nerve root may be obtained in those patients clinically suspected of root avulsion by having paralysis of the ipsilateral hemidiaphragm demonstrated by fluoroscopy or inspiration-expiration chest radiographs. Since the accessory phrenic branch of C5 and any contribution to the phrenic

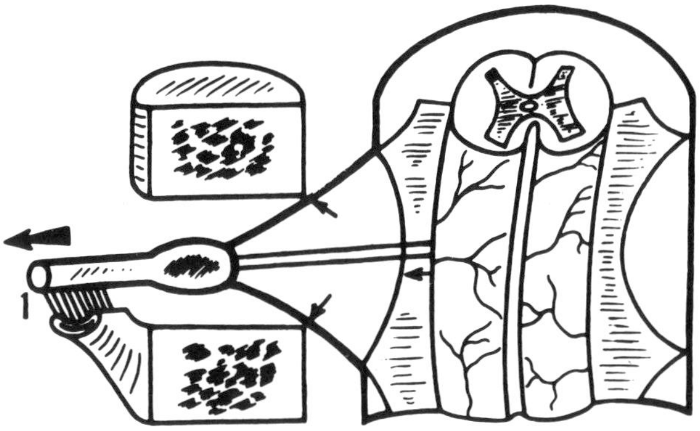

Fig. 4.5. Note the attachment of the spinal nerve to the transverse process, indicated by "1." (Reproduced from Sunderland S: Mechanisms of cervical root avulsion in injuries of the neck and shoulder. J Neurosurg 41:705, 1974, with permission.)

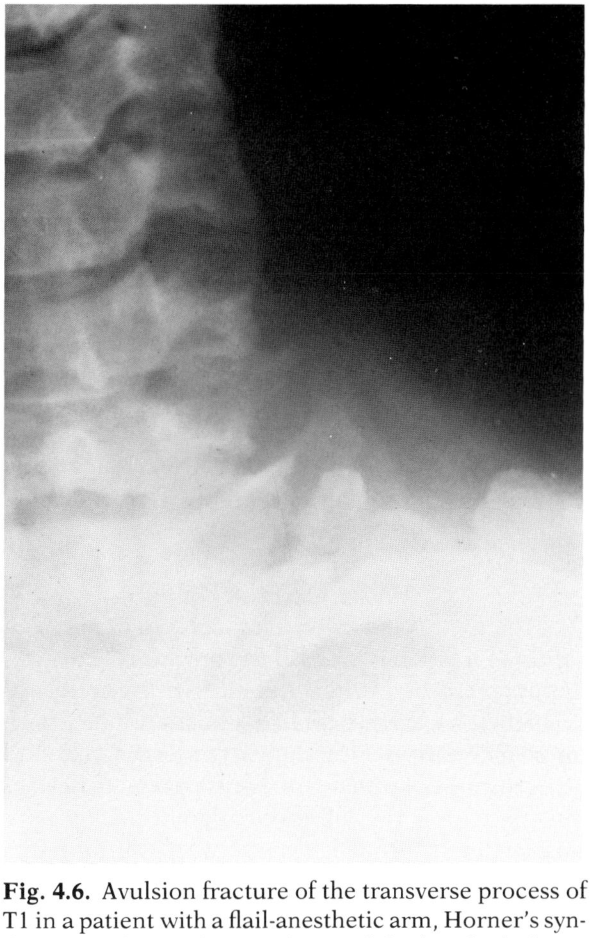

Fig. 4.6. Avulsion fracture of the transverse process of T1 in a patient with a flail-anesthetic arm, Horner's syndrome, and complete avulsion of the brachial plexus following traction injury.

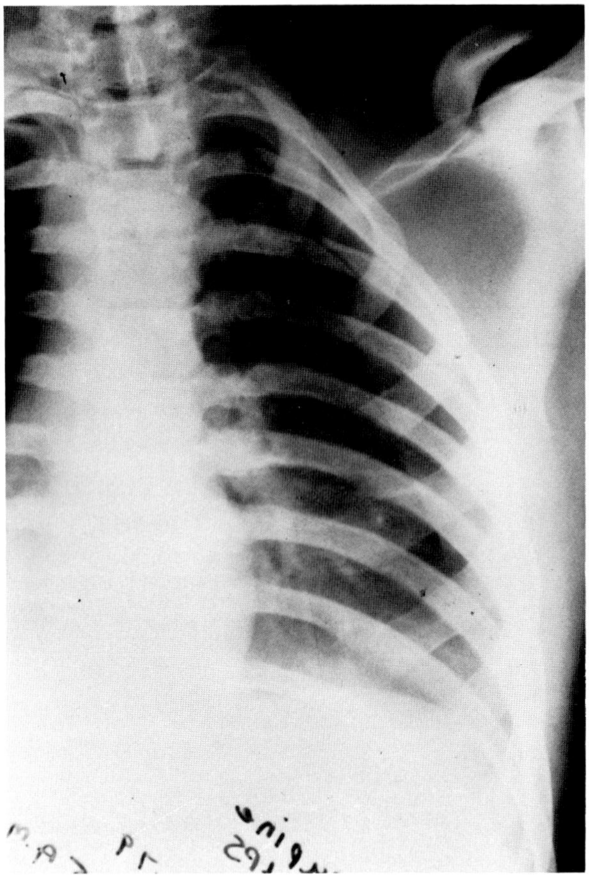

Fig. 4.7. Fracture of the clavicle with massive avulsion of the brachial plexus. Note the lateral position of the scapula relative to the thorax.

nerve from C5 is a root collateral, a supraganglionic lesion at this level will result in diaphragmatic paralysis.

MYELOGRAPHY

The use of cervical myelography in the investigation of traction injuries of the brachial plexus was first reported by Murphey et al.[24] In the course of evaluating a patient who had a traction injury with intractable pain, they attempted to rule out a cervical disk protrusion by means of a myelogram. Instead of disk herniation, they observed migration of the contrast material through the intervertebral foramina into extraspinal diverticula. They called these pouches "traumatic meningoceles" and concluded that these myelographic findings represented nerve root avulsion. In 1949 Murphey and Kirklin[25] described seven patients, three of whom were verified as having avulsions by extraspinal exploration. Additional papers appeared in the next few years with similar findings.[22] In 1954 White and Hanelin[36] reported three additional cases, one of which was explored intradurally, thus confirming the myelographic diagnosis of root avulsion. The lining of the pouches was described as meningeal in nature, thus legitimizing the term meningocele. In the same year Tarlov and Day[33] reported two cases of root avulsion documented by myelography and confirmed by laminectomy. The myelographic findings in a third case, clinically diagnosed as avulsion, differed in that, instead of protrusions of the dye column, there were concave defects at the affected roots. At operation the explanation for these variations was found to be avulsion with meningeal scar tissue that obliterated the arachnoidal and dural apertures at the level of the avulsed roots. Further experience with the use of myelography established that it was an extremely useful adjunct to clinical evaluation of traction injuries of the brachial plexus.[7,26]

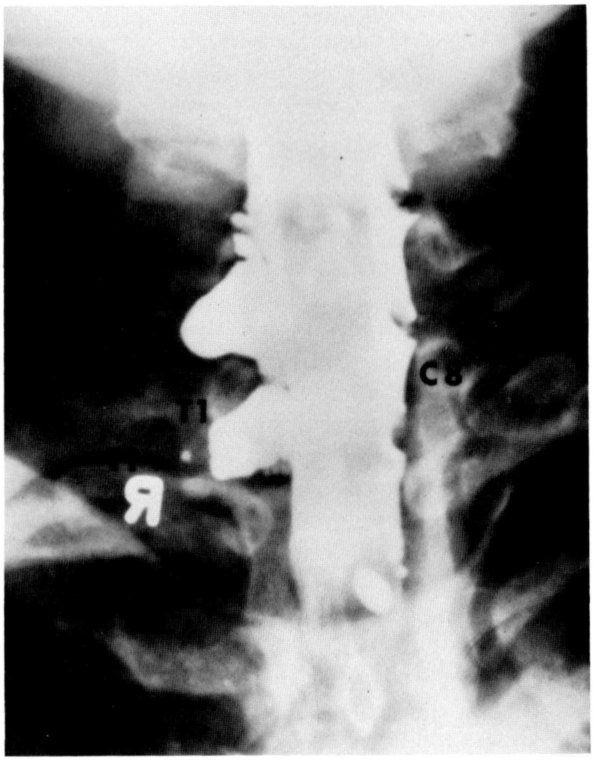

Fig. 4.8. Pantopaque myelogram showing traumatic pseudomeningoceles at C8 and T1 of a patient with a severe traction injury of the brachial plexus.

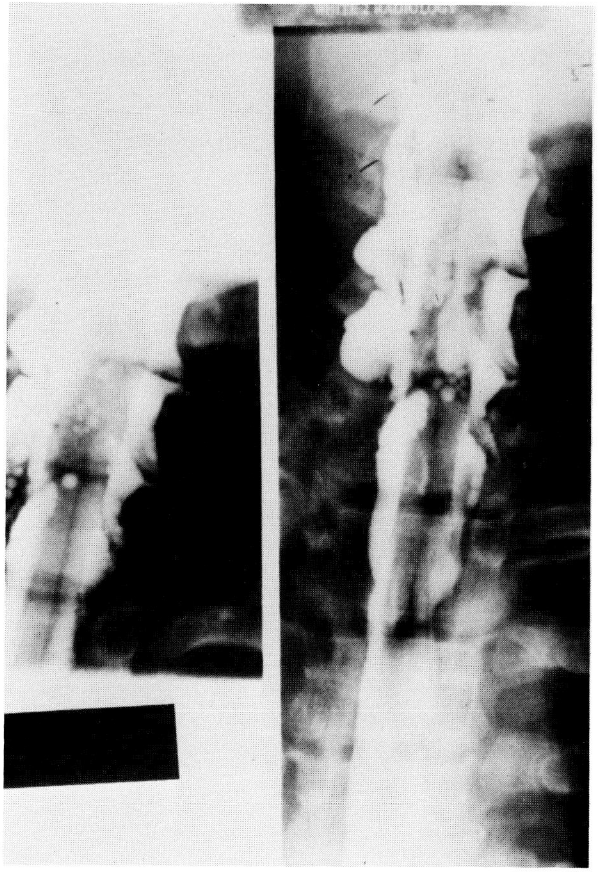

Fig. 4.9. Pseudomeningoceles of C8, C7, and C6. The detail of C5 is not clearly seen, but the insert on the left shows the detail of the contralateral nerve roots.

Accordingly, the technique that we currently employ can be summarized as follows: In the average patient with a severe traction lesion, myelography is done at about one month post injury when there is total paralysis or sensory loss in the peripheral distribution of any portion of the plexus, indicating the possibility of avulsion or distal rupture. Historically, and in our department, Pantopaque was the contrast material of choice, introduced by lumbar puncture, with the patient fluoroscoped on a tilting table in the prone position. In order to facilitate the flow of the contrast medium into the pseudomeningoceles, should they be present, the patient could be turned on either side or semilateral, while the neck was maintained hyperextended to prevent flow into the basal cisterns (Figs. 4.8, 4.9). As a general rule, it is best to avoid the procedure within the first two weeks following injury, when there is a possibility of fresh hemorrhage into the subarachnoid space with increased risk of arachnoiditis. In addition, detail could be obliterated or disguised by the changes caused by the fresh injury.

With the evolution of water-soluble contrast material, the definition that can be documented has improved significantly. The Neuroradiology Section at the Massachusetts General Hospital has evolved through several different techniques in an attempt to enhance resolution. Although polytomography was thought to be of significant advantage, the logistics of combining that with the safe performance of a myelogram have made it less desirable for them when evaluated against the ultimate result (Fig. 4.10). The technique using Metrizamide is to premedicate the patient on the day before the study with two divided

(Text continues on p. 86)

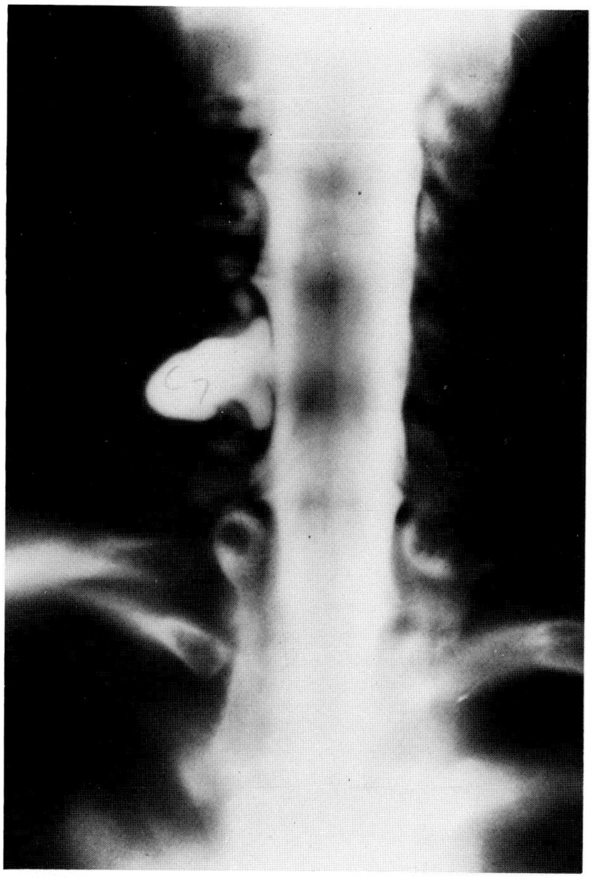

Fig. 4.10. Metrizamide myelogram combined with polytomography. Note the obvious dye-pouch at C7 and the detail of the relatively normal C8 nerve root below it in which there is some bulging of the meninges, but the shadows of the root may still be seen.

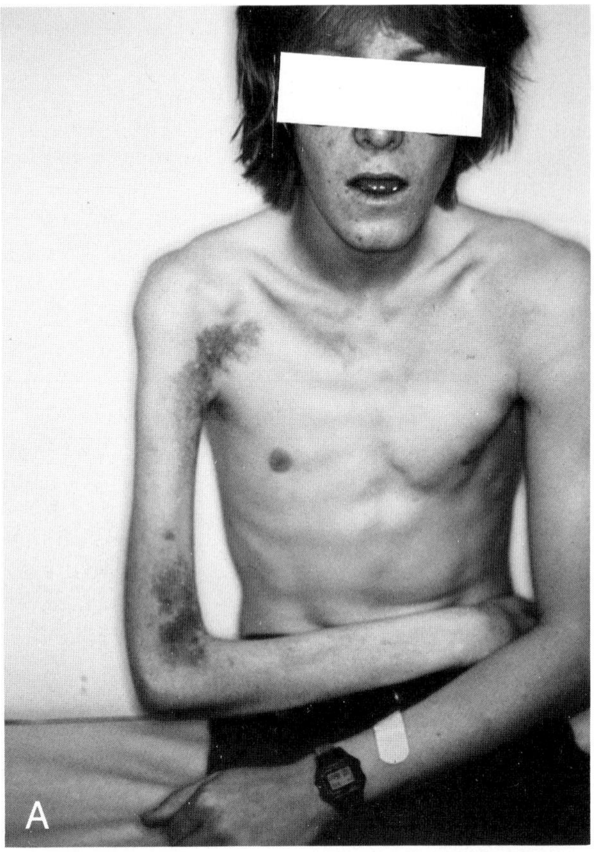

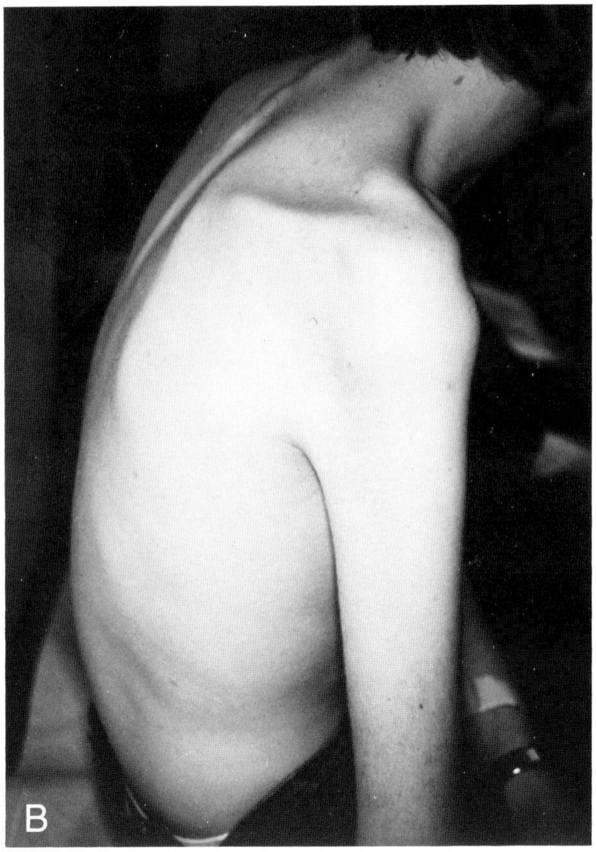

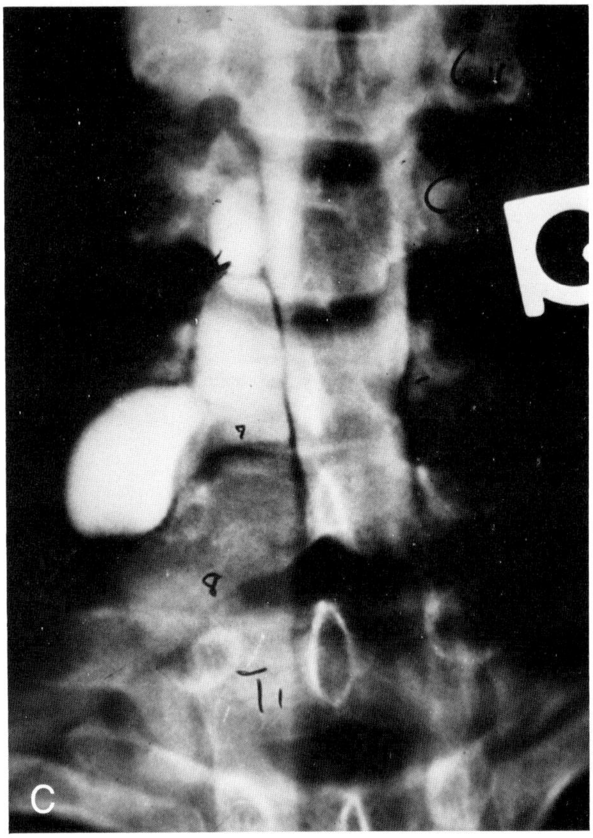

Fig. 4.11. A: 17-year-old patient with flail-anesthetic arm due to traction injury of the brachial plexus. **B:** Note the winging of the scapula and atrophy of muscles, which include serratus anterior and rhomboids. **C:** Metrizamide myelogram showing multiple pseudomeningoceles.

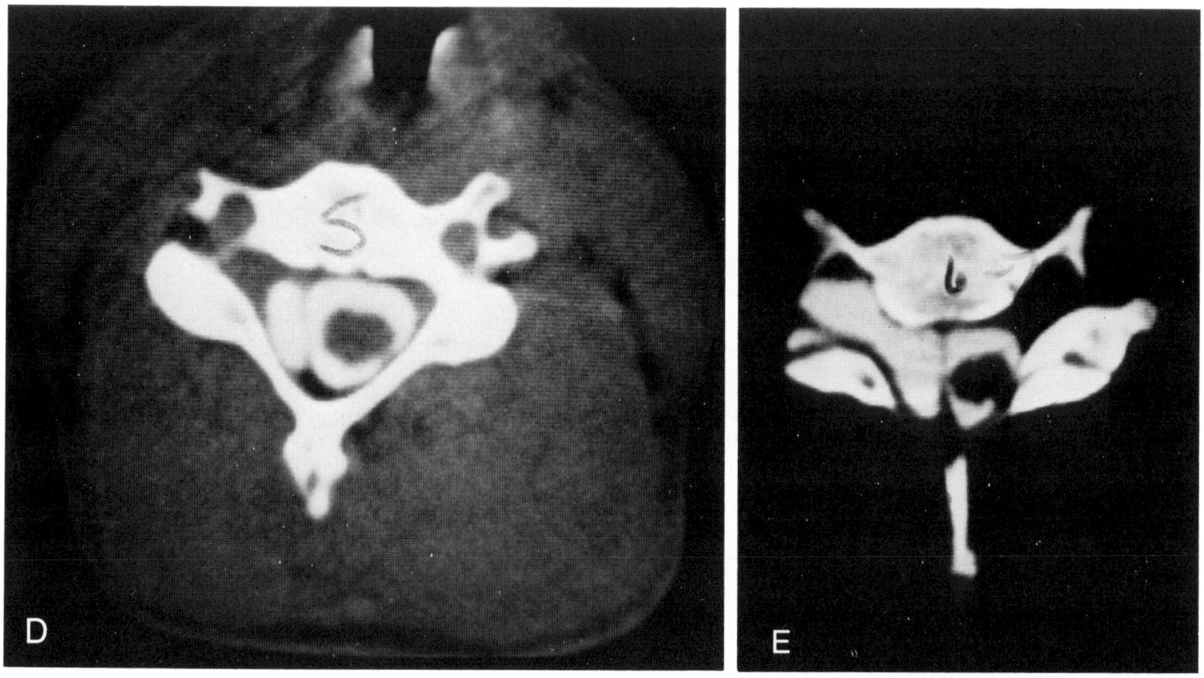

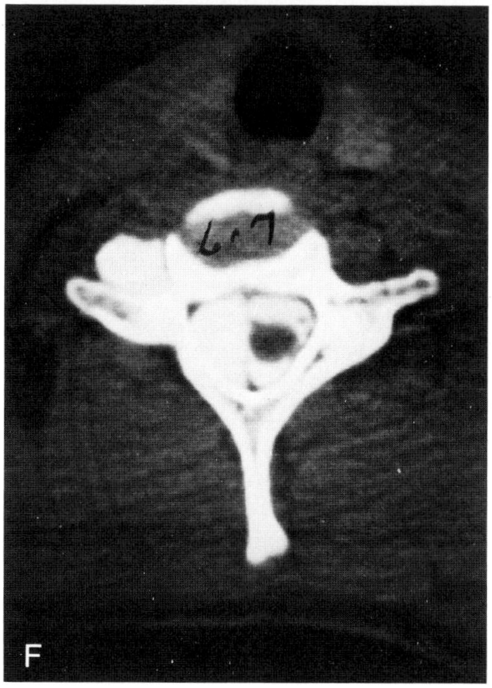

Fig. 4.11. *(continued)* **D – F:** Selected cuts from CT scan showing meningeal diverticulum as it appears at each level. Note the displacement of the spinal cord.

doses of 60 mg of phenobarbital and 100 mg on-call to the radiology department. The patient is not fasted and every effort is made to encourage hydration. A C1–2 puncture, using a 22-gauge short-bevel needle, is performed under local anesthesia. This is markedly facilitated by the use of fluoroscopy or a C-arm to guide the needle puncture to the posterior third of the interspace. The patient is in the prone position with the neck hyperextended and loosely held by a padded clamp. Then 9 ml of the contrast material containing 220 mg/ml of iodine is used. The position of the patient is stationary during the procedure and no tilt or turning is necessary. The optimal position on the table is determined by the anatomy of the cervical spine, and the head is maintained with the chin up to avoid spillage into the basal cisterns. The major potential complication of the use of this agent is generalized seizures, which have been seen in none of the patients that I have referred to the department. Some of the patients have had postmyelographic headaches, which we believe can be minimized by keeping the head of the bed elevated 30 degrees and encouraging fluids by mouth.

This is an evolving field with technological advances making better and better resolution possible. Studies employing computed tomography can provide significantly more information if combined with myelography (Fig. 4.11). The General Electric 9800 scanner is capable of 1 mm definition, which would certainly demonstrate the presence of nerve roots, and even the confluence of the rootlets as they come off the cord.

The advent of nuclear magnetic resonance (NMR) brings up the possibility of even greater resolution, and this will certainly have to be evaluated in the future. For the present time, however, it is not available on a general basis.

It should be noted, however, that myelography, being an indirect method of evaluation, cannot be relied upon without qualification to indicate the presence of root avulsion and to define it from distal rupture. Historically, this was corroborated by the following observations:

1. Root avulsion could occur in the presence of a normal myelogram.[13] Sunderland[32] has graphically summarized this phenomenon.
2. Intact roots can be found at operation within a meningeal diverticulum seen on myelography. In 1965 Heon[10] reported three patients with traumatic meningoceles on myelography in whom the nerve roots within the meningoceles were intact at operation. Thus the meninges could be torn without avulsion of the accompanying nerve root.
3. Functional restitution can occur after cervical avulsion injury with "typical" myelographic findings. This course of events was documented by Jelasic and Piepgras[14] in 1974 in two patients whose myelograms indicated extensive avulsion and who made excellent clinical recoveries at multiple levels.
4. Differential avulsion of both anterior and posterior roots can occur. Tarlov and Day[33] in 1954 and others have demonstrated this by laboratory and clinical operative means. According to Sunderland,[32] the anterior nerve root is thinner than the posterior root, and it has a lower tensile strength and a thinner dural sheath.
5. Variation in innervation and specific composition of the roots contributing to the plexus could result in errors in identification of the exact roots involved in particular patient's injury.
6. Cervical nerve root "cysts" have been demonstrated radiographically on only one occasion, by Smith[30] in 1962. Although these "cysts" have been reported in the lower levels of the spinal column and have been shown to exist in about half of 120 cervical spines examined at random in the anatomy laboratory by Holt and Yates[12] as small pouches projecting laterally into the dorsal root ganglion and connected medially with the subarachnoid space, they are unlikely to fill during the course of myelography and cause confusion in evaluation of brachial plexus injury.

Yeoman's[37] experience with myelography in traction injuries of the brachial plexus is of interest. In 1968 he correlated it with axon responses elicited in a large series of patients. The 60 patients in the series were selected because they had all sustained severe traction injuries. From this group 78 pseudomeningoceles were outlined. Most of them occurred in the lower roots of the brachial plexus, and they appeared as single, double, or treble meningoceles. Table 4.1 summarizes the findings. Eight myelograms were normal, and the patients made a slow, steady recovery.

The experience of Frot[8] and his colleagues in

Table 4.1. Combinations of Traumatic Meningoceles*

Singles		Doubles		Trebles	
C6	1	C6–C7	2	C5–C6–C7	1
C7	9	C7–C8	2	C7–C8–T1	6
C8	7	C8–T1	11	C5–C8–T1	1
T1	7				
Totals	24	15 × 2 =	30	8 × 3 =	24

* C = cervical; T = thoracic.

An isolated meningocele was rare in the upper roots. Of the treble combinations, one occurred at C5, C8, and T1, and the other seven involved adjacent nerve roots, mostly at the levels of C7, C8, and T1.

From Yeoman, PM: Cervical myelography in traction injuries of the brachial plexus. J Bone Joint Surg 50B-25, 1968

Paris, published in 1977, is also extensive and carefully documented. In addition, correlations between radiographic and surgical findings were described. In Table 4.2, the myelograms are tabulated according to the number and level of roots involved.

Forty-one patients were surgically explored anteriorly, and five of these were also explored posteriorly by laminectomy. Thus 153 roots were studied radiographically and surgically (Table 4.3).

Frot[8] summarized his experience in great and useful detail. He described two cases in which pseudomeningoceles were wrongly diagnosed. On the basis of subsequent clinical recovery, these were probably pedunculated nontraumatic cysts. Of the 90 abnormal roots myelographically, 70 were true avulsions, while 16 were distal lesions. Thus, avulsions were most frequently depicted by myelography. There were four false positives in which the myelogram showed pseudomeningoceles and the surgeon found a root in continuity. Two of these were entirely normal and two had partial lesions clinically.

It should be emphasized, therefore, that myelography is a very useful, but by no means infallible, technique of evaluating the status of the roots in traction injury to the brachial plexus.[10] Certainly it does not seem reasonable to advocate routine cervical laminectomy for diagnosis, nor can I agree with Millesi,[23] who no longer employs myelography in

Table 4.2. Myelograms

		Roots Involved					
	No. of Cases	C4	C5	C6	C7	C8	T1
6 levels							
(1 case)	1	+	+	+	+	+	+
5 levels	1	+	+	+	+	+	
(7 cases)	6		+	+	+	+	+
4 levels	1	+	+	+	+		
(13 cases)	2		+	+	+	+	
	10			+	+	+	+
3 levels	3		+	+	+		
(18 cases)	7			+	+	+	
	8			+	+	+	+
2 levels	2		+	+			
(9 cases)	4			+	+		
	1				+	+	
	2					+	+
1 level	2			+			
(9 cases)	2				+		
	4					+	
	1						+

From Frot B: La myelographie cervicale opaque dans les paralysies traumatiques du plexus brachial. Rev Chir Orthop 63:67, 1977, with permission.

Table 4.3. Myelographic-Radiographic-Surgical Correlation (41 Patients, 153 Roots)

Myelograms (State of the Roots)		Surgical Exploration (Anterior & Posterior)		
		Normals	Distal Lesions	Avulsion
Normals	63	24	34	5
		(38%)	39 (62%)	
M, m, r, d, l	90	4	16	70
		(5%)	86 (95%)	

M = large pseudomeningocele (typical finding), m = small pseudomeningocele, r = minimal abnormality of one root, d = picture of "defect," l = gap

From Frot B: La myelographie cervicale opaque dans les paralysies traumatiques du plexus brachial. Rev Chir Orthop 63:67, 1977, with permission.

these patients because he considers it of little value. Until a totally noninvasive means of investigation is developed, I believe that myelography, which is tolerably invasive, should be retained.

AXON REFLEX TESTING

Although axon reflexes had been intensively studied by Lewis and his coworkers,[18-20] it was George Bonney[2-4] who applied these principles to formalized and systematic testing in a clinical situation of patients with traction injuries of the brachial plexus. His observations and documentations of his patients in these two papers are well worth reading in detail because they are classics. Simply stated, if a drop of 1% acid histamine phosphate is pricked into normally innervated skin, the following sequence of events occurs: first there is local vasodilation, then a wheal, and finally a spreading flare. If the skin has been denervated by interruption of continuity between the neuronal cell and its axon (infraganglionic), then the flare will not occur. If the denervation results from a supraganglionic lesion, there will be no disturbance of the normal axon reflex, even though there is no sensibility in the involved dermatome. Bonney formulated his thesis after examining nerve biopsies in patients known to have complete brachial plexus injuries when he found myelinated fibers present in the denervated limbs long after the injury.

From a practical point, the test can be applied only to those dermatomes represented by several clear centimeters of flat skin, which includes the C5, C6, C8, and T1. However, C7 cannot be assessed because it is represented by the skin of the middle finger, where the test would be difficult to interpret. To allow for testing in the hand, Bonney made use of the cold vasodilatation test, which was a thermoelectric measurement of heat elimination from the fingertip, using heat-flow disks. In a normally innervated finger immersed in water at 50°C, there is a rapid cooling, followed within 5 to 10 minutes by reactive vasodilatation and a rise with local temperature. The finger denervated by an infraganglionic lesion would, after the time required for Wallerian degeneration to occur, fail to exhibit this response. As in the axon reflex done on a supraganglionic lesion, the latter would display a normal response. While this test does facilitate evaluation of the axon response in the hand, it is still subject to the same reservations that detract from its usefulness and specific reliability. Because it is ultimately an indirect method, there is no assurance that a supraganglionic lesion is not accompanied by an infraganglionic one at the same level, or that a prefixed or postfixed plexus is not present, making determination of the root level of the lesion difficult. These problems were enumerated by Yeoman[37] in 1968 in his careful study of cervical myelograms and axon responses in 40 patients with severe traction injuries (see above). Although there was a fairly close correlation in the inferences of the two methods, a number of disparities occurred, and these were of great importance. Eighteen traumatic meningoceles were demonstrated at the level of nerve roots in which infraganglionic responses were obtained from histamine and cold vasodilator tests. This verified Bonney's contention that infraganglionic lesions could occur in the same root that had been avulsed from the cord. Obviously, it is of great significance, since surgical exploration of the neck in these cases might lead to the mistaken diagnosis of an uncomplicated distal lesion with a potential for recovery or surgical reconstruc-

Table 4.4. Disparities between Postganglionic Responses and the Presence of Traumatic Meningoceles

Level	Postganglionic Response	Traumatic Meningocele
C6	38	1
C7	21	3
C8	19	9
T1	16	5

From Yeoman PM: Cervical myelography in traction injuries of the brachial plexus. J Bone Joint Surg 50B:25, 1968, with permission.

tion. There were 14 instances of supraganglionic response without an associated meningocele. In eight of these there was a meningocele in the root above the one showing a supraganglionic response. In two there were meningoceles below the one showing a supraganglionic response, and in the remaining four there were doubtful protrusions in one or two nerve roots. Table 4.4, taken from Yeoman's article, details the disparities.

It is apparent then, as all of the indirect methods of documentation of the level and extent of traction injuries of the brachial plexus are reviewed in detail, that none of them can or should supplant clinical evaluation and the application of neurodiagnostic logic. The information derived from these evaluations must be interpreted and weighed according to the limitations that have been noted and described. At the present time it is my practice to defer myelography and electrodiagnostic studies for a month from the time of injury in a fresh case. Because of the difficulties of interpreting the axon responses in the hand and the fact that allergically susceptible patients may react adversely to intradermal histamine, I no longer use this method of evaluation.

REFERENCES

1. Aminoff MJ: Electromyography in Clinical Practice. Addison-Wesley, Menlo Park, CA, 1978
2. Bonney G: The value of axon responses in determining the site of lesion in traction injuries of the brachial plexus. Brain 77:588, 1954
3. Bonney G, Gilliat RW: Sensory nerve conduction after traction lesion of the brachial plexus. Proc R Soc Med 51:365, 1958
4. Bonney G: Prognosis in traction lesions of the brachial plexus. J Bone Joint Surg 41B:4, 1959
5. Bufalini C, Pesatori G: Posterior cervical electromyography in the diagnosis and prognosis of brachial plexus injuries. J Bone Joint Surg 51B:627, 1969
6. Copeland S, Landi A: Value of the Tinel sign in brachial plexus lesions. Ann R Coll Surg 61:470, 1979
7. Davies ER, Sutton D, Bligh AS: Myelography in brachial plexus injury. Br J Radio 39:362, 1966
8. Frot B: La myelographie cervicale opaque dans les paralysies traumatiques du plexus brachial. Rev Chir Orthop 63:67, 1977
9. Henderson WR: Clinical assessment of peripheral nerve injuries. Tinel's test. Lancet 11:801, 1948
10. Heon M: Myelogram: A questionable aid in diagnosis and prognosis in avulsion of brachial plexus components by traction injuries. Conn Med 29:260, 1965
11. Highet WB: Grading of motor and sensory recovery in nerve injuries. p 356. In Seddon HJ (ed): Peripheral Nerve Injuries. Medical Research Council Report Series No. 282, HMSO, London, 1954
12. Holt S, Yates PO: Cervical nerve root "cysts." Brain 87:481, 1964
13. Jaeger R, Whitley WH: Avulsion of the brachial plexus. JAMA 153:633, 1953
14. Jelasic F, Piepgras U: Functional restitution after cervical avulsion injury with "typical" myelographic findings. Eur Neurol 11:158, 1974
15. Jones S: Investigation of brachial plexus traction lesions by peripheral and spinal somatosensory evoked potentials. J Neurol Neurosurg Psychiatry 42:107, 1979
16. Jones SJ, Wynn-Parry CB, Landi A: Diagnosis of brachial plexus traction lesions by sensory nerve action potentials and somatosensory evoked potentials. Injury 12:376, 1981
17. Kendall HO, Kendall FP, Wadsworth GE: Muscles—Testing and Function. 2nd Ed. Williams & Wilkins, Baltimore, 1971
18. Lewis T: Observations upon the reactions of the vessels of the human skin to cold. Heart 15:177, 1930
19. Lewis T: Observation upon the vascular axon reflex in human skin, as exhibited by a case of urticaria, with remarks upon the nocifensor nerve hypothesis. Clin Sci 4:365, 1942
20. Lewis T, Landis EM: Some physiological effects of sympathetic ganglionectomy in the human being and its effects in a case of Raynaud's malady. Heart 15:151, 1930
21. Licht S: Electrodiagnosis and Electromyography. 3rd Ed. E. Licht, New Haven, CN, 1971
22. Mendelsohn RA, Weiner IH, Keegan JM: Myelographic demonstration of brachial plexus root avulsion. Arch Surg 75:102, 1957
23. Millesi H: Surgical management of brachial plexus injuries. J Hand Surg 2(5):367, 1977
24. Murphey F, Hartung W, Kirklin JW: Myelographic

demonstration of avulsing injuries of the brachial plexus. Am J Roentgenol 58:102, 1947
25. Murphey F, Hartung W, Kirklin JW: Myelographic demonstration of avulsion injuries of the brachial plexus. Clinical Congress of the American College of Surgeons, Chicago 1949 (quoted by RJ Jaeger and WH Whitley in Ref. 13)
26. Murphey F, Kirklin JW: Myelographic demonstration of avulsing injuries of the nerve roots of the brachial plexus—A method of determining the point of injury and the possibility of repair. Clin Neurosurg 20:18, 1972
27. Omer GE Jr: Sensation and sensibility in the upper extremity. Clin Orthop 104:30, 1974
28. Roaf R: Lateral flexion injuries of the cervical spine. J Bone Joint Surg 45B:36, 1963
29. Seddon H: Surgical Disorders of the Peripheral Nerves. 2nd Ed. Churchill Livingstone, New York, 1975
30. Smith DT: Multiple meningeal diverticula (perineurial cysts) of the cervical region disclosed by pantopaque myelography. Report of a case. J Neurosurg 19:599, 1962
31. Smorto MP, Basmajian JV: Clinical Electroneurography: An Introduction to Nerve Conduction Tests. 2nd Ed. Williams & Wilkins, Baltimore, 1979
32. Sunderland S: Mechanisms of cervical root avulsion in injuries of the neck and shoulder. J Neurosurg 41:705, 1974
33. Tarlov IM, Day R: Myelography to help localize traction lesions of the brachial plexus. Am J Surg 88:266, 1954
34. Thompson LL: The Electromyographer's Handbook. Little, Brown Boston, 1981
35. Warren J, Gutmann L, Figueroa AF, Bloor BM: Electromyographic changes of brachial plexus root avulsion. J Neurosurg 31:137, 1969
36. White JC, Hanelin J: Myelographic sign of brachial plexus avulsion. J Bone Joint Surg 36A:113, 1954
37. Yeoman PM: Cervical myelography in traction injuries of the brachial plexus. J Bone Joint Surg 50B:25, 1968
38. Zalis AW, Oester YT, Rodriguez AA: Electrophysiological diagnosis of cervical root avulsion. Arch Phys Med 51:708, 1970

5

Congenital Brachial Palsy

Since the first report by Smellie[38] in 1764 of paralysis of both arms following a difficult delivery, congenital brachial paralysis has continued to be a problem (Fig. 5.1). Sever[33] in 1916 collected a total of 457 cases from 58 authors, beginning with Duchenne in 1872.[8] He contributed a personally studied series of 470 additional cases, which grew to 1100 by 1925.[34,36] Fortunately, with improvements in obstetrical management, the incidence of this disorder has diminished considerably. For example, The Hospital for Special Surgery in New York saw 491 new cases from 1928 to 1939, whereas in the next 23 years there were 123 patients. In 1967 Adler and Patterson[1] reported these statistics as well as those of the Obstetrical Service at the New York Hospital, where the incidence of this complication decreased from 1.56 per 1000 live births in 1938 to 0.3 per 1000 in 1962. Yet, despite these improved statistics, such patients are still seen by pediatricians and orthopedic surgeons. In 1981 Hardy[15] reported statistics from the National Women's Hospital in Aukland, New Zealand and gave an incidence of 0.87 per 100 live births.

In 1983 Tassin[40] reported in his thesis at the University of Paris on 110 infants with obstetrical brachial palsy who underwent reconstructive surgery on the plexus by Gilbert at Trousseau Hospital. These patients came from 230 obstetrical palsies seen at that hospital between October 1977 and October 1982 as part of a study requiring nationwide cooperation, and in 20% of the cases, the patients were from foreign countries. In order to compare the results of surgery with a control group, 44 infants were followed conservatively at Saint Vincent de Paul Hospital. This most valuable study will be referred to later in this chapter.

PATHOGENESIS

Although there is little doubt today that obstetrical paralysis is due to a supraclavicular traction lesion of the brachial plexus incurred during delivery, a historical survey reveals that considerable controversy surrounded the etiology in the past. Smellie[38] believed that the condition was due to prolonged intrauterine pressure on the arm. Duchenne,[8] who described four cases in 1872, attributed it to pressure during delivery by forceps or fingers in the axilla. He further realized that the lesion could occur during obstetrical manipulation of the fetus, thus recognizing the possible role of traction. Two years later, Erb[9,10] described the picture of upper trunk paralysis in adults, and attributed the condition in infants to a combination of traction and compression of the brachial plexus. Stransky was quoted by Sever[33] in 1916 as having reviewed the literature up to 1902. He reported 94 cases from various authors, most of whom believed that traction and/or compression of the nerves was the cause. Justner's theory, quoted by Sever, that it was not the nerves but the shoulder joint or humerus that was the site of the primary pathology, was rejected by most. However, Thomas[44] of Philadelphia advanced a theory wherein the shoulder injury actually caused a secondary lesion of the adjacent plexus. He postulated that compression of the shoulder in utero by the maternal pelvis caused local capsular injury that resulted in joint exudate. This fluid then tracked into the supraclavicular fossa to involve the previously uninjured nerve roots and trunks and produced scarring. According to Platt,[28] in 1905 Clarke, Taylor, and Prout[5] of New York had attempted to reproduce cadaver lesions of the brachial plexus by traction on the head with the shoulder fixed. They showed that the upper trunk was the first to fail in traction and that further force affected the remainder of the plexus. In an attempt to resolve this issue, Sever[33] repeated these experiments in 1916 and found that considerable force was needed to rupture the C5 and C6 and that the suprascapular nerve was prone to rupture before the roots. In most cases he found that the nerve sheath tore, but that the nerve bundles themselves tended to fray without being transected. An important observation made during these experiments was that in order to place great tension on the lower trunk of the plexus, the arm had to be abducted. Sever was unable to rupture the shoulder joint capsule, dislocate the humerus, or separate its proximal epiphysis. Injection of methylene blue into a lacerated shoulder joint capsule caused tracking into the axilla rather than into the supraclavicular fossa as Thomas had reported. Finally, Pratt's repetition of these experiments on infant cadavers brought him to the similar conclusion that the lesions were most likely to be in the spinal roots themselves or in the anterior primary rami.

Why such confusion should have persisted among these investigators is understandable when one considers the almost universal association of secondary shoulder lesions with significant congenital brachial plexus injury. As late as 1936, Scaglietti[31] of Bologna maintained that obstetrical shoulder lesions could be either obstetrical joint trauma, paralysis due to nerve injury, or a mixed form.

The first of these, which he stated was the most frequent lesion observed, was not the result of nerve injury, but was, in reality, a proximal humeral epiphyseal separation. Differentiation between this and the second and lesser group, true brachial plexus injury, could be made by electrodiagnosis and roentgenograms.

Despite the fact that improved obstetrical care has drastically reduced the incidence of obstetrical palsy, long-term review of a series of such patients is revealing. Adler and Patterson[1] in 1967 reported a series of 88 patients seen at The Hospital for Special Surgery in New York from 1939 to 1962 and followed for an average of 18 years. Their obstetrical history was of interest. Only 13 of the 123 patients were said to have had a normal delivery, while 56 had what were called difficult deliveries, and in 54 there was no indication of the difficulty. The incidence of breech presentation was 9%, which was twice the normal expected rate. All four patients with bilateral involvement were breech presentations. As a reflection of the cephalopelvic disproportion that usually underlies a birth palsy, the birth weight of these infants was considerably higher than normal —9 pounds, 8 ounces (4318 g), compared with the average United States mean of 7 pounds, 8 ounces (3400 g).

In 1982 Rossi and coworkers[30] reported in detail on a series of 34 patients with a total of 36 pareses studied at The Children's Hospital and the Department of Neurology of the University of Bern between 1965 and 1975. Six patients had been born by breech presentation, while in the others the birth was reported as normal. Five of the 30 infants with known birth weight were heavier than 4 kg. Two babies had had a hematoma of the sternomastoid muscle, three had fracture of the clavicle, and two had experienced perinatal anoxia.

Of the patients operated upon by Gilbert and reported by Tassin[40] in 1983, the birth weight varied from 2500 to 6000 g. Sixty-seven of these infants were born by cephalic presentation, and 37 weighed between 4000 and 4750 g; 13 weighed less than 4000 g. By contrast, in the 10 breech presentations where the birth weight was known, none exceeded 4000 g.

The observations of Sever on 471 patients with obstetrical palsy are presented in Table 5.1.

Table 5.1 Conditions Existing at the Time of Birth

Boys	235
Girls	236
Total	471
Right arm affected	272
Left arm affected	186
Both arms affected, upper arm type	2
Both arms affected, lower or whole arm type	1
Both arms affected, type not noted	6
Upper arm type	400
Lower or whole arm type	64
Difficult labor	418
Ether used	363
Forceps used	317
Normal labor	32
Asphyxiation of child	102
Head presentation, including face	219
Breech presentation, including foot and version	66
Position not known	186
Fractured clavicle	14
Arm broken	3
Cord around neck and arm	2
Cord around neck	2
Pupils unequal	16

From Sever JW: Obstetrical paralysis—Its etiology, pathology, clinical aspects and treatment, with report of four hundred and seventy cases. Am J Dis Child 12:541, 1916.

CLINICAL PRESENTATION AND DIFFERENTIAL DIAGNOSIS

The diagnosis of brachial plexus injury must be suspected in any neonate with asymmetrical upper extremity motion, especially if passive range is retained (Fig. 5.1). This may become evident from the resting position of the limb, or from lack of active motion, as when eliciting the Moro reflex. Since pseudoparalysis resulting from fracture of the clavicle, humerus, or forearm, or local injury to the shoulder joint, such as dislocation or epiphyseal separation, may be present, an attempt to rule them out by means of radiographs must be made. It should be noted, however, that x-ray films taken in the early stages of the shoulder lesion may be entirely negative, and only with the appearance of periosteal callus around the upper end of the humerus will the diagnosis become apparent. This may occur within eight to ten days, according to Truesdale,[45] who considered it diagnostic of epiphyseal separation. Scaglietti[31] pointed out that, since the proximal humeral epiphysis could be observed radiographically at three months, its position and size could be used to determine the presence of epiphysealysis, with or without displacement of the upper end of the humerus, but that prior to this time, such determinations could be very difficult.

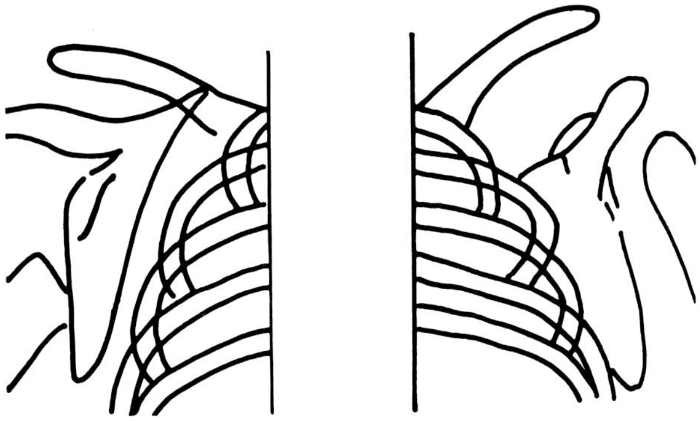

Fig. 5.2. Diagram of an infant with right-sided Erb's paralysis. The humerus is farther from the glenoid on the affected side. (Reproduced from Kattan KR, Spitz HB: Roentgen findings in obstetrical injuries to the brachial plexus. Radiology 91:462, 1968, with permission.)

According to Kattan and Spitz[18] in the young infant with a brachial plexus injury (Fig. 5.2), the metaphysis of the humerus is further from the glenoid than normal. The development of the epiphysis of the humeral head is retarded, and atrophy of the soft tissues about the shoulder joint is present. The scapula may be elevated and rotated outward. Later, the ossification center of the humeral head may lie lateral to that of the greater tuberosity because of the

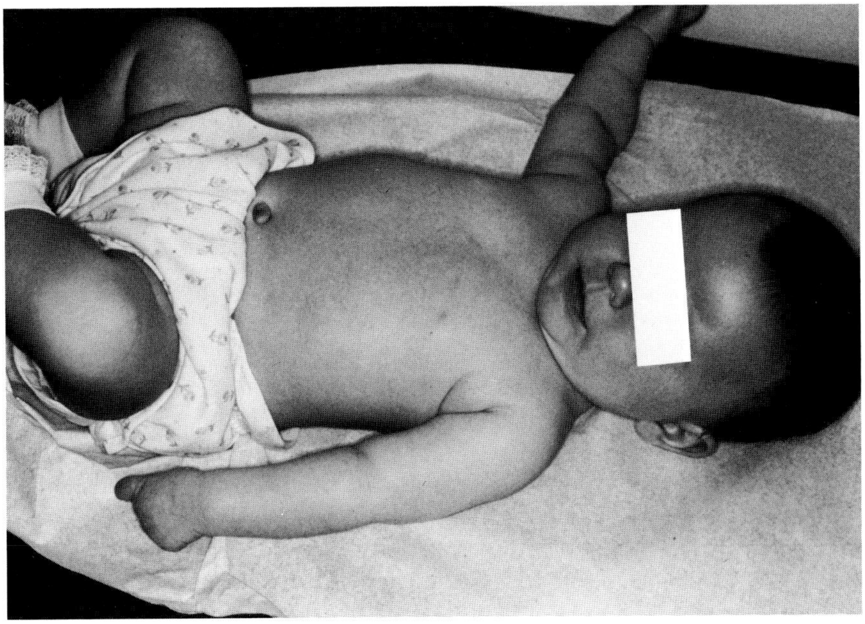

Fig. 5.1. A typical infant with obstetrical palsy. Note the adducted, medially rotated arm and the pronated forearm on the left.

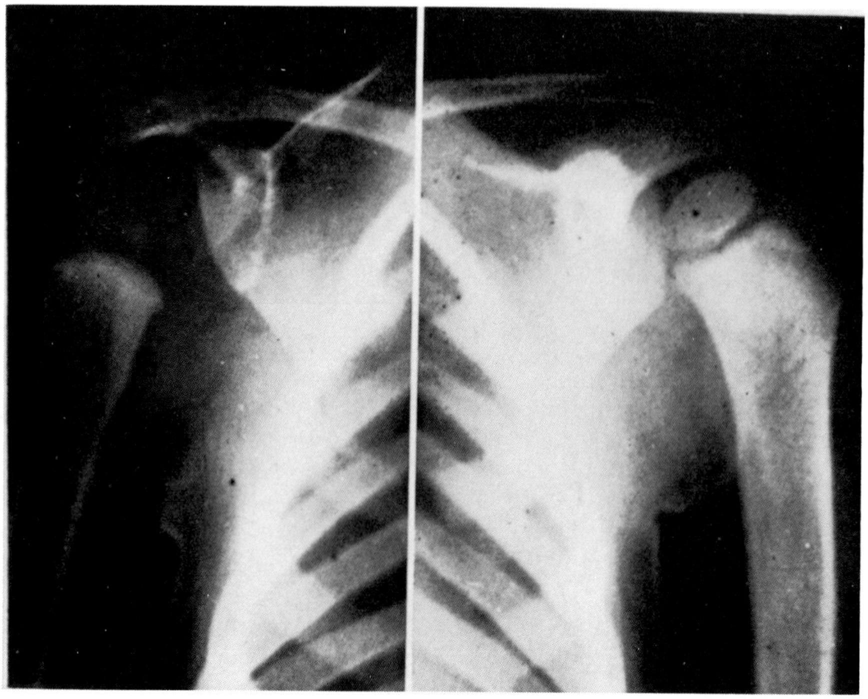

Fig. 5.3. Infant with right-sided Erb's paralysis. The space between the humerus and glenoid is abnormally wide. The development of the right humeral epiphysis and metaphysis is retarded. The scapula is elevated and underdeveloped. (Reproduced from Kattan KR, Spitz HB: Roentgen findings in obstetrical injuries to the brachial plexus. Radiology 91:462, 1968, with permission.)

internal rotation of the humerus (Fig. 5.3). They point out that the child with Sprengel's deformity may also present with a small scapula that is congenitally high in position, and that this must be considered in the differential diagnosis. However, the presence of hemivertebrae and an omovertebral bone extending between the scapula and the cervical spine will correctly identify the patient with Sprengel's deformity.

Since, as has been illustrated by the brief historical review of this condition, there has been considerable confusion between its neurological and musculoskeletal manifestations, I shall first describe the common patterns of paralysis as seen in the newborn, and then the secondary phenomena, which develop with time in the bones and joints.

There are three major types of neurological deficit observed in obstetrical palsy. The first, described in infants by Duchenne[8] in 1872 and adults by Erb[9,10] two years later and commonly referred to as Erb-Duchenne palsy, is the most common. According to Colonna,[6] this type appears four times more often than the other two types combined. Seventy-five of Sever's 1100 patients were of this distribution. It represents a lesion of the C5,6 or upper trunk outflow. The muscles affected, therefore, are those responsible for lateral rotation and abduction of the shoulder as well as elbow flexion. The supraspinatus, infraspinatus, deltoid, biceps, brachialis, coracobrachialis, and brachioradialis may be paralyzed or weak, resulting in an arm which is maintained adducted and medially rotated and the elbow held extended. The wrist extensors and, less frequently, the finger extensors may also be weak. Pronated forearm and flexed wrist result in a classical "waiter's tip position" (Fig. 5.4).

The second most common type results from involvement of the entire brachial plexus. The upper extremity may be totally flail. The scapula may be winged, and all motor activity absent in the limb. In addition, Horner's syndrome may be present, depending on involvement of T1. Lessor degrees of severity of this extensive lesion may be seen (Fig. 5.5).

The least common variety of birth palsy (Klumpke's paralysis[7,22] results from injury to the C7, C8, T1 outflow. Therefore, the hand and finger long flexors and extensors as well as the intrinsics are weak and Horner's syndrome is invariably present. Isolated C8, T1 lesions are not usually seen.

In terms of nerve lesions, 87 children treated by Wickstrom[47] from 1944 to 1958 had the following

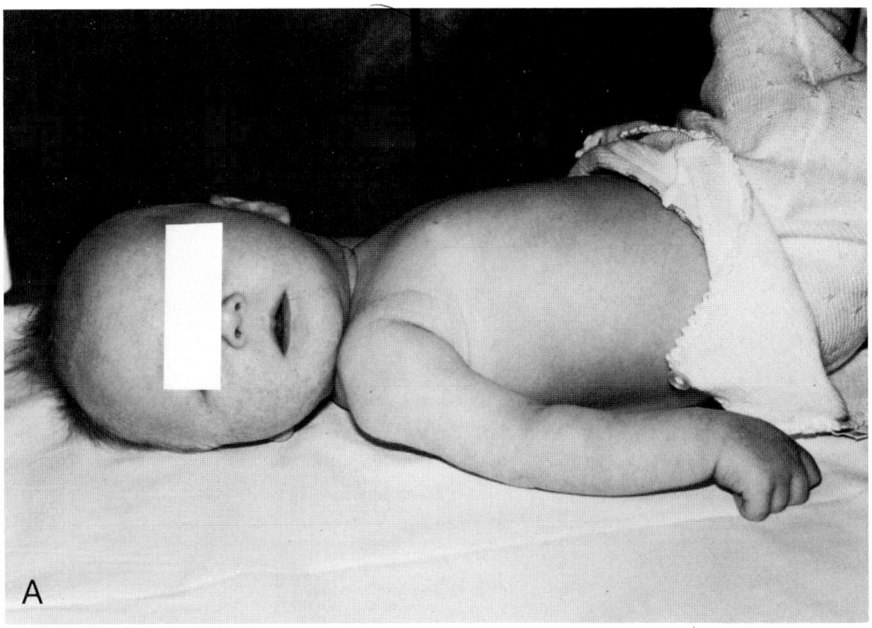

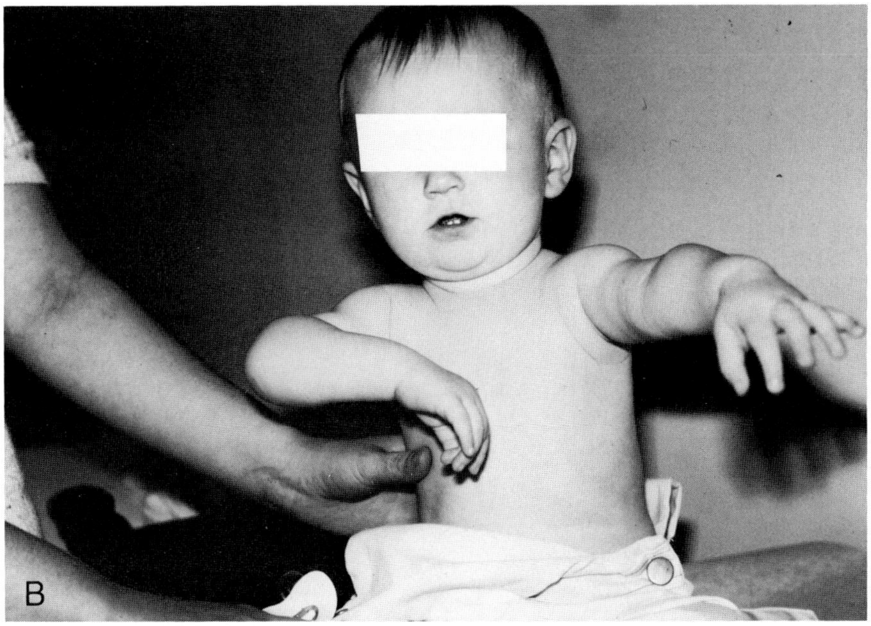

Fig. 5.4. A: Two-month-old infant with Erb's palsy. **B** and **C**: Spontaneous recovery at one year of age. Abduction of the humerus and active lateral rotation are still slightly weak, but elbow flexion and wrist extension are normal. *(Figure continues on next page.)*

distribution: There were 54 patients with evidence of injury to the fifth and sixth cervical nerve roots (62.1%), 22 with some involvement of all components of the plexus (25.3%), and 11 with evidence of damage to C8 and T1 (12.6%).

The lesions that were described as a result of Gilbert's 100 operated cases are most interesting. Lesions of C5 and C6 were most frequent, 51%. Root avulsions were found 11 times, while 27 cases had neuroma in continuity, including Erb's point, and four gross ruptures at Erb's point were found, and these were the rarest. Other lesions, located between Erb's point and the intervertebral foramen, were not associated with lesions of the subjacent roots.

(Text continues on p. 100.)

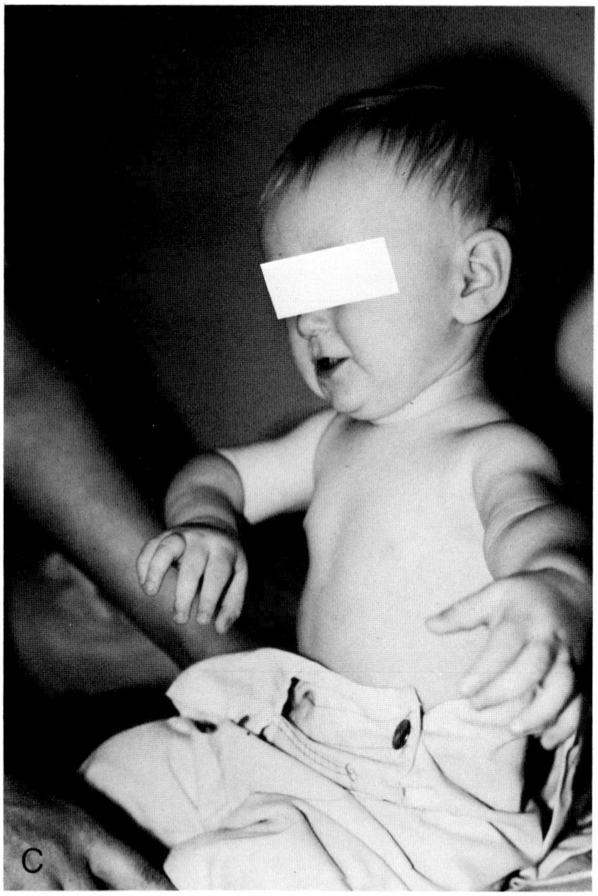

Fig. 5.4. *(continued)* **C:** Same as **B. D**: Further improvement by age two.

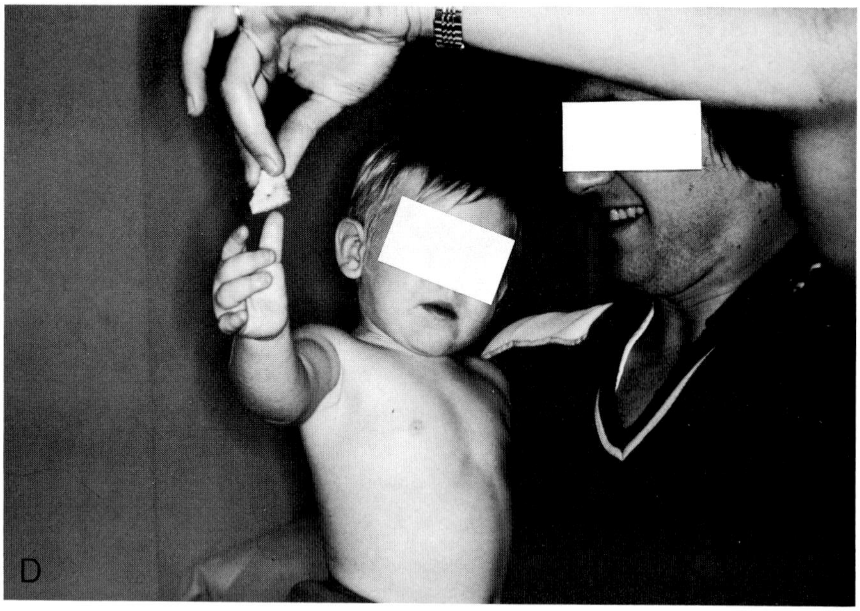

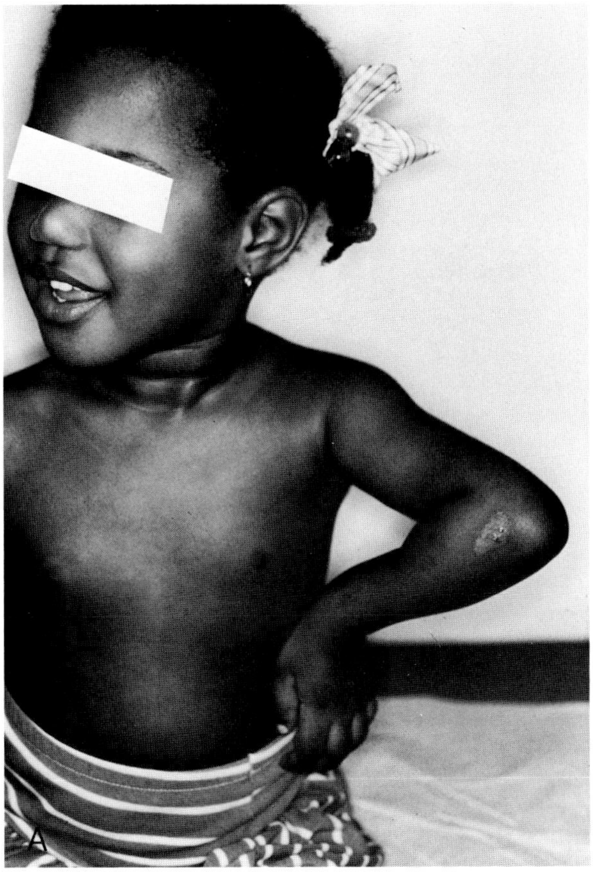

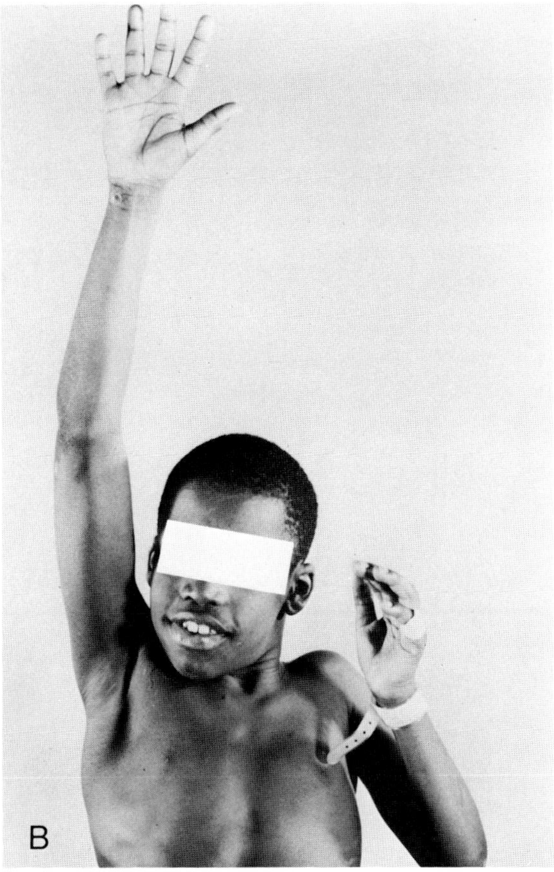

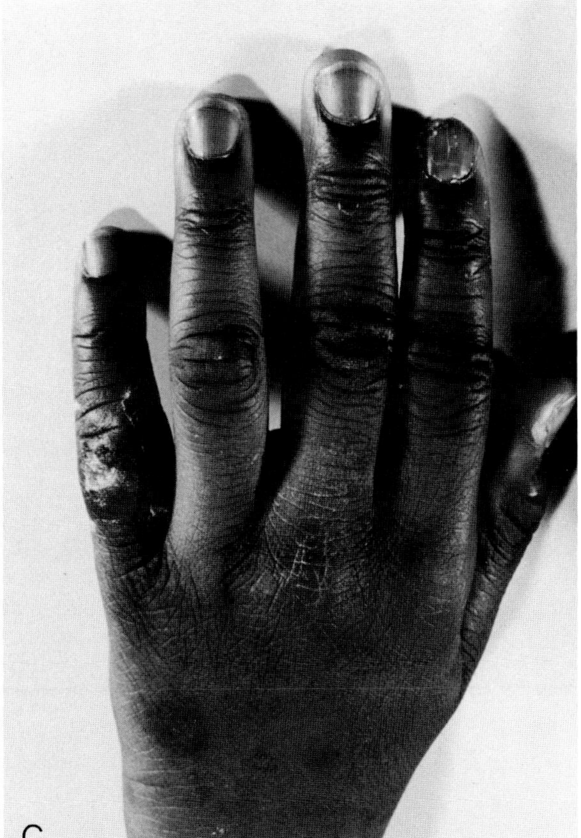

Fig. 5.5. A: Diffuse left brachial palsy from birth. Although the deltoid and biceps are moderately strong, lateral rotation of the humerus is poor, and there is no voluntary control of the wrist or hand. **B** and **C**: Ten-year-old boy with diffuse brachial palsy. Shoulder function is poor and intrinsic muscles of hand are moderately weak. Because of poor sensibility in the little finger and ulnar side of his hand (T1), he has skin ulcerations.

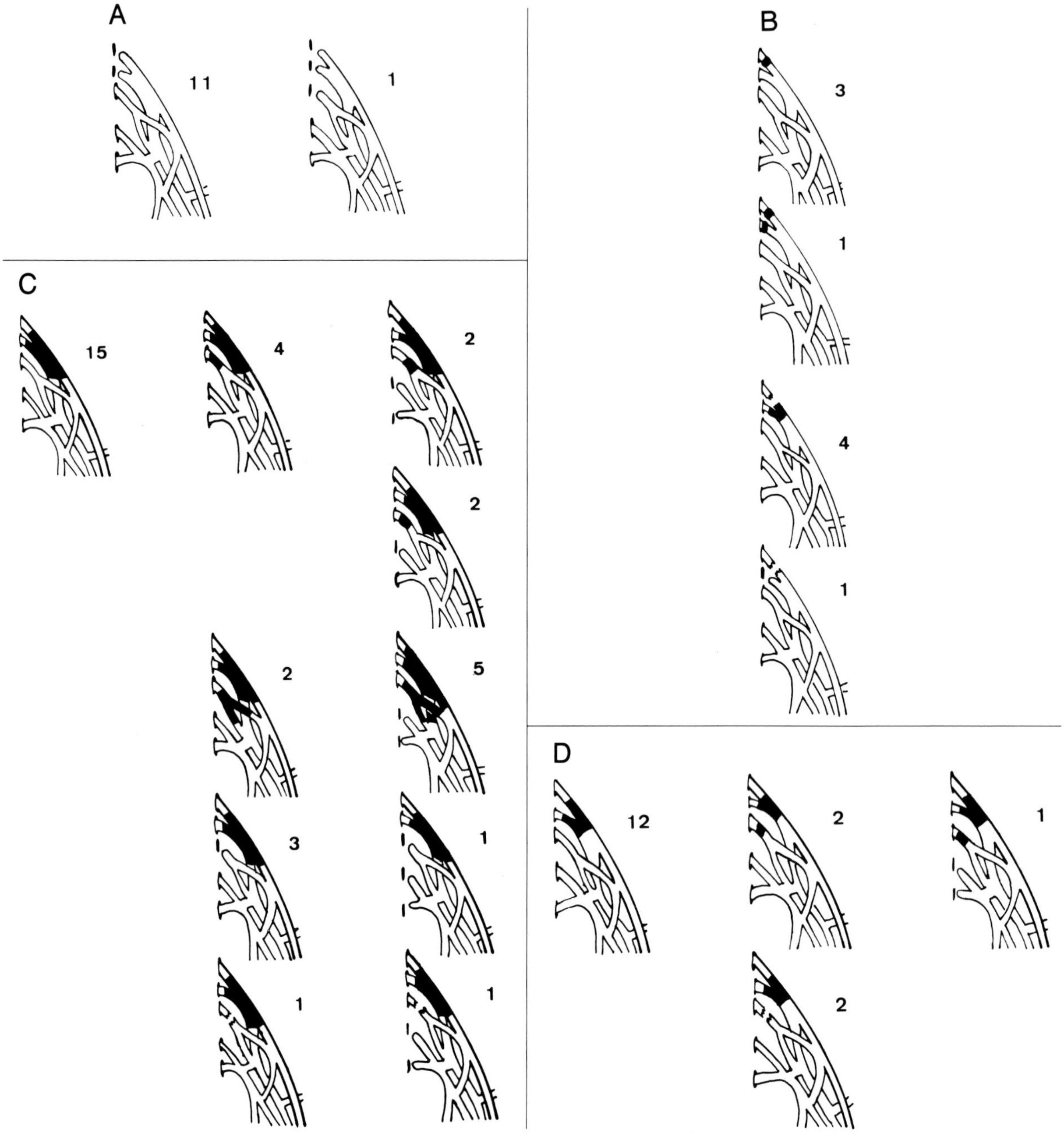

Fig. 5.6. In all cases, the number corresponds to the number of cases of each type seen by Gilbert. **A**: Isolated avulsion of upper roots. **B**: Lesions of C5 and C6, nerve associated with lesions of subjacent roots. **C**: The most frequent lesion, neuroma-in-continuity of C5, C6, the upper trunk and its branches, and the lesions that can be associated with it—neuromatous rupture of C7; avulsions of C8 and T1. **D**: Neuroma-in-continuity not affecting the branches of the upper trunk, rarity of involvement of C7, C8, and T1.

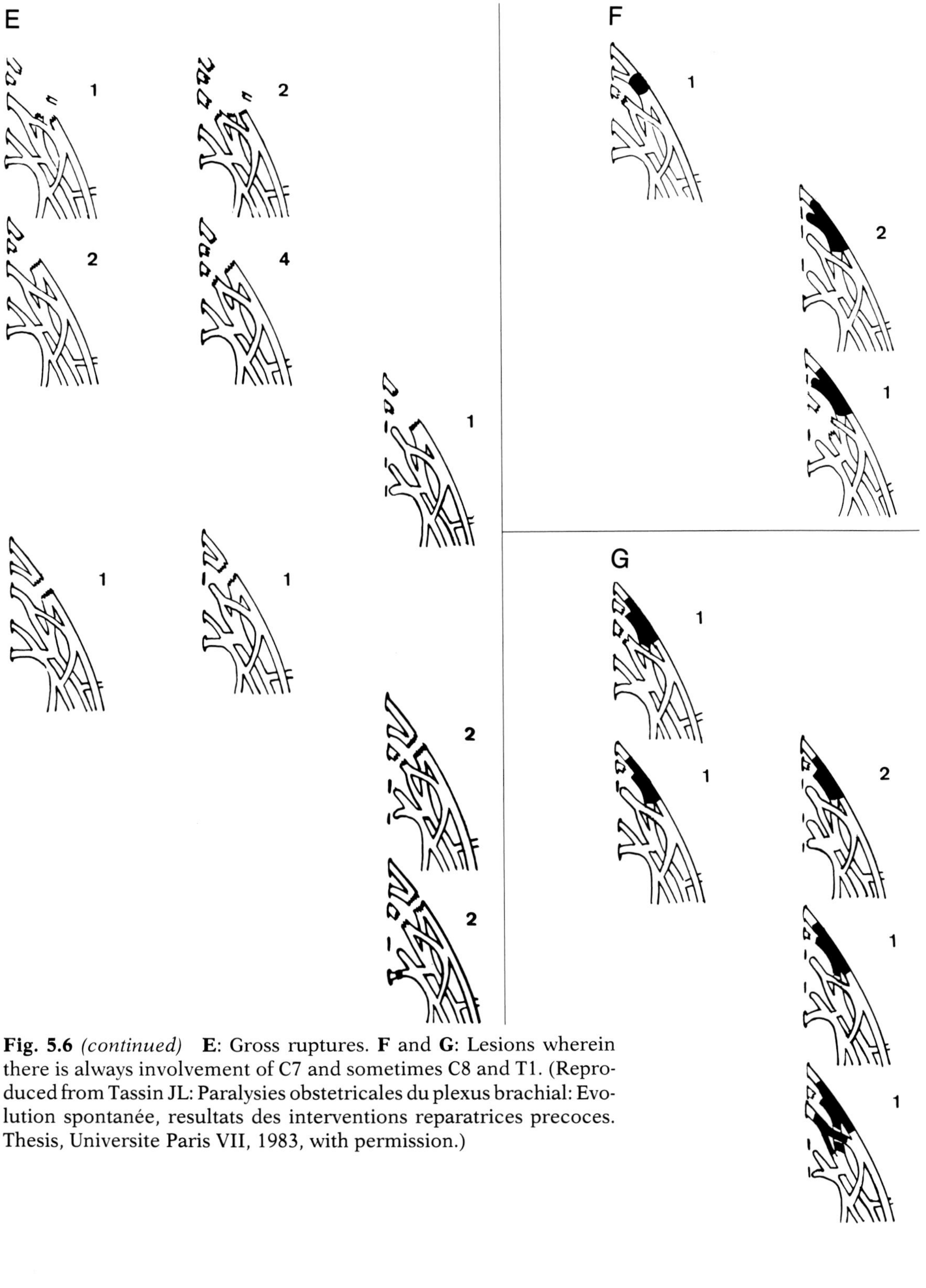

Fig. 5.6 *(continued)* **E**: Gross ruptures. **F** and **G**: Lesions wherein there is always involvement of C7 and sometimes C8 and T1. (Reproduced from Tassin JL: Paralysies obstetricales du plexus brachial: Evolution spontanée, resultats des interventions reparatrices precoces. Thesis, Universite Paris VII, 1983, with permission.)

In this same series, lesions of C5, C6, C7 constituted 25%, while complete lesion of the plexus represented 24% of the cases.

The details of the pathological findings at operation of Gilbert's patients are reproduced in Figure 5.6. Gilbert concluded the following:

1. There was never a double level injury (of the same root).
2. There was no isolated lower trunk palsy.
3. Root avulsion in C5–C6 was rare, sometimes associated with C7 avulsion, but never with lower root (C8, T1 avulsion).
4. Upper roots are usually ruptured; lower roots are always avulsed.
5. Complete lesions are always an association of ruptures and avulsions.

In all of these infants it may be extremely difficult to make an early accurate assessment of sensation. Years later, when they are able to cooperate and communicate fully, it will be found that, even in the presence of significant motor loss, sensation will be surprisingly much less defective than would be found in a corresponding adult injury.

MUSCULOSKELETAL CHANGES

Although it is now universally acknowledged that the primary pathology in obstetrical palsy is neurogenic, it is the secondary effects of growth, muscular imbalance, and dyskinesia that produce the characteristic pattern of deformity we observe in the older child. Before any consideration can be given to the question of spontaneous recovery or management, we must explore in detail those changes and their evolution.

Primary pathology at the shoulder girdle due to obstetrical trauma has already been discussed. Aside from such reports as those of Scaglietti[31] in 1936, there have been few such recent references in the literature. The pathogenesis of the secondary changes in the shoulder have been well-documented to result from the persistent adduction and medial rotation of the humerus in the untreated patient. Since the deltoid and lateral rotators are weak or paralyzed, the more massive and relatively normal pectoralis major, teres major, and latissimus dorsi as well as the subscapularis develop myostatic contracture with time. Whereas the neonate lacks only active motion, the older child loses passive motion as well. Attempts at normal abduction or forward flexion are further hampered by dyskinesia affecting reciprocal motion of the shoulder joint complex. Scapular rhythm is lost, and motion tends to consist of scapulothoracic shrugging. As the arm is brought forward to the horizontal, its own weight along with muscle imbalance causes medial rotation of the humerus (Fig. 5.7). Control of hand placement is severely compromised as it involuntarily drops toward the waist. It is this dynamic abnormality as well as the static imbalance that results first in significant anterior and inferior capsular contracture and then modification of normal development of the involved osseous structures. The scapula itself is generally smaller than normal and the glenoidal neck is foreshortened. The glenoidal cavity remains small and underdeveloped and may become flattened or even convex. The acromial and coracoid processes become elongated and hooked downward, probably from the unsupported weight of the arm. Humeral head dysplasia makes it conical, rather than spherical, and may produce a flattened side that faces the glenoid (Fig. 5.8). In addition to this deformity, there is torsion of the humerus in response to unequal muscle pull, and the head faces more posteriorly than normal (Fig. 5.9). It may subluxate posteriorly or dislocate with time if the factors producing it are sufficiently unbalanced. The downward prolongation of acromion and coracoid may actually serve as a bony block to repositioning of the posteriorly displaced head in a patient with established deformity. With attempts to use the shoulder, the articular incongruity may eventuate in painful and disabling traumatic arthritis. The occurrence of anterior, subcoracoid dislocation of the shoulder associated with obstetrical paralysis is a rare condition. In 1953 a case was reported by Liebolt and Furey,[25] and this was presumed to have resulted from treatment in abduction of the newborn's shoulder. However, despite its rarity, it should be kept in mind to avoid missing the diagnosis in an older patient whose condition could be significantly worsened by an operation designed to correct posterior dislocation (Fig 5.10).

Abduction contracture at the shoulder is thought by Tachdjian[39] to result from constant abduction required to compensate for limited lateral rotation of the shoulder. In 1939 Milgram[27] pointed out that it results from treatment with abduction

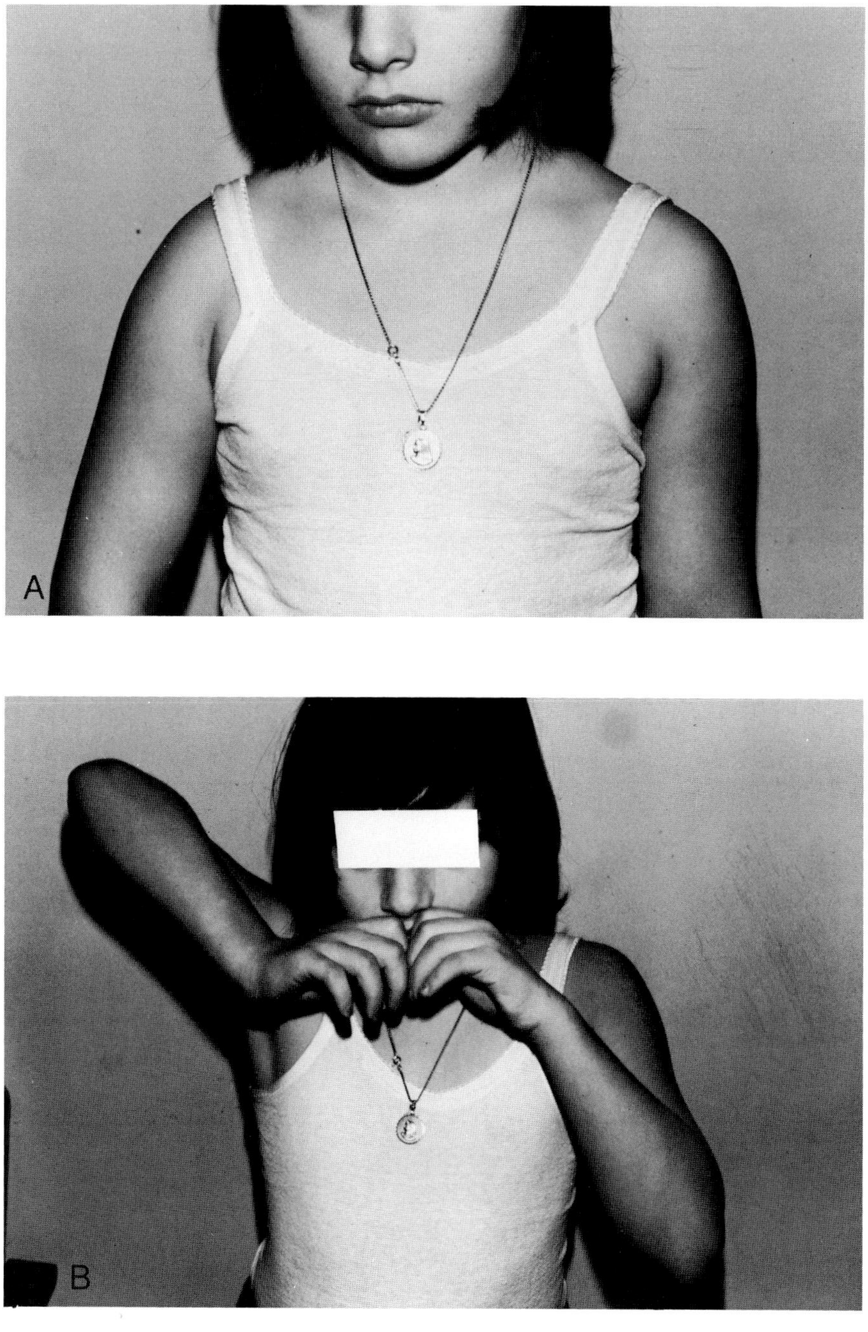

Fig. 5.7. Older child with persistent medial rotation of humerus on the right.

braces. He stated that 16 of his 23 patients had this as a persistent and disabling deformity. In Alder and Patterson's series[1] of 123 patients 71 were given braces and 42 were not. Of these 71 who were braced, 14 had no additional physiotherapy, and all had significant abduction-external rotation contractures.

Contractures and deformity of the elbow as a result of obstetrical palsy is well documented, and must be considered as distinct from direct trauma to the joint at birth, according to Sever.[36] In Aitken's[2] study of 107 cases of Erb's palsy there were 33 with bony deformity of the elbow, an incidence of 30.8%.

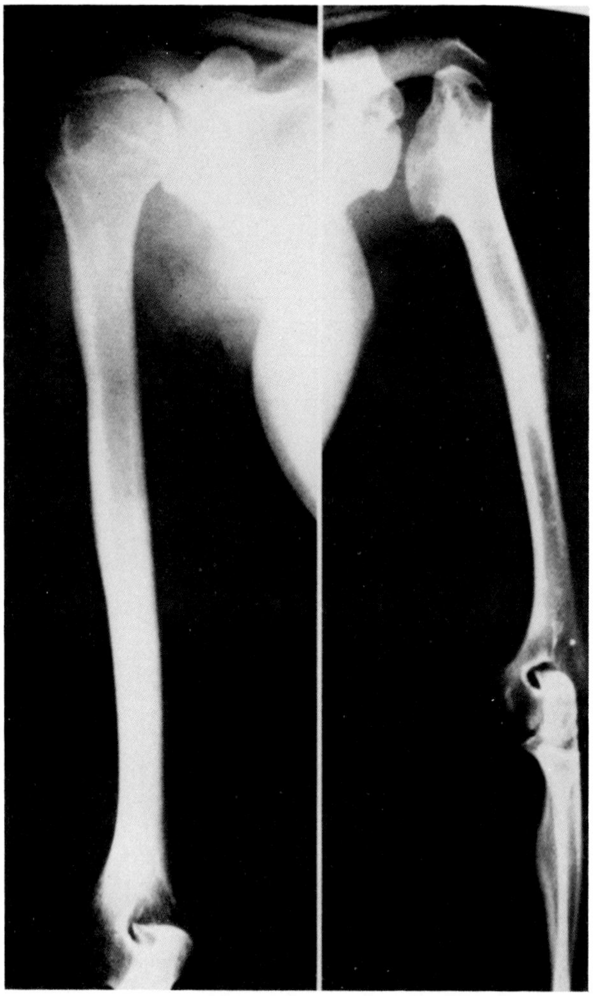

Fig. 5.8. Radiograph of a 17-year-old patient with Erb's palsy on the left. (Reproduced from Kattan KR, Spitz HB: Roentgen findings in obstetrical injuries to the brachial plexus. Radiology 91:462, 1968, with permission.)

Adler and Patterson's[1] series of 88 patients had an incidence of 42.3%. There were flexion contractures of less than 45 degrees in 13 patients and more severe contractures in 11. Radial head posterior dislocation was found in 14 patients (16%). Aitken's[2] extensive study of the problem revealed a 25.4% incidence of posterior radial head dislocation and a 5.6% incidence of anterior dislocation, which he characterized as simple dislocation not necessarily associated with Erb's paralysis. Early subluxation may, with growth, eventuate in complete dislocation. Aitken explained in great detail the pathogenesis of the lesion as resulting from muscle imbalance and rigid splinting of the elbow in the Fairbanks type of splint. The radiographic findings of clubbing of the proximal radial metaphysis may be seen before two months of age, and this as well as bowing of the ulna may be followed as they progress with growth (Figs. 5.11–5.14). According to his analysis, the contracture of the pronator teres and the interosseous membrane also contributes to the deformity.

Adler and Patterson[1] characterized the most severe problem about the elbow as "a relentlessly progressive disruption of the entire elbow joint — a medial sliding dislocation of the ulna and dislocation of the radial head." Fortunately this was uncommon, since they could not suggest any means of prevention or treatment.

The deformities that eventuate in the forearm and hand depend on the distribution of the imbalance of paralyzed or weakened muscles. Pronation of the forearm is common, but paralysis in the arm may also result in a supination contracture. The hand may be considerably smaller than normal. Wrist position will depend on the imbalance of those muscles crossing it. In the Klumpke variety of paralysis, the wrist may be maintained hyperextended, the transverse arch may be obliterated from the palm, and the fingers maintained in a gentle claw attitude. Lack of intrinsic thenar musculature positions the thumb in the adducted plane of the palm where it is of little use. Often such a deformed and nonfunctional limb is kept covered by clothing, or the patient develops elaborate maneuvers to avoid having it exposed to view.

PROGNOSIS

Once the diagnosis of obstetrical palsy is established in the infant, the question most often asked by the parents, and probably the most difficult for the physician, is: "Will the baby recover?" Obviously, as with corresponding plexus injuries in adults, the prognosis for spontaneous recovery depends to a large degree on the distribution and severity of the lesion. In 1883 Duchenne[8] wrote that early treatment with electrical stimulation could result in complete recovery. Clark and coworkers[5] noted a recovery rate of 26 percent of patients with palsy. Sever[34] made a distinction between lesions of the upper trunk, which had a relatively good outlook, and those of the whole arm or lower trunk type, in which

(Text continues on p. 106.)

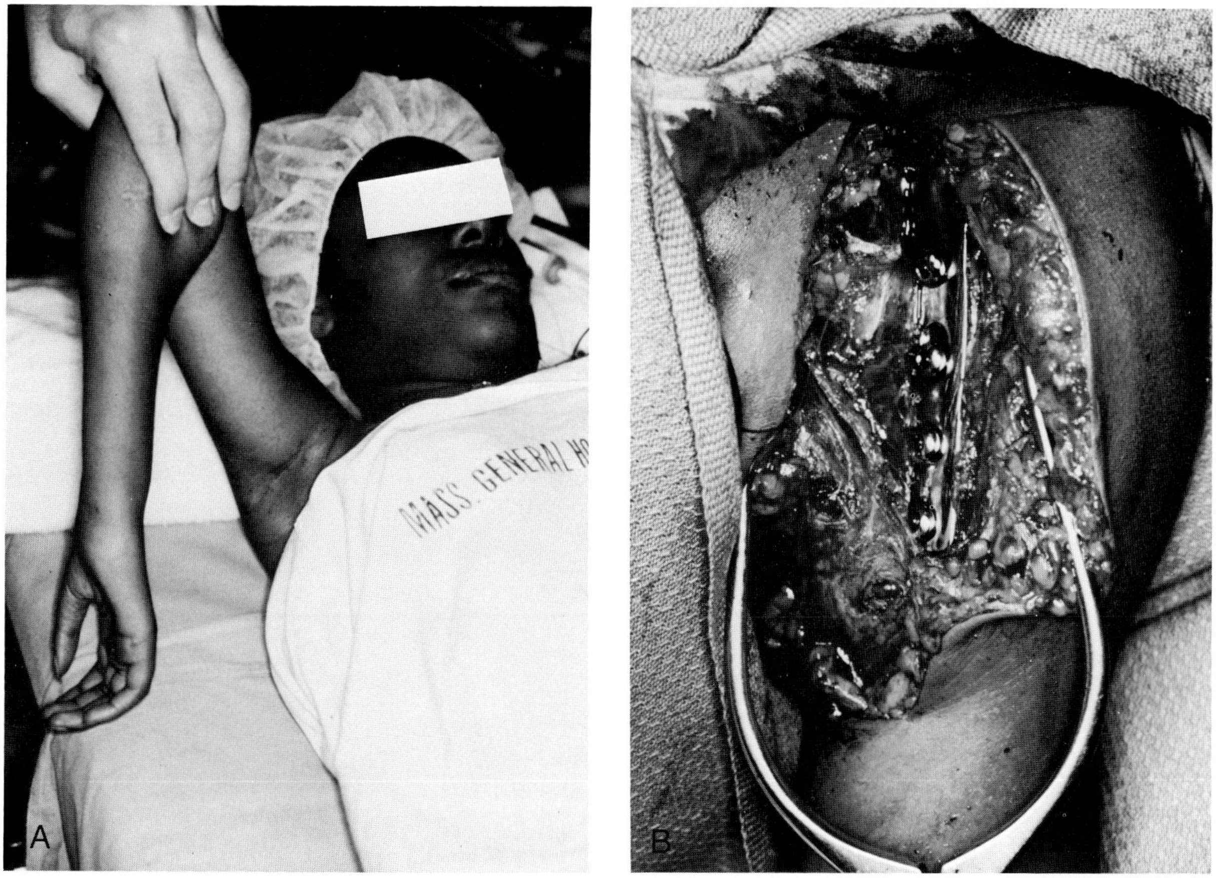

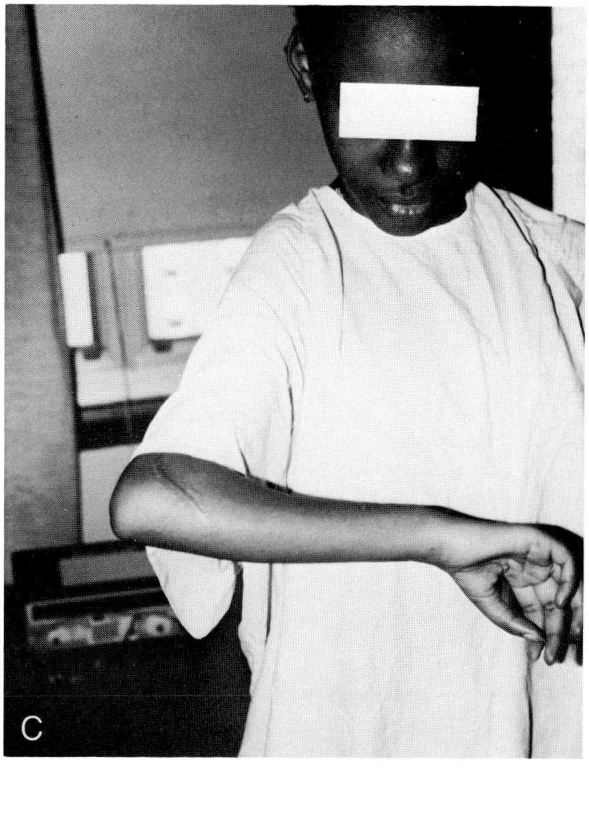

Fig. 5.9. **A**: Extreme medial rotation of the humerus. **B**: Correction by humeral osteotomy. **C**: Clinical improvement. The forearm had been previously treated by osteotomy elsewhere. Another osteotomy was done in the forearm after this picture was taken.

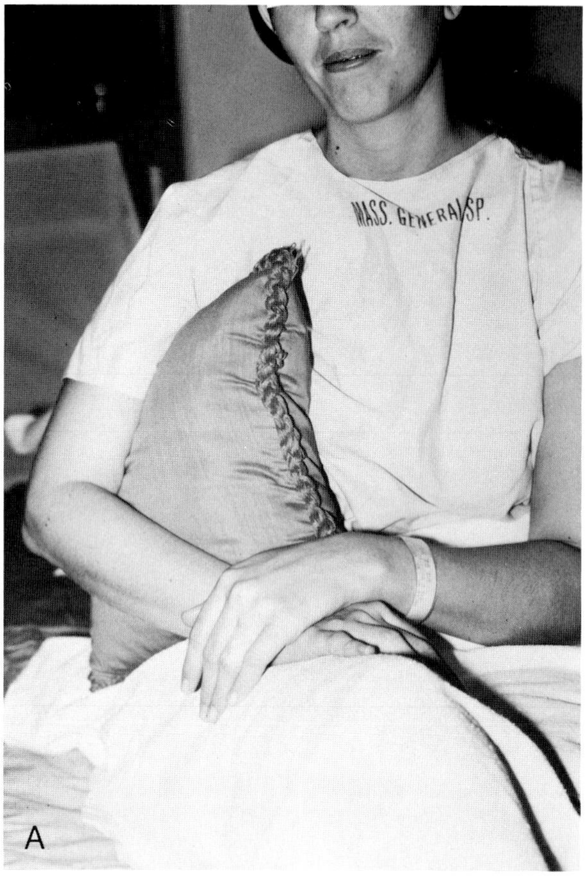

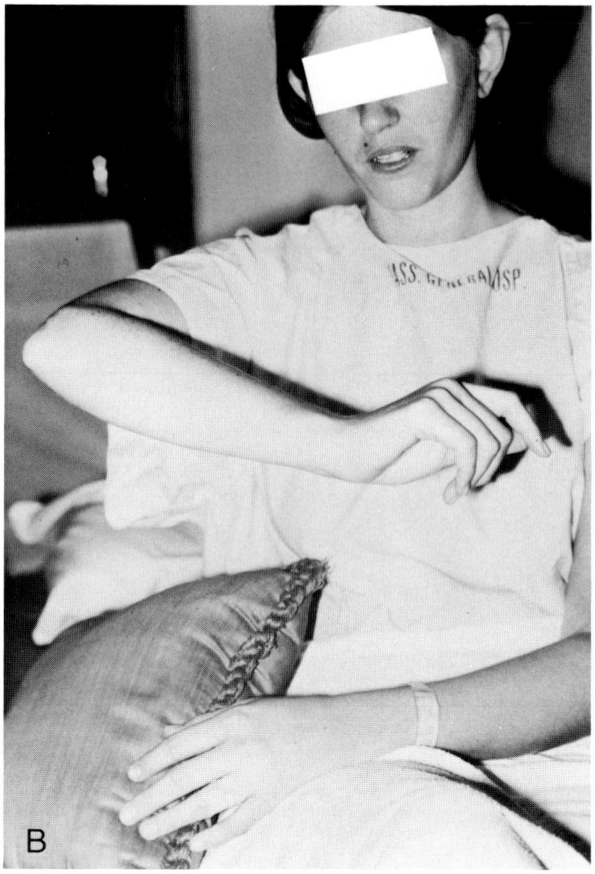

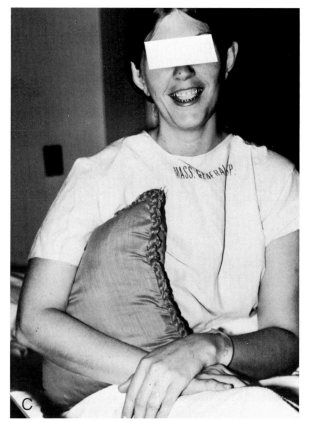

Fig. 5.10. A: Adult patient with right shoulder dysfunction due to obstetrical palsy. She had to support her arm with a pillow to prevent dislocations, which were thought by her referring doctor to be posterior. Examination with fluoroscopy demonstrated that the dislocations were anterior. **B**: Attempt to abduct the laterally rotate her arm to reach her mouth results in significant apprehension for impending dislocation. **C**: Replacement of arm on pillow restores stability.

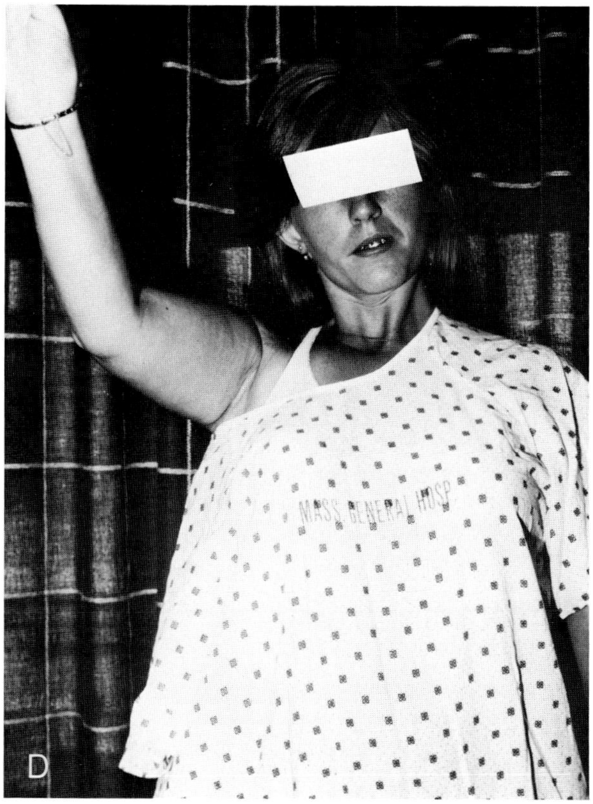

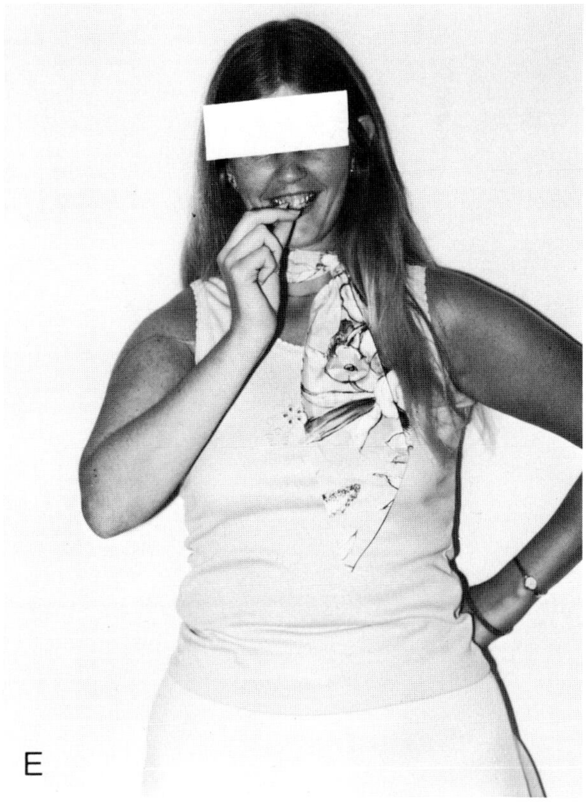

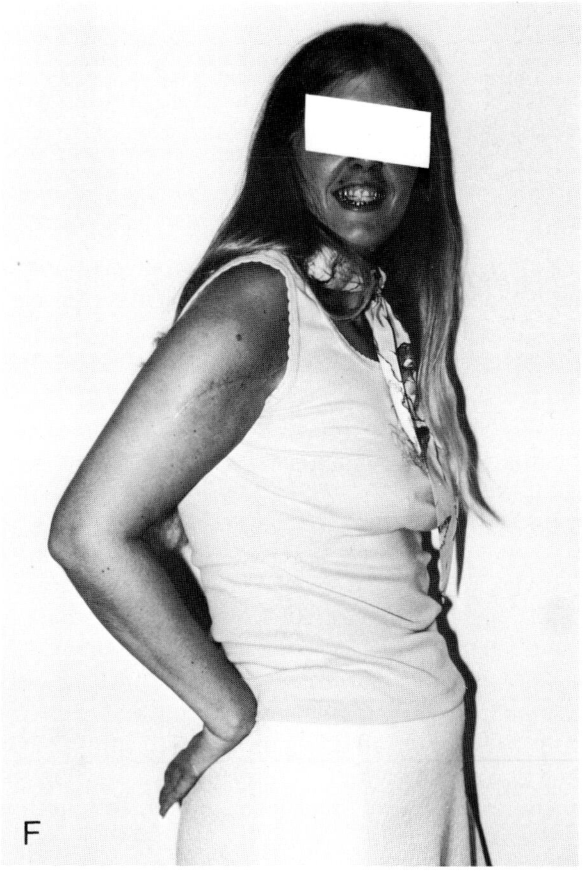

Fig. 5.10. *(continued)* **D**: Two years following operative procedure which consisted of Putti-Platt and lateral rotation osteotomy at surgical neck of humerus. Patient able to abduct and laterally rotate humerus. **E**: She is able to get her right hand to her mouth. **F**: Allowable medial rotation following osteotomy.

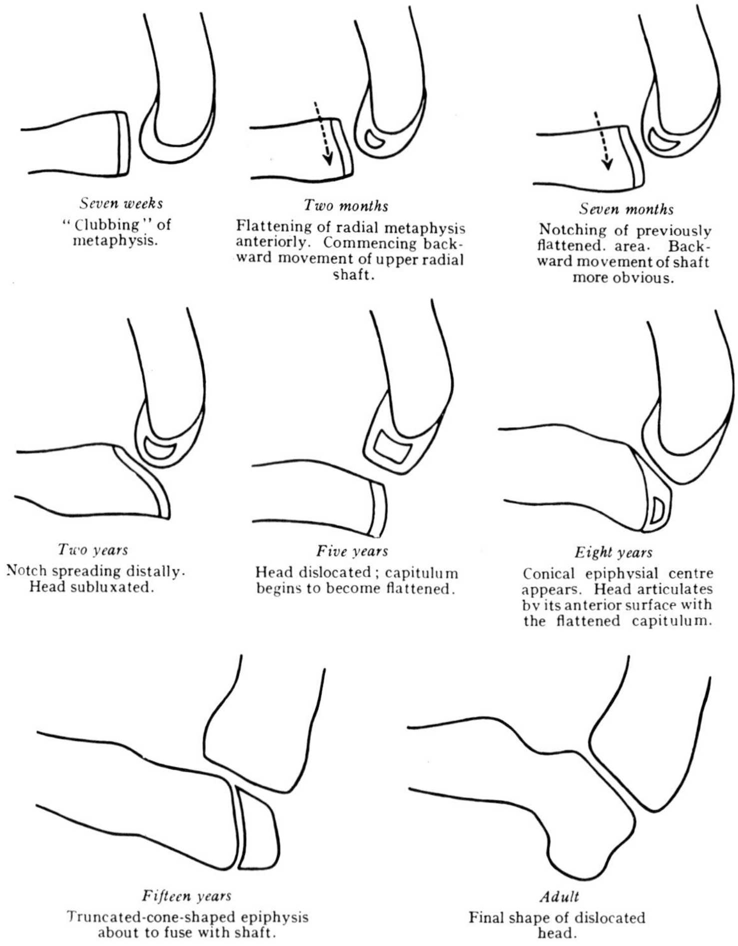

Seven weeks
"Clubbing" of metaphysis.
Two months
Flattening of radial metaphysis anteriorly. Commencing backward movement of upper radial shaft.
Seven months
Notching of previously flattened. area. Backward movement of shaft more obvious.
Two years
Notch spreading distally. Head subluxated.
Five years
Head dislocated; capitulum begins to become flattened.
Eight years
Conical epiphysial centre appears. Head articulates by its anterior surface with the flattened capitulum.
Fifteen years
Truncated-cone-shaped epiphysis about to fuse with shaft.
Adult
Final shape of dislocated head.

Fig. 5.11. Serial diagrams showing the changes of the head of the radius as age advances. (Reproduced from Aitken J: Deformity of the elbow joint as a sequel to Erb's obstetrical paralysis. J Bone Joint Surg 34B:352, 1952.)

the prognosis was distinctly poorer. Wolman's series[48] demonstrated that the outlook was considerably improved by early conservative treatment. In 1952 Aitken[2] focused on recovery of the elbow, but he concluded that if recovery were to be complete, it would come about in three to six months, while those patients who required up to 12 months of treatment would get fair recovery and those who needed more would obtain minimal improvement.

Wickstrom's series[46,47] correlated the degree of recovery with the severity and extent of the damage to the brachial plexus. No patient noted to have a moderate-to-severe injury at birth was seen to recover completely. Of his entire series of 75 patients treated from early infancy by splinting and exercise, only 10 (13.4%) had no significant deformity or dysfunction of the shoulder. Thirty-two (42.6%) had abduction in excess of 90 degrees and some limitation of lateral rotation. Thirty-three (44%) never acquired motor function of the shoulder, forearm, or hand.

Adler and Patterson[1] reported an incidence of 7% spontaneous recovery in their series. They stated that the time required for maximal recovery varied from one to 18 months.

Of the 36 babies with birth injuries to the brachial plexus reported by Hardy[15] in 1981, nearly 80% of these children had made a complete recovery by the age of 13 months, and none of those with significant residual defects had severe sensory or motor defect of the hand.

Tassin's series[40] of 44 patients observed over the five-year period 1977–1982 provides us with further data on the natural history of spontaneous recovery of obstetrical palsy.

Twelve newborns experienced complete recovery. Of these, seven had paralyses of shoulder and

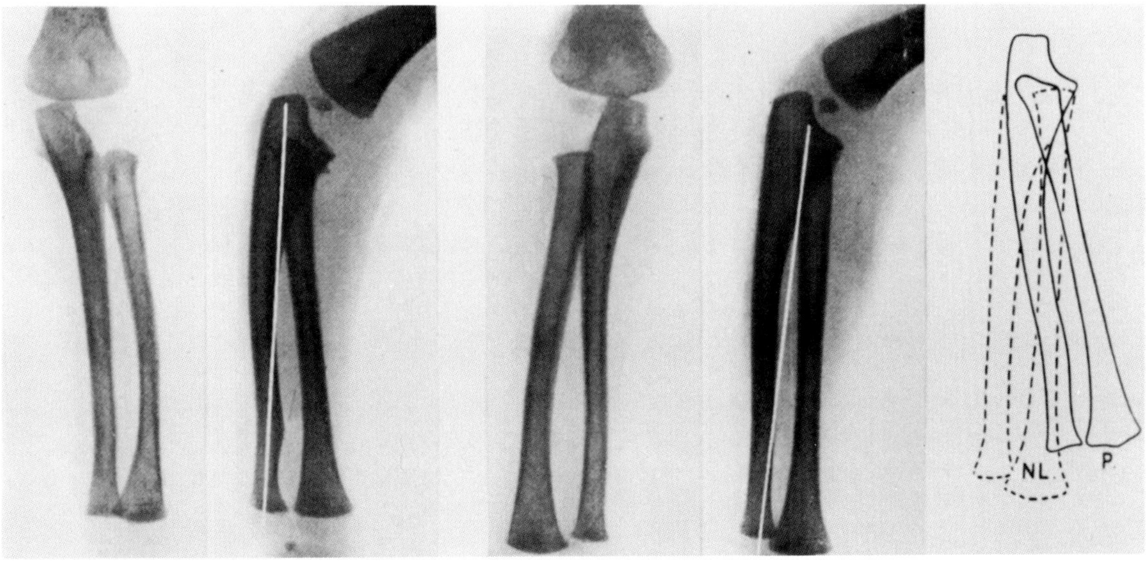

Fig. 5.12. Radiographs of the forearm and elbow of a child with a right Erb's palsy. The two illustrations on the left show posterior displacement of the axis of the radius and a curve of the distal third of the ulna. The middle plates show the normal side, and the drawing on the right superimposes both forearms for comparison. (Reproduced from Aitken J: Deformity of the elbow joint as a sequel to Erb's obstetrical paralysis. J Bone Joint Surg 34B:352, 1952.)

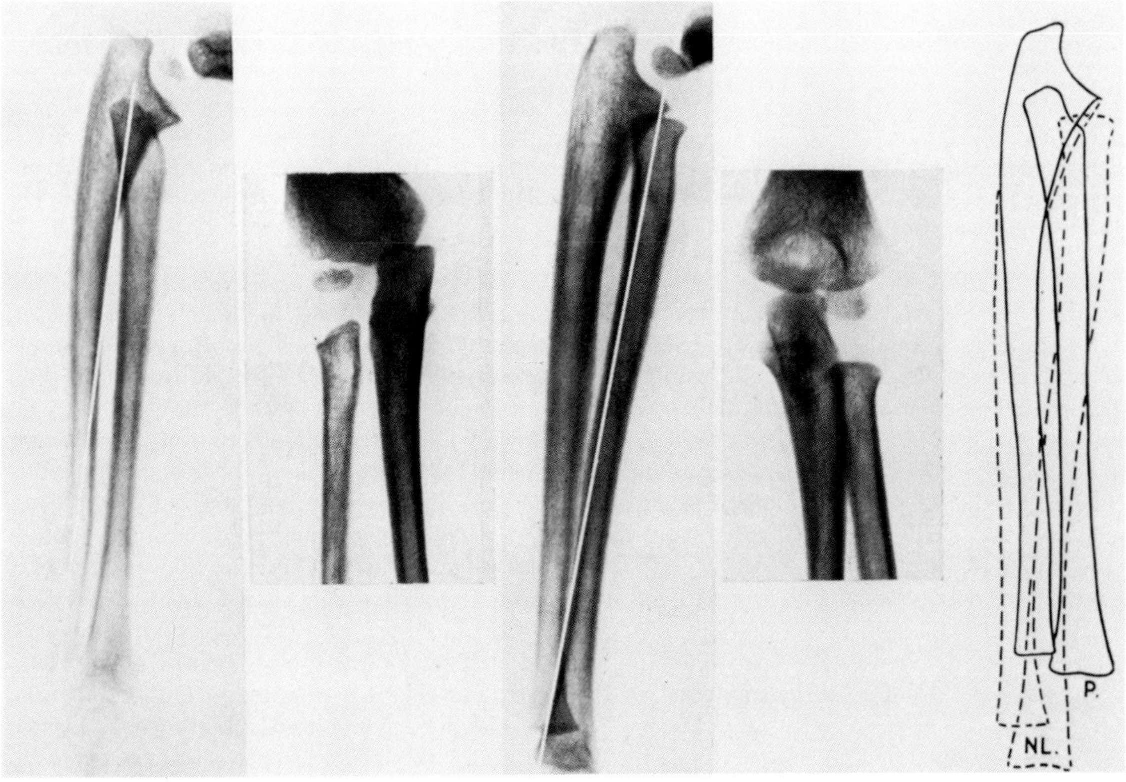

Fig. 5.13. Left Erb's palsy in a five-year-old child. The axis of the radius is displaced as before. The two central plates are of the normal forearm, and the tracing on the right superimposes the films for comparison. (Reproduced from Aitken J: Deformity of the elbow joint as a sequel to Erb's obstetrical paralysis. J Bone Joint Surg 34B:352, 1952.)

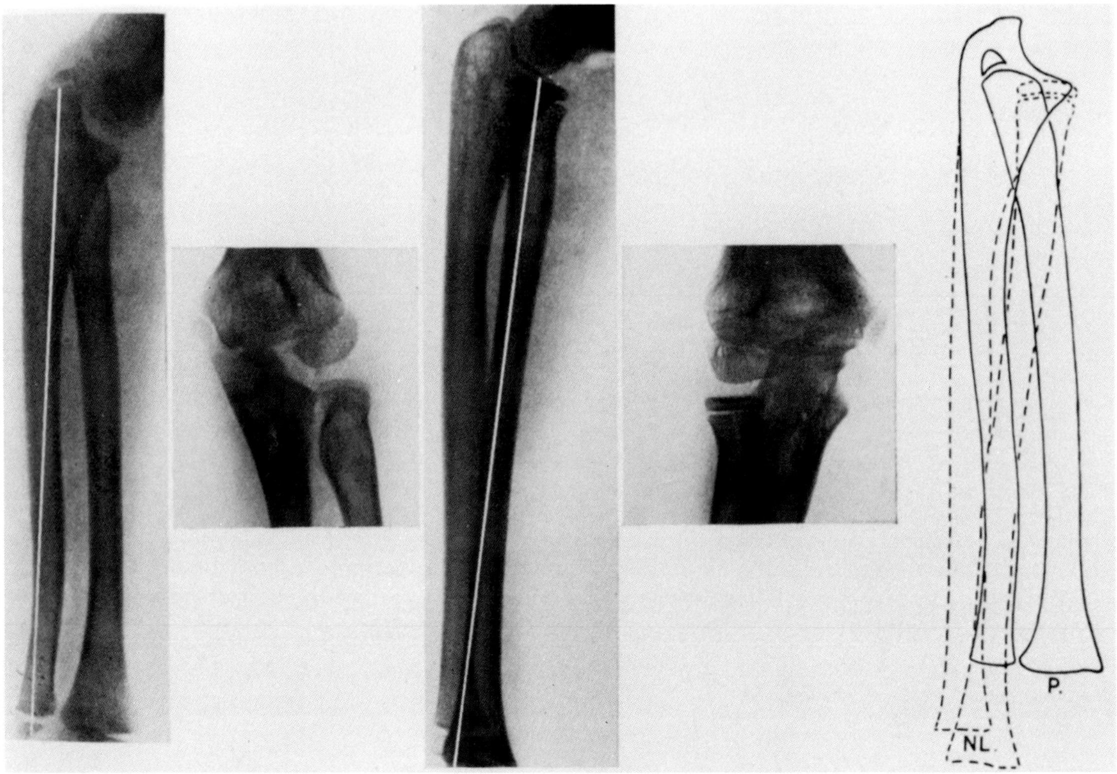

Fig. 5.14. Appearance of the deformity in an eight-year-old child with right Erb's palsy. Axis of radius displaced as before. The central plates are of the normal left forearm. The tracing on the right superimposes the films for comparison. (Reproduced from Aitken, J: Deformity of the elbow joint as a sequel to Erb's obstetrical paralysis. J Bone Joint Surg 34B:352, 1952.)

elbow, and five had paralysis of shoulder, elbow, and hand. It should be noted that four out of five in the last group had intact flexors in the hand, while only one had a total paralysis of the limb at birth which resolved completely.

If complete recovery occurs, the musculature will have recovered power to contract against gravity at the latest:

1 1/2 month for triceps, wrist, and finger extensor
2 months for deltoid and biceps
2 months for thumb extensor and long abductor
3 months for lateral rotators of the humerus

Tassin[40] also documented, by means of histograms, the progress of incomplete recovery. He found that after 10 to 20 months, no further significant recovery takes place in the shoulder.

In order to understand the method of reporting used by Tassin, it is necessary to reproduce his diagram of the notation of Mallet,[26] which incorporates both shoulder and elbow motion as a functional unit, appreciated in three major groups (Fig. 5.15). According to Tassin, when the shoulder does not recover, it is because of lateral rotators; these were later treated by anterior release and tendon transfers.

In order for a shoulder to reach level IV in these patients with incomplete recovery, both deltoids and biceps are able to contract against gravity by 5 months. For shoulders ultimately in groups III and II, the chronology of recovery was more variable in that the deltoid could contract against gravity before 1 year for class III shoulders, but certain class II shoulders have a deltoid at that level at 11 months. Although the biceps usually cannot contract against gravity until 18 months in the class III shoulders, in one class II, it had recuperated at 7 months. Those patients who attain Mallet Class II do not recover biceps and deltoid capable of contraction against gravity.

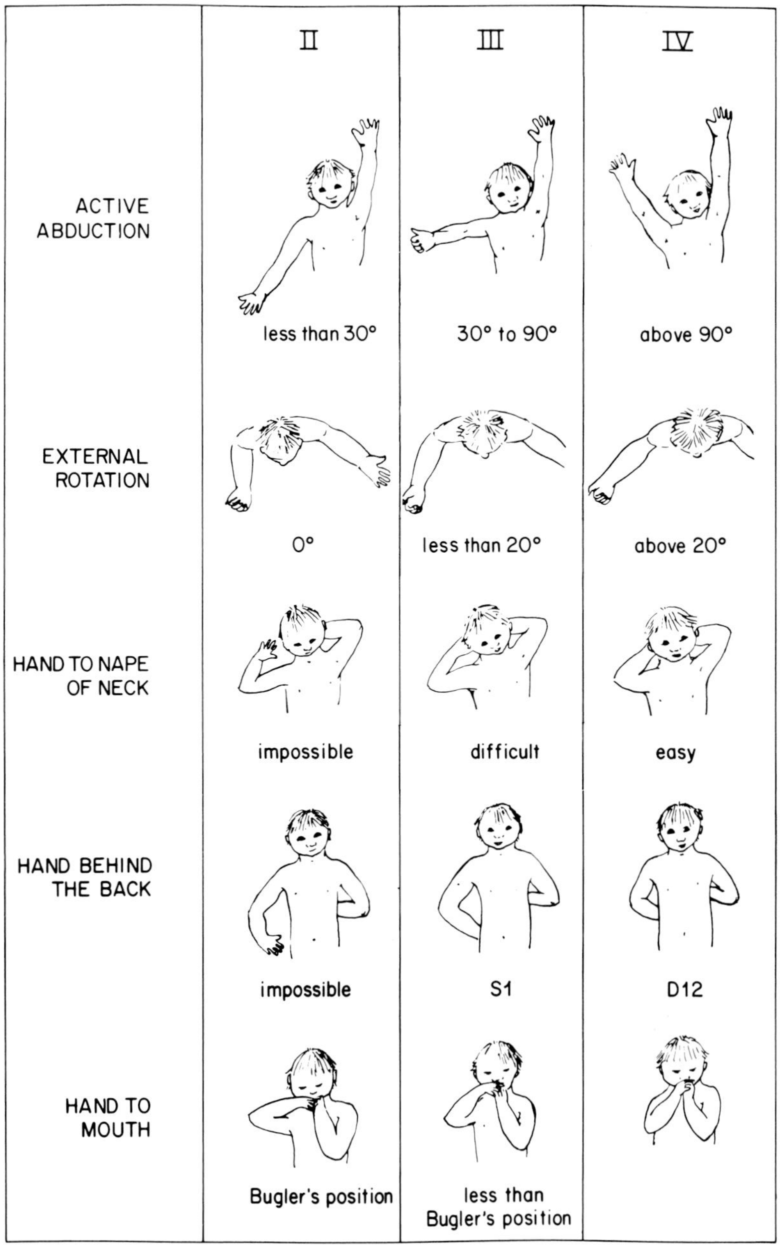

Fig. 5.15. Functional classification of Erb's palsy according to Mallet. (Reproduced from Tassin JL: Paralysies obstetricales du plexus brachial: Evolution spontanée, resultats des interventions reparatrices precoces. Thesis, Universite Paris VII, 1983, with permission.)

It is important to remember in interpreting these data that the functional classification of the shoulder depends on the recovery of elbow flexion. Furthermore, Tassin noted that, as the rating for the shoulder decreased, the fixed flexion contracture at the elbow increased.

In describing the course of recovery in the hand, Tassin noted that normal hands were achieved when at the initial examination the paralysis was confined to the extensors of fingers and thumb, with power to contract fingers and thumb against gravity by

6 months for the finger extensors
10 months for the wrist extensors
14 months for the thumb extensors and long abductor

Those hands remaining with mild motor involvement, mostly in terms of slow voluntary contraction but no sensory loss were usually of two types on initial examination. The first involves complete paralysis in the hand with rapid recovery of the wrist and finger flexors by three weeks and then proceeding as in the previous group. The second is those with paralysis initially limited to the extensors of wrist and fingers that recover slowly and incompletely.

The patients who ultimately have some but poor motor control accompanied by significant contractures and sensory changes do not attain motor power sufficient to contract against gravity by 18 months.

In summary, of the 44 infants treated conservatively, 32 followed for three years ultimately had residua of their obstetrical brachial plexus injury.

Twelve infants (4 C5, C6; 8 C5, C6, C7) had a Mallet class IV shoulder and elbow. Although all had normal or near-normal hands and eight had no difficulty with forearm rotation, four lacked active supination.

Twelve infants (2 C5, C6; 5 C5, C6, C7; 5 C5, T1) ultimately attained Mallet Class III. They had residua in elbow flexion and extension, as well as rotation, and although five had normal hands at last evaluation, seven had significant deficits of hand function.

Eight infants ultimately attained shoulders and elbows classified as Mallet II. These all had complete paralysis initially and regained no active forearm rotation. Four had moderately impaired hands, and four had severely impaired hands as a final result.

TREATMENT

Just as the pathophysiology of obstetrical palsy remained controversial for many years, even when the neurogenic mechanism was accepted, there remained a wide divergence of opinion as to treatment. Surgeons in the first two decades of the twentieth century were neither hesitant to operate on the plexus of these infants, nor particularly obsessed by the necessity of objectively reporting their results. As early as 1903, Kennedy[19,20] of Glasgow reported suture of the brachial plexus in three cases of birth paralysis of the upper extremity, of which two were infants and one was 14 years old. The results in the first case were said to be excellent, and the other two were not followed long enough for final assessment.

Sharpe[37] of New York published his surgically treated series of 56 cases of obstetrical palsy in 1916. He advised in cases where there was complete paralysis of the arm, hand, and fingers at birth to explore the plexus at 1 month. His reasons for this advice were as follows:

1. The child would stand the operation better than earlier and as well as any time later: little if any anesthesia needed to be used at that age.
2. The earlier the anastomosis *[sic]* of the nerve roots, the better the ultimate improvement.
3. The scarring would be less than later.
4. The nerve ends would not have retracted significantly.

In reporting his results, Sharpe indicated that only within the previous year had he had the opportunity to operate on children three months old or younger, and that prior to 1915, the majority of his patients were between four and six years of age. He stated that the children operated on at three months of age made excellent recoveries and explained that in them, there was not a complete tear of all the roots of the plexus, whereas in the 1-month-old children, the damage was always more severe. About half of the children in this latter group were said to have shown marked improvement, and in four, he predicted the possibility of a normal arm. The children operated on at three months showed more constant improvement. There were two superficial infections and no deaths in this series.

By 1920, Taylor[41–43] of New York had reported on a 16-year operative experience that encompassed 70 patients. He concluded that surgical repair of the nerves was indicated in the great majority of cases and that the best results followed operation at about three months of age. Of the 70 operative cases, there were three deaths attributable to surgery. The functional results were reported as follows:

> . . . there has been no perfect anatomical and physiological recovery. With a few exceptions, in which the damage has been found to be irremediable, these children have made marked improvement and many of them have obtained almost perfect function in the extremity.

Platt's[28] experience of 23 personal cases of birth paralysis was presented to the British Orthopaedic Association in November 1919 as part of a discussion on birth paralysis, at which Fairbank also spoke. He considered the pathology as well as the musculoskeletal consequences of the nerve lesions with time and growth and urged strict attention to these important deformities. His series of five cases of nerve exploration had indifferent results. The discussion and the remarks that followed were most illuminating.

In 1925 Sever[36] of Boston stated:

> In regard to operation on the brachial plexus, we are not taking quite the radical stand that we have taken in the past. . . . We have had no very brilliant results from the plexus repair. Many of the plexuses that have been operated on have shown absolutely nothing in the way of functional recovery, and nothing could be expected from the type of injury found at the time of operation.

Jepson's[17] opinion in 1930 was to condemn surgery on the nerves. Thus, the early enthusiasm for direct attack on the plexus gave way to a program of conservative management of the nerve lesions, supplemented by orthopaedic surgical correction of the peripheral musculoskeletal manifestations.

Recently, however, there has been renewed interest in the direct surgical treatment of the nerves in neonates with obstetrical palsy. The series of patients operated upon by Gilbert and documented by Tassin[40] provides us with a carefully controlled population upon which to evaluate the efficacy of neurological reconstruction of the plexus in infancy. It should be noted that the majority of these patients were seen immediately at birth or shortly thereafter, when an initial gross muscle and sensory examination was performed. The presence or absence of Horner's syndrome was noted, and the lower extremities were examined as well, since in apparent bilateral brachial palsy the possibility of obstetrical tetraplegia must be ruled out. In fact, his series revealed two such neonates. Radiographs of the chest included the shoulder girdles and diaphragms to rule out fractures and lesions of the phrenic nerve, although Tassin commented on the problem of interpretation of the radiographs of the proximal humeral injuries prior to the two weeks required for the appearance of callous. Electromyograms were done at three weeks, by which time in some infants recovery will have begun or even have been complete. In those without signs of recovery and with Horner's syndrome, the prognosis for recovery was considered nil, and plans were made for operative exploration at two months. If the hand had recovered, but the shoulder had remained paralyzed, there was a chance of recovery, but the inclination was to prepare the family for surgery. A baseline EMG was done, to be repeated at three months, at which time the decision was made regarding surgery. At three weeks, gentle physical therapy was begun. No braces were used.

At three months the final evaluation for those infants with residual paralysis consisted of a new manual muscle test, an electromyogram, and a myelogram. A paralyzed biceps at three months was considered an indication for surgery. Repeat EMG of previously examined muscles was done in addition to an EMG of the diaphragm, using an esophageal electrode, although it was admitted that this last examination was often difficult to correlate with clinical findings. The myelogram was done on 118 patients, 108 of whom were less than 124 days of age. Most often it required general anesthesia, sometimes only sedation. Amipaque was used, and the significant complications were one aseptic meningitis, which resolved, and two seizures.

Seventy-nine studies were judged to be of sufficient quality for interpretation. There were 14 considered to be "false positives," of which four had a meningocele without a clinical lesion at that level, nine had a meningocele and a nonvisualized root at that level with an avulsion clinically *present* and *not* confirmed at surgery. In one case, there was no pseudomingocele but the roots were not seen. Of the total of 495 roots studied, there were three false negatives, wherein the myelogram was normal, and three roots were found avulsed at surgery.

Gilbert then discussed the accumulated evidence with the parents, giving the clinical findings the greatest weight. For example, if the biceps was clinically paralyzed, even in the face of an encouraging electromyogram, surgery was advised. Furthermore, the existence of the meningoceles did not negate the operative indication because of the possibility of false positives.

Surgery was performed a few days after the myelogram under halothane endotracheal anesthesia with monitoring equipment to allow the measurement of somatosensory evoked potentials intraoperatively. These were helpful in defining pathology in the presence of traumatic pseudomeningoceles, but since it is possible to have a partial root avulsion (motor rootlets avulsed, sensory preserved), the author felt that if there was disagreement between clinical findings and evoked potentials, they preferred to abort the surgical procedure rather than proceeding.

The findings at surgery were carefully documented to serve as the basis for generalization for neurological reconstruction. C8 and T1 lesions virtually assured avulsion at these levels, and, although C7 was sometimes additionally avulsed, avulsion of all the roots was not encountered. If C5, C6, C7 were ruptured distally, the stumps could be used to reinnervate the three cords and suprascapular nerve. If only C5 and C6 remain, one must choose. Since some hand function can be retrieved in the newborn, according to Tassin, one should use C5 and C6 to neurotize the lateral cord and ulnar nerve. The posterior cord is abandoned. If possible, the suprascapular nerve is reinnervated, with later transfer of trapezius to the deltoid. If C5 only remains, the prognosis is very poor. This root is used to graft the musculocutaneous and suprascapular nerve and perhaps the lateral root of the median nerve. Intercostal nerves T2–T5 are used to graft the medial root of the median nerve. Isolated C5 and C6 avulsions were treated by neurotization of the musculocutaneous nerve by one of the nerves to the pectoralis major. Tassin also described cross-pectoral neurotization.

Tassin's analysis of Gilbert's first 100 cases of surgical reconstruction of the plexus revealed that the timing and quality of recovery are variable—very good for the biceps, with 75% of the muscles able to contract through full range against gravity at two years, a bit less good for the deltoid and external rotators. The results were said to be especially good if paralysis was less extensive in the plexus. Supinators recovered poorly, and the children retained abnormalities of forearm rotation. Recovery of the triceps was stated to always be excellent. However, 25% of those with paralyses of C5–C7 and C5–T1 have wrist extension against gravity at two years. Finger extensors do not recover in the C5–T1 lesions, but do so in the C5, C6, and C7. Recovery of finger flexion was very poor. The functional level of shoulder and elbow at two years using Mallet's classification to evaluate 38 infants who had undergone surgery was

17–class IV
16–class III
5–class II

Tassin concluded that the type of surgical intervention demonstrated by Gilbert improves the prognosis of obstetrical paralysis by increasing the number of good shoulders and diminishing the number of very bad ones.

The precise detail of this unique experience of surgery in the neonate with obstetrical palsy may be found in Tassin's thesis.[40]

EARLY ADDITIONAL MANAGEMENT

Those surgeons concerned with the treatment of obstetrical paralysis in the first 20 years of the twentieth century were almost universally agreed that splinting, massage, and exercise were to be employed for the neonate with an upper type of palsy. In 1913 H. A. T. Fairbank[11] stated:

> Relaxation of the paralyzed muscles is the keynote of treatment; it is, in my opinion, far more important than anything else. Put the joints of the paralyzed limb in the erect position and order massage, and nature will do the rest unless the nerve lesion is beyond recall. Electricity may be allowed if the friends desire it.

In 1916 Sever[33] recommended holding the arm in a plaster cast or a light wire splint in an abducted and externally rotated position with the hand supinated between massage and exercise treatments. A number of splints were used to position the limb.[11,12]

Despite the fact that the use of splints continues to the present time, it would be unfair to conclude that their complications were unappreciated by these earlier surgeons. They did not continue to advocate unrelieved splinting. In 1925 Sever[36] wrote:

> We are not as insistent on the use of splints from the very start as we were at first, and the reason for the change is this: we have found that in certain cases the use of the splint seems to cause a certain amount of swelling about the wrist and elbow, and makes the exercise treatment, when the splint is removed, painful and difficult. . . . We have found also that the use of the splint in certain children leads to a lower convalescence and a less free use of the arm, even with adequate treatment, so that we discard the splint, even in the face of increasing muscle contractures, and in this way

give the child a free and better use of the arm then it would have with the constant wearing.

The findings of Milgram[27] as well as Adler and Patterson[1] that injudicious splinting actually causes contractures of the type opposite to the ones that develop without treatment have already been detailed, Wickstrom,[46,47] who noted similar deformity in children kept uninterruptedly in a protective splint for an excessive period of time, modified both the position of the arm and the length of the time the arm was kept in the splint. He advised use of the splint with the arm in full external rotation, forward flexed 45 degrees, and abducted 70 degrees, with the elbow flexed 120 degrees.

In light of the uncertainty and difficulty of supervision in use of appliances for treating the arm, I believe it is far safer to avoid splints altogether. A regular program of range-of-motion exercises is instituted after the first postnatal week, with the parents doing them at each diaper change. It is particularly important that gentle passive motion of the shoulder be performed to maintain lateral rotation and abduction in the absence of active muscle control so that medial rotation and adduction contractures do not develop. Regular visits to the physician, the physicial therapist, or the clinic nurse will help to prevent deformity and usually obviate the necessity of later muscle release operations. If the child begins to regain active motor control of the limb, every attempt ought to be made to encourage its normal use by means of structured play. Under no circumstances should the normal extremity be restrained to encourage use of the paretic one. If there is a significant residual weakness, this limb is destined to be assistive rather than dominant, no matter what is done.

LATER MANAGEMENT

As the child grows and becomes better able to communicate and cooperate, the degree of functional impairment will become apparent even before formal testing is done. Ordinarily, handedness does not become manifest before 18 months of age, so that if the infant uses both hands interchangeably, there is unlikely to be significant deficit.

Even in the presence of significant residual weakness, if the passive range of motion has been maintained by diligent exercise, the problem of reconstruction for optimal function is very much simplified. It is those children who have not had the benefit of medical supervision or who are seen late and who have developed contractures that present the most difficult management problems. The characteristically adducted and internally rotated shoulder has already been described. With growth of contractures, bony changes will compound the problem. A radiograph of both shoulders is mandatory before planning treatment, realizing that in the infant there may be notable limitations in the information derived. The uncomplicated medial-rotation adduction contracture must be relieved before any active tendon transfer can be performed.

In 1913 Fairbanks[11] advocated anterior release of the contracted shoulder through a deltopectoral groove incision which allowed release of the contracted anterior capsule as well as the overlying subscapularis. The pectoralis major was "nicked" but not totally divided. The dislocation, when present, was then reduced. Postoperatively the humerus was maintained in abduction and lateral rotation by a plaster cast for three months, following which intensive exercise was employed.

Sever's operation[35] was similar to that of Fairbanks. Using the same anterior approach, the pectoralis major tendon and subscapularis were divided, but the joint capsule was not opened for fear of later adhesion of the capsule to the joint cartilage with consequent loss of motion. If the coracobrachialis or biceps were found to be tight, they were partially divided as well. If the head of the humerus was blocked by the downward hooking of the acromion, an osteotomy was done. In rare cases, where an anterior subluxation of the joint was present, the pectoralis major was the only muscle to be divided, since to divide the subscapularis as well would only tend to increase the deformity. Postoperatively the arm was held in the corrected position for only two weeks, followed by intensive physical therapy.

Although both of these authors reported favorable results of their operations, they were described anecdotally rather than statistically, making assessment difficult.

Wickstrom's[47] experience with the Sever procedure demonstrated a loss of correction with time. Five patients were examined six years after the operation. Two of them retained correction of the internal rotation deformity, while in three there was significant loss of correction and recurrence of internal rotation contracture.

In an attempt to provide a static check-rein to prevent recurrence of the internal rotation deformity, in 1932 Kleinberg[21] of New York presented the results of an operation which he called "reattachment of the capsule and external rotators of the shoulder." In this procedure, the subscapularis tendon was detached and the lateral capsule and rotator cuff attachments brought anteriorly on the humerus to act as a strong check ligament that would theoretically maintain the lateral rotation and increase the efficiency of weakened lateral rotators. Ten patients with good results were reported without mention of length of follow-up. The operation has not achieved popularity. It is of interest that one of the discussants of this paper, when it was presented before the American Medical Association meeting in Philadelphia in 1959, was J. W. Sever. He criticized the procedure for not dividing the pectoralis major and coracobrachialis and for opening the capsule. Finally, he concluded that the use of the weakened rotators as check ligaments must inevitably result in their stretching, with recurrence of the internal rotation deformity.

In an attempt not only to correct the deformity, but to restore muscle balance about the paretic shoulder of patients with the upper type of obstetrical palsy, L'Episcopo[23] in 1934 reported an important modification of the release procedures. As in the Fairbanks' operation, the capsule and subscapularis were released as was the pectoralis major. In late cases with torsion of the upper end of the humerus, a high derotation osteotomy of the humerus was done. For the earlier case, the release was then followed by a transfer of the tendon teres major posterolaterally. The tendon was identified through the anterior incision and tagged with sutures before being detached from their insertions. Then a posterior incision was made and tendon passed posteriorly around the humerus to be reattached under an osteoperiosteal flap just above or at the origin of the lateral head of the triceps. Subsequently, he included the latissimus dorsi in the transfer. Of the 15 patients operated upon by L'Episcopo between 1934 and 1939[24] for obstetrical palsy, all were reported to "have been definitely improved functionally."

Zachary[49] subsequently modified the procedure slightly in 1947 as have Green and Tachdjian[13] and Hoffer et al.[16]

The L'Episcopo procedure has been quite successful, in that it not only removes a deformity force, but converts it into a corrective one. Thus the tendency to recurrence following release of the contracted anterior structures alone is negated, and the patient actually has increased voluntary control in addition to the gain in passive range of motion. It does not produce a strong shoulder, but in the 24 cases that I have done over the past 20 years, there has been significant patient and parent satisfaction in virtually all cases (Fig. 5.16). It has been necessary to attempt to eliminate the exaggerated truncal movements that have been present with abduction preoperatively lest they persist postoperatively, even in the presence of marked improvement in glenohumeral motion and control of lateral rotation. This has required several months of physiotherapy for some patients. If a young child is seen with a minimal contracture, often the parents, with the guidance of a therapist, can overcome it, but unless there is at least some active power of lateral rotation, the contracture will recur, and the movements of forward flexion of the arm will always be accompanied by an annoying tendency to medial rotation. Such patients, as well as those with established contractures, will usually require surgery, which I rarely do before four or five years of age. It is mandatory to obtain adequate radiographs of the shoulder joint preoperatively to insure that the glenohumeral joint is congruous and does not require bony correction in addition to soft-tissue surgery.

In 1916 Rogers[29] advocated proximal humeral osteotomy with lateral rotation of the distal fragment to correct persistent internal rotation deformity when the humerus was neither retroverted nor subluxated. Wickstrom[46] used this in nine shoulders in which the humeral head was flattened and fixed in internal rotation with satisfactory results, and this has remained the primary rationale for the operation. It cannot be overemphasized that soft tissue correction alone is inadequate in the presence of joint subluxation or dislocation. Then osteotomy may be combined with anterior release to obviate the adverse effect of the retroverted humeral head. The technique of Scaglietti[32] used a Sever anterior release followed eight weeks later by a rotational osteotomy

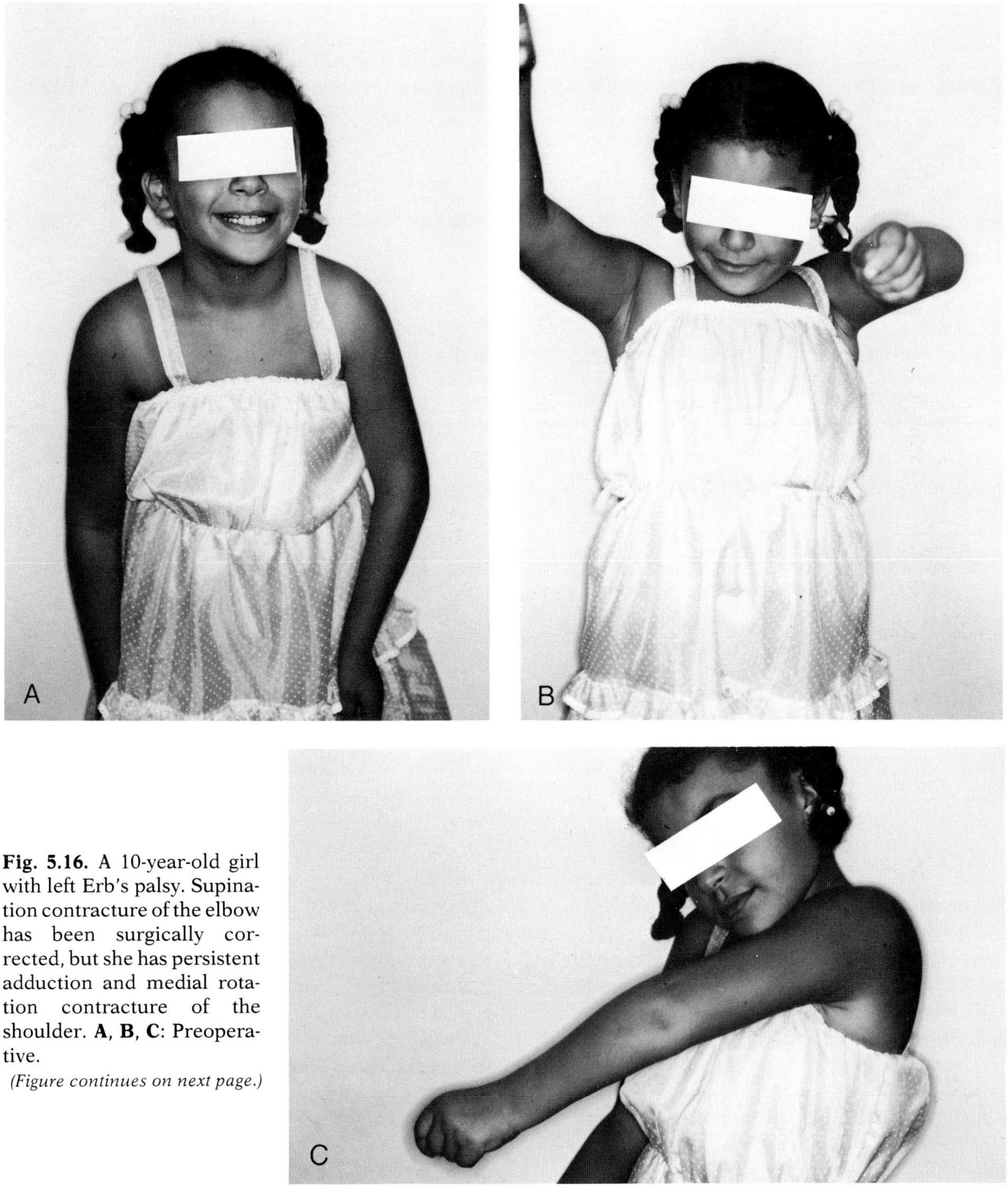

Fig. 5.16. A 10-year-old girl with left Erb's palsy. Supination contracture of the elbow has been surgically corrected, but she has persistent adduction and medial rotation contracture of the shoulder. **A**, **B**, **C**: Preoperative.

(Figure continues on next page.)

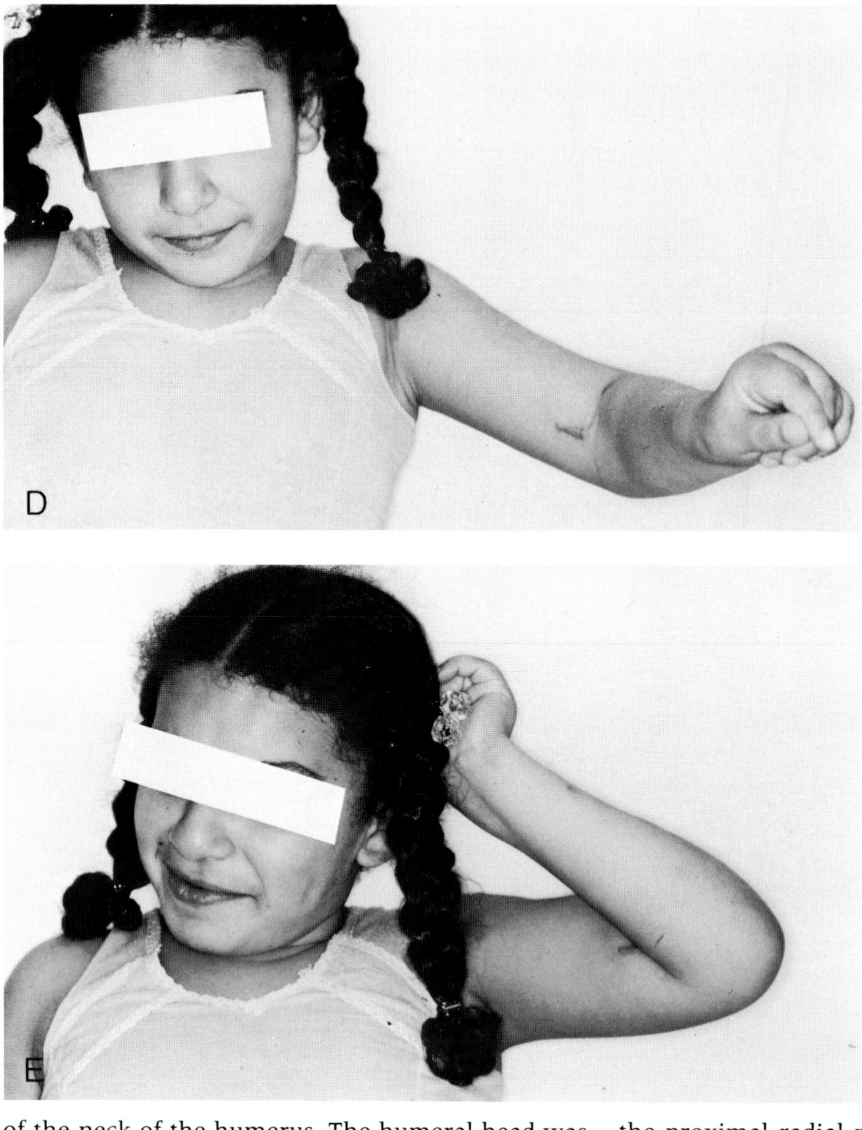

Fig. 5.16 *(continued)* **D**, **E**: Following L'Episcopo transfer.

of the neck of the humerus. The humeral head was held in normal relationship with the glenoid and the distal fragment of the humerus was rotated internally. It may be held by means of a small compression plate.

The deformities of the elbow have already been described. In the upper type of palsy they are particularly common, and Aitken's[2] paper in 1952 is valuable in clarifying the pathogenesis of production of the deformity as well as its avoidance by not using rigid splinting. In his series of 107 patients, 33 (30.8%) had osseous deformity of the elbow. Six had anterior dislocations, thought to be present at birth. The remaining 27 patients with posterior dislocation could be identified very early because of clubbing of the proximal radial metaphysis associated with increasing bowing of the ulna. The radial head went on to dislocate posteriorly between ages five and eight. Radial head excision at any time during the growth period was ineffective in increasing supination of the forearm or extension of the elbow. It was therefore recommended by Aitken that osteotomy through the upper third of the ulna was necessary to reposition the radial axis.

In addition to the static deformity of the elbow, the lack of active elbow flexion may be a significant disability in the upper trunk or Erb's type of paralysis. For those patients with good flexor-pronator muscles, a Steindler flexorplasty may be quite useful. The occasional patient will exhibit the curious phenomenon of dyssynergia at the elbow so that attempts at elbow flexion will result in strong contraction of the triceps and elbow flexors, resulting in an elbow that is locked and unable to function. Whether this phenomenon is due to confused reinnervation in the peripheral nerves or disturbance at the spinal or cortical level is unknown. Milgram[27] in 1939 reported several cases, including one successfully treated by triceps tenotomy after a preliminary test of Novocain block. An alternative method for treating this problem would be anterior transfer of the triceps.

Disturbances of forearm rotation due to muscle weakness and development of contractures can result in further disability in patients who have already had serious functional loss. In 1963 Zaoussis[51] reported on 150 patients with obstetrical paralysis. The forearm was fixed in pronation in 14% and in supination in 10%. These deformities were treated by rotation osteotomy of the proximal one third of the radius. The results were reported in six patients, with good results in five. Although two patients developed proximal radioulnar synostosis, their function and appearance were said to be improved by the operation.

A number of other surgeons have contributed to our ability to manage the persistant supination deformity due to obstetrical palsy. Blount[3] recommended manual osteoclasis of the middle one third of the radius and ulna in patients with insufficient potential motors for tendon transfer, but restricted it to those under the age of 12. Occasionally a second osteoclasis was necessary because of loss of correction with growth.

In 1956 Burman[4] discussed the triple deformity of shoulder, elbow, and wrist in obstetrical palsy. He stated that the first step in reconstruction was to return the shoulder to neutral, then correct the supination deformity of the forearm with osteotomy, and finally to do a wrist fusion. The rerouting of the biceps tendon to convert it from a supinator to a pronator was originally described by Grilli.[14]

In 1967 Zancolli[50] described the results of treatment of 14 patients with supination contractures of the forearm due to paralysis of the pronators. The functional deficit of this paresis is particularly disabling, since many common activities of daily living such as dressing, eating, and writing require simultaneous elbow flexion and pronation. With weak or absent pronators, the unopposed biceps supinates the forearm, putting the hand in a disadvantageous position. Zancolli therefore combined a surgical release of the contracted structures preventing passive pronation of the forearm with a Z-lengthening of the biceps tendon, which is rerouted posterolaterally around the neck of the radius to change its action from that of a supinator to pronator. It is an extensive procedure, requiring an incision on the dorsum of the forearm from elbow to wrist. The interosseous membrane must be carefully released from the ulna deep to the plane of the muscles to avoid injury to the posterior interosseous nerve, and if either the distal or proximal radioulnar joints are contributing to the supination contracture, they too must be released by capsulotomy. Further care must be taken to protect the posterior interosseous nerve from injury when the biceps tendon is rerouted, and this can be done by passing the tendon around the radial neck in contact with the bone at all times.

Although this procedure has proved to be extremely useful, and most patients are very gratified with the result (Fig. 5.17), it should be carefully noted preoperatively and pointed out to the patient and his parents that if weakness of wrist or finger extension is present preoperatively, it is not as apparent with the forearm supinated, since gravity will reinforce these actions, and the dorsum of the wrist and hand are hidden from view. Once the forearm is pronated, these deficits will become much more obvious, and may even necessitate bracing or surgical correction.

Zancolli stated that, since the operation was described for patients with contractures of varied etiologies, those with obstetrical palsy tended to achieve somewhat less active motion than those with polio or quadriplegia. Still, the resulting correction that is usually maintained in the birth palsy group as well as those with deformity due to childhood-acquired brachial plexus injury make this a useful and dependable procedure.

The treatment of the paralytic hand due to obstetrical palsy must be highly individualized with due regard for the realistic goals of surgery as understood by both surgeon and patient. Tendon transfers are usually not indicated before the age of four or five years, when active cooperation of the patient can be assessed and secured for the necessary rehabilitation program. It must be remembered that the patient may have a significant psychological or neurophysiological bias against habitual use of the hand, even in the face of what the surgeon might view as an excel-

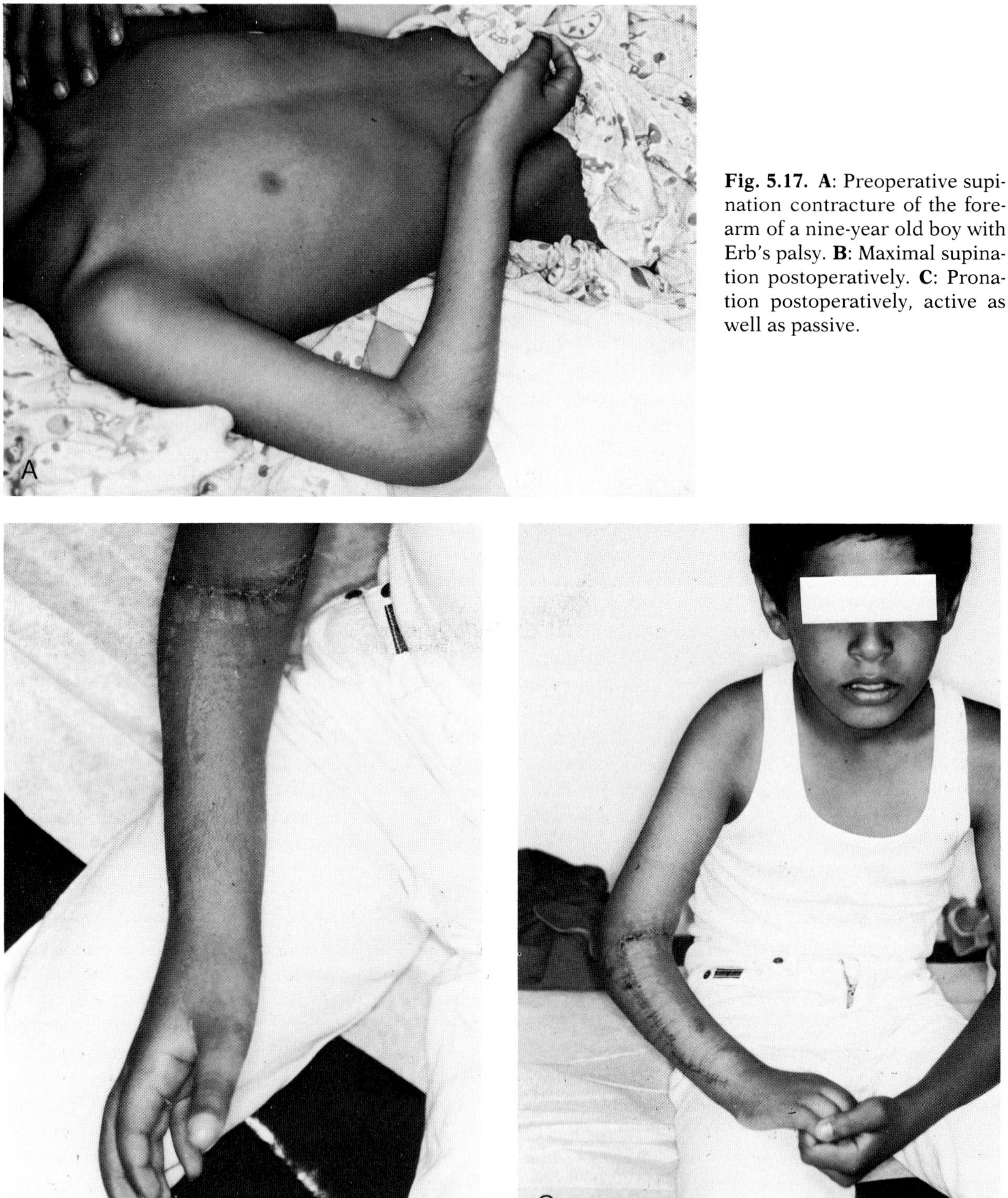

Fig. 5.17. **A**: Preoperative supination contracture of the forearm of a nine-year old boy with Erb's palsy. **B**: Maximal supination postoperatively. **C**: Pronation postoperatively, active as well as passive.

lent anatomic result. Furthermore, the older patient may have a totally unrealistic picture of what the surgery is to accomplish, often accompanied by false hopes that with operation, all that is not satisfactory in his life will suddenly improve. This type of magical thinking is particularly likely to occur in the adolescent and young adult who is finding competition in the social or vocational spheres difficult. It is prudent for the surgeon to make a sincere effort to attempt to determine the patient's motivation and needs in several preoperative conferences and carefully explain what can be expected from surgical reconstruction.

Finally, to return to the consideration of nerve repair in obstetrical palsy, it is evident from review of the convoluted literature of treatment of obstetrical palsy that early and accurate evaluation of the neonate is mandatory if any attempt is to be made to modify the natural history of the disease by means of neurological reconstruction. These children should be seen immediately after birth by those physicians and surgeons who are prepared to employ any of the techniques available, based on accurate record-keeping and unbiased reporting of functional results.

Because of the referral pattern of my clinical practice and the general reluctance on the part of parents and physicians caring for newborns to consider a major neurosurgical procedure for the treatment of obstetrical palsy, I have no personal experience in the neurological reconstruction of these lesions. Nevertheless, I believe that those patients who show no evidence of recovery by 3 months should be systematically evaluated with a view towards surgical exploration. Furthermore, patients whom I see with obstetrical palsy within the first decade of life often have established contractures and some have bony deformity. These conditions can be ameliorated and sometimes avoided altogether if they can be seen by physical therapists and physicians who are knowledgeable in the treatment of this entity.

REFERENCES

1. Adler JB, Patterson RL: Erb's palsy: Long-term results in treatment in eighty-eight cases. J Bone Joint Surg 49:1052, 1967
2. Aitken J: Deformity of the elbow joint as a sequel to Erb's obstetrical paralysis. J Bone Joint Surg 34B:352, 1952
3. Blount WP: Osteoclasis for supination deformities in children. J Bone Joint Surg 22:300, 1940
4. Burman M: Paralytic supination contracture of the forearm. J Bone Joint Surg 38A(2):303, 1956
5. Clark LP, Taylor AS, Prout TP: A study on brachial birth palsy. Am J Med Sci 130:670, 1905
6. Colonna P: Regional Orthopedic Surgery, p 521. Saunders, Philadelphia, 1959
7. Dejerine-Klumpke A: Paralysie radiculaire totale du plexus brachial avec phénomènes oculo-pupillaires autopsiée trente-six jours après l'accident. Rev Neurol 16:637, 1908
8. Duchenne GB: De l'électrisation localisée et de son application a la pathologie et à la thérapeutique. 3rd Ed. p 357. Baillière, Paris, 1872
9. Erb W: On a characteristic site of injury in the brachial plexus. (Transl. by Brody & Wilkins). Arch Neurol. 21:443, 1969
10. Erb W: Ueber eine eigenthumliche Lokalisation von Lahmunger in Plexus Brachialis im Nov. 1874. Verh Histor Med Vereins, Heidelberg (1874–1877). p 130. Carl Winter's Universitatsbuchandlung.
11. Fairbank HAT: Birth palsy: Subluxation of shoulder joint in infants and young children. Lancet 1:217, 1913
12. Gilmour J: Notes on the surgical treatment of brachial birth palsy. Lancet 696, 1925
13. Green WT, Tachdjian, MO: Correction of the residual deformities of the shoulder in obstetrical palsy. J Bone Joint Surg 45A:1544, 1963
14. Grilli FP: Il trapianto del bicipite brachiale in lunzione pronatoria. Arch Putti Chir Organi Mov 12:359, 1959
15. Hardy AE: Birth injuries of the brachial plexus, incidence and prognosis. J Bone Joint Surg 63B:98, 1981
16. Hoffer MM, Wickenden R, Roper B: Brachial plexus birth palsies, results of tendon transfers to the rotator cuff. J Bone Joint Surg 60A:691, 1978
17. Jepson PN: Obstetrical paralysis. Ann Surg 91:724, 1930
18. Kattan KR, Spitz HB: Roentgen findings in obstetrical injuries to the brachial plexus. Radiology 91:462, 1968
19. Kennedy R: Suture of the brachial plexus in birth paralysis of the upper extremity. Br Med J 1:298, 1903
20. Kennedy R: Further notes on the treatment of birth paralysis of the upper extremity by suture of the fifth and sixth cervical nerves. Br Med J 2:1065, 1904
21. Kleinberg S: Reattachment of the capsule and external rotators of the shoulder for obstetrical paralysis. JAMA 98:294, 1932
22. Klumpke A: Contribution a l'etude des paralysies radiculaires du plexus brachial. Paralysies radiculaires totales. Paralysies radiculaires inferiennes. De la participation des filets sympatheiques oculo-pupillaries dans C5 paralysis. Rev Med 5:591, 1885

23. L'Episcopo JB: Tendon transplantation in obstetrical paralysis. Am J Surg 25(1):122, 1934
24. L'Episcopo JB: Restoration of muscle balance in the treatment of obstetrical paralysis. NY State J Med 39:357, 1939
25. Liebolt F, Furey JG: Obstetrical paralysis with dislocation of the shoulder. A case report. J Bone Joint Surg 35A:221, 1953
26. Mallet J: Paralysies obstetricales du plexus brachial traitement des sequellae. Rev Chir Orthop 5(Suppl 1):166, 1972
27. Milgram JE: Discusion of L'Episcopo's presentation. Restoration of muscle balance in treatment of obstetrical paralysis. NY J Med 39:357, 1939
28. Platt H: Opening remarks on birth paralysis. J Orthop Surg 2:272, 1920
29. Rogers MH: An operation for the correction of the deformity due to "obstetrical paralysis." Boston Med Surg J 174:163, 1916
30. Rossi LN, Vassella F, Mumenthaler M: Obstetrical lesions of the brachial plexus. Eur Neurol 21:1–7, 1982
31. Scaglietti O: Obstetrical lesions of the shoulder. Chir Organi Mov 22:183, 1936
32. Scaglietti O: The obstetrical shoulder trauma. Surg Gynecol Obstet 66:868, 1938
33. Sever JW: Obstetrical paralysis — Its etiology, pathology, clinical aspects and treatment, with report of four hundred and seventy cases. Am J Dis Child 12:541, 1916
34. Sever JW: A research on obstetrical paralysis, its causation and anatomy. Boston Med Surg J 174:327, 1916
35. Sever JW: The results of a new operation for obstetrical paralysis. Am J Orthop Surg 16:248, 1918
36. Sever JW: Obstetrical paralysis: Report of eleven hundred cases. JAMA 85:1862, 1925
37. Sharpe W: The operative treatment of brachial plexus paralysis. JAMA 66:876, 1916
38. Smellie W: Collection of preternatural cases and observations in midwifery compleating the design of illustrating his first volume on that subject. Vol III. p 504. London, 1764
39. Tachdjian MO: Pediatric orthopedics. Vol 2. Ch 5. Saunders, Philadelphia, London, Toronto, 1972
40. Tassin JL: Paralysies obstetricales du plexus brachial: Evolution spontanée, resultats des interventions reparatrices precoces. Thesis, Université Paris VII, 1983
41. Taylor AS: Results from the surgical treatment of brachial plexus palsy. JAMA 48:96, 1907
42. Taylor AS: Conclusions derived from further experience in the surgical treatment of brachial birth palsy (Erb's type). Am J Med Sci 146:836, 1913
43. Taylor AS: Brachial birth palsy and injuries of similar type in adults. Surg Gynecol Obstet 30:494, 1920
44. Thomas TT: The relation of posterior subluxation of the shoulder-joint to obstetrical palsy of upper extremity. Ann Surg 59:197, 1914
45. Truesdell EO: Skeletal birth injuries. In Bancroft FW, Marble HC (eds): Surgical treatment of the motor skeletal system. 2nd Ed. Part 1, p 1239. Lippincott, Philadelphia, 1951
46. Wickstrom J, Haslam ET, Hutchinson RH: The surgical management of residual deformities of the shoulder following birth injuries of the brachial plexus. J Bone Joint Surg 37A:27, 1955
47. Wickstrom J: Birth injuries of the brachial plexus: Treatment of defects in the shoulder. Clin Orthop 23:187, 1962
48. Wolman B: Erb's palsy. Arch Dis Child 23:129, 1948
49. Zachary, RB: Transplantation of teres major and latissimus dorsi for loss of external rotation at shoulder. Lancet 2:757, 1947
50. Zancolli E: Paralytic supination contracture of the forearm. J Bone Joint Surg 49A:1275, 1967
51. Zaoussis AL: Osteotomy of the proximal end of the radius for paralytic supination deformity in children. J Bone Joint Surg 45B:523, 1963

6

Postanesthetic Brachial Plexus Palsy

Postanesthetic palsy results from injury to the brachial plexus of a patient undergoing either general or regional anesthesia for the performance of a surgical procedure that is unrelated to the plexus. In the case of general anesthesia, the injury is usually due to the patient's position on the operating table and is not directly caused by the surgical manipulation. It is ordinarily a preventable entity, but one which is often unsuspected or unanticipated by both surgeon and anesthesiologist preoperatively. In the postoperative period it is sometimes misdiagnosed. It is for these reasons that the actual incidence of postanesthetic palsy is impossible to determine. Nevertheless, it is a well-known and described complication of anesthesia.[20,27,28,32,34] For example, in 1950, Dhuner[7] from the Karolinska Institute in Stockholm reviewed the records of 30,000 patients who received an anesthetic in the period of 1940–1945 and reported 31 patients who suffered from paresis of one or more nerves in the postanesthetic period. Of the 26 involving the upper extremities, 11 were in the brachial plexus. In 1973 Parks[26] analyzed 50,000 operative procedures and found 28 brachial plexus lesions.

Historically, brachial plexus palsy following anesthesia was first described by Konrad Budinger,[3] who in 1894 was an assistant in Bilroth's clinic. He attributed it to compression of the nerves between the clavicle and first rib. Krumm,[17] a year later, postulated compression between the clavicle and cervical transverse processes as the cause. Halstead's[11] analysis in 1908 resulted in multiple possible etiologies, including compression and traction. In 1942 Clausen[4] concluded that unusual positions associated with complete muscular relaxation during anesthesia may result in abnormal tension on and stretch of the brachial plexus. He emphasized that the arm should never be abducted beyond 90 degrees and when the arm is abducted at all, the head and neck must be held in neutral position so as to diminish the tension on the plexus. He also cautioned about the Trendelenburg position and the use of shoulder braces. In 1950 Dhuner[7] considered both traction and direct compression by the clavicle as potential causes and performed roentgenographic studies on the displacement of the plexus as outlined by contrast medium when the arm was abducted. He stated that abduction of the arm 90 degrees or more with external rotation and extension was a significant cause of injury, as was the use of shoulder braces with the patient in steep Trendelenburg position. In 1965 Jackson and Keats[14] investigated the mechanism of injury by cadaver dissection and by simulation of position on the operating table, and demonstrated that stretch was the most likely mechanism leading to injury.

To summarize, it would appear that traction on the plexus of an unconscious, and therefore unguarded, patient is the most significant etiological factor in the production of postanesthetic palsy, with compression playing a lesser role. The retropulsion of the clavicle that takes place both in abduction of the arm and in a relaxed patient in the supine position, with or without shoulder braces, is a contributing factor to injury. The displaced clavicle may create a point of fixation in the plexus and thereby decrease the amount of potentially safe elongation of the nerves further distally. This restriction predisposes them to traction injury rather than direct pinching between the clavicle and first rib or cervical transverse processes. If, as several authors have shown, the arm is abducted and the head and neck deviated

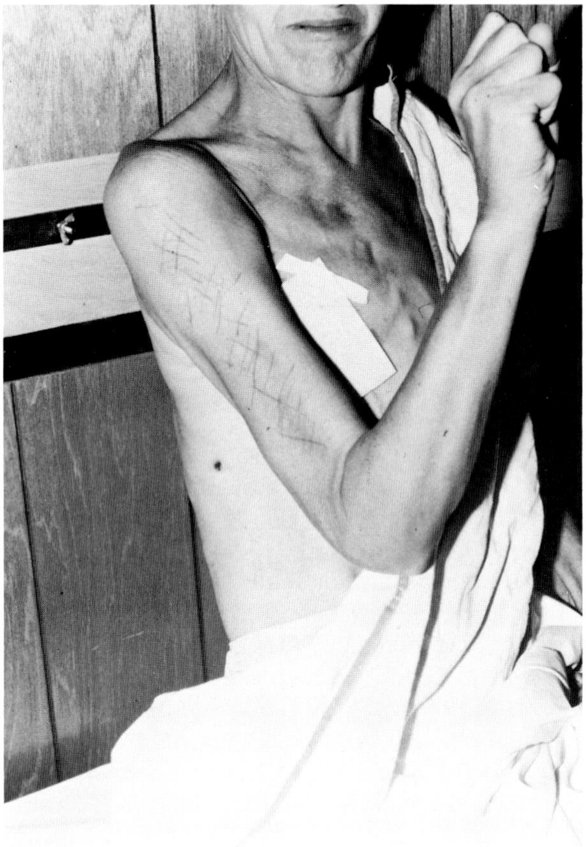

Fig. 6.1. A woman with diabetes who sustained an intraoperative brachial plexus injury during the performance of a mastectomy. The upper trunk lesion resolved within a month.

to the contralateral side, this position increases the tension on the ipsilateral plexus. Backward extension and lateral rotation of the humerus increases the tension even more. The "hands-up" position often preferred for thoracic and abdominal operations may produce significant tension on the brachial plexus that can be markedly alleviated by simply bringing the elbows up 5–6 inches in front of the plane of the body, as demonstrated by Jackson and Keats.[14] With the patient in the lateral decubitus position, even with the arms at the side, significant tension in the plexus may be developed on the "up" side if the head and neck are allowed to laterally deviate as they sink into a pillow or blanket.

The use of an "axillary roll" has been the subject of some debate. If, as is sometimes done, a folded sheet is merely stuffed into the dependent axilla of an anesthetized patient, it not only does not serve as a protection against direct pressure injury to the plexus, but may actually cause it. Alternatively, a folded sheet or pad beneath the "downside" hemithorax will relieve pressure of the axilla and thereby protect the plexus.

There is a distinctive subgroup of postanesthetic palsy that occurs following cardiac surgery done through a median sternotomy. Several groups have called attention to this entity, which is not due to the effects of position on the operating table,[10,13,16] but rather is a result of spread of the sternal retractors, which push the clavicles backward and rotate the first ribs superiorly. The result is abnormal tension on the brachial plexus, which can be worsened by turning the head and abducting the arm. Although the prognosis for recovery is usually good, it may be protracted and sometimes incomplete.

It should be noted that there are identifiable predisposing factors in patients at risk of developing postanesthetic palsy. Well-padded individuals seem more resistant to stretch injury than those who are spare or cachectic. Possibly the latter group is also more likely to suffer from clinically manifest neuropathy or subclinical neuropathy. Patients with toxic-metabolic abnormalities, diabetes, or cancer are often in this group (Fig. 6.1).

PREVENTION OF POSTOPERATIVE BRACHIAL PLEXUS PALSY FROM GENERAL ANESTHESIA

From the mechanisms of injury described in the previous section, a list of precautions can be suggested to reduce the incidence of postoperative palsy.

1. All prospective candidates for general anesthesia should have a careful history and physical examination to determine whether there are increased risk factors, such as a prior history of palsy or any of the conditions associated with neuropathy.
2. The surgeon and anesthesiologist should cooperate in planning and maintaining a position of the head, neck, shoulder girdle, and upper extremity that will safeguard against development of a palsy.
3. Steep Trendelenburg position with shoulder braces should be avoided. If braces are used, they

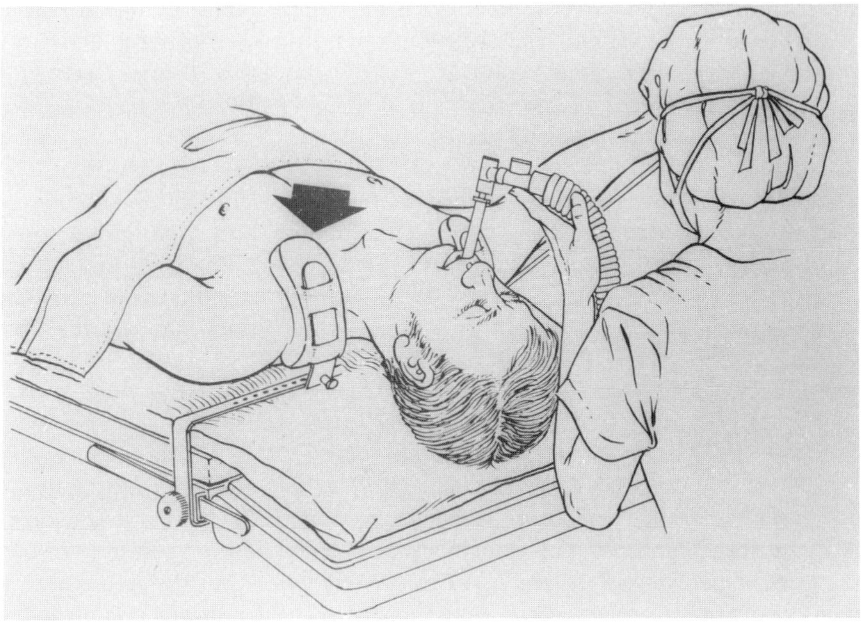

Fig. 6.2. If the braces are medially placed, as indicated by the arrow, there is significant danger of injury to the plexus if the patient is in Trendelenburg position.

should be well padded and located as far laterally as possible[35] (Fig. 6.2).

4. Armboards should be modified so that the arm cannot be abducted more than 90 degrees (Fig.6.3). Backward extension of the arm behind the plane of the body should be avoided. It is preferable to have the abducted arm actually slightly forward flexed by building up the height of the armboard. If the elbows are located in a plane 5 inches forward of the chest, considerable slack is conveyed to the brachial plexus.
5. The head and neck should be maintained in neu-

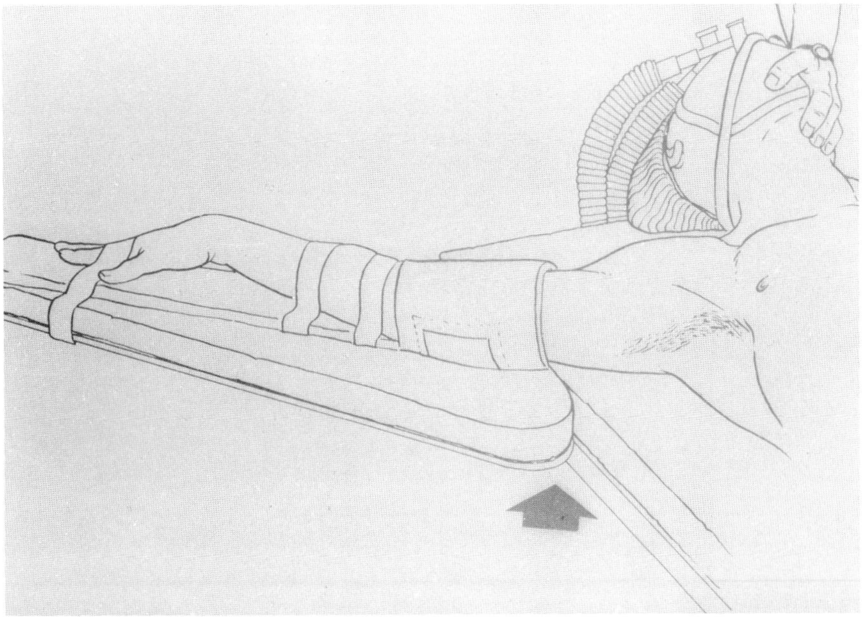

Fig. 6.3. This position is likely to produce a traction injury of the lower trunk outflow of the brachial plexus.

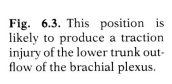

tral position, even when the patient is in the lateral decubitus position. These cautions obviously also pertain to the prone position.

6. In the lateral decubitus position, a pad that lifts the downside hemithorax off the table will protect against pressure injury to the contents of the axilla. This effect is easily demonstrated and monitored by observing the effect on the facility of flow of intravenous fluid in that arm and the lack of distention of the veins.

CLINICAL PRESENTATION, EVALUATION, AND PROGNOSIS FOR BRACHIAL PALSIES FOLLOWING GENERAL ANESTHESIA

It has generally been observed that cases of postoperative brachial plexus palsy are most likely to involve the upper roots of the plexus. Considerably less common is involvement of the entire plexus. The least common is the Klumpke type of paralysis involving the lower roots. Of the 11 patients reported by Dhuner,[7] 10 had upper root involvement and one had lower. Parks'[26] 28 postoperative brachial plexus injuries had a predominance of upper plexus lesions. A compilation of 39 cases by Kwaan and Rappaport[19] in 1970 is reproduced in Table 6.1.

The length of time recorded in cases of postoperative palsy has varied from as short as 40 minutes in one of Dhuner's cases to the times recorded in Kwaan and Rappaport's[19] compilation. Although the shortest period for Parks' cases was 2 hours, most of the patients were on the operating table for at least 6 hours.

The upper trunk lesions are clinically expressed as weakness of shoulder abduction, lateral rotation, and forward flexion as well as elbow flexion. It is more common to have paresis rather than paralysis, and the motor deficit is generally greater than the sensory loss. Probably this distribution results from

Table 6.1. Reported Cases of Postoperative Brachial Plexus Palsy

Author	No. of Cases	Type of Operation	Arm Position	Operation Time	Injury	Recovery Period
Stephens[33]	3	Intracardiac procedure, cardiopulmonary bypass	Abduction at shoulder	Not stated	Upper roots	Not stated
Ewing[9]	3	Abdomino-perineal resection	Abduction, Trendelenburg	2–3.5 hr	Upper roots or bilateral total paralysis	3–9 months
Ewing[9]	2	Cholecystectomy and sigmoid resection	Bilateral arm abduction	1.5–2.5 hr	Upper roots	1–5 months
Cotton and Allen[5]	4	Appendectomy, hip operation	Bilateral arm abducton	0.75–2 hr	Total paralysis	Several months
Kiloh[15]	4	Cholecystectomy	Bilateral arm abduction, 90 degrees	1.5–2 hr	Total/partial paralysis	4–7 months
Raffan[29]	2	Hysterectomy	Arm abduction 90 degrees, Trendelenburg	1–1.5 hr	Total paralysis	2–4 months
Wood-Smith[36]	1	Cystectomy	Arm abduction 90 degrees, Trendelenburg	3 hr	Upper roots	3 months
Clausen[4]	8	Abdomino-perineal resection	Arm abduction, Trendelenburg	2–3 hr, some not stated	Mostly upper roots	6 weeks to 11 months
Clausen[4]	1	Chest lobectomy	Arm abduction (marked)	2.5 hr	Upper roots	7 months
Dhuner[7]	11	Not stated	Mostly bilateral, abduction 90 degrees	40 min and not stated	Upper roots	Few weeks to 3 months

From Kwaan JHM, Rappaport I: Postoperative brachial plexus palsy. Arch Surg 101:612. Copyright 1970 American Medical Association.

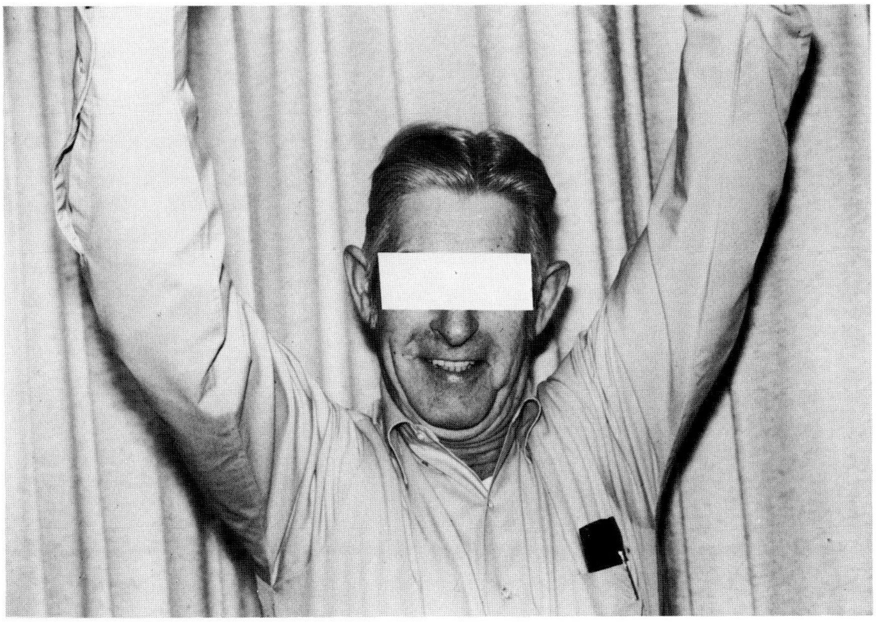

Fig. 6.4. This man awoke from his vascular surgery with bilaterally paralyzed arms. He recovered almost totally.

the preponderance of neurapraxias or first-degree lesions of which this disparity is characteristic. Furthermore, unless there is an element of axonotmesis or degenerative change, there will be no fibrillations observed if electromyography is performed three weeks postoperatively. If electromyographic examination is done immediately postoperatively in a patient with what would appear to be a postanesthetic palsy and there are fibrillations present at rest, this indicates a preexisting neurological lesion, since it ordinarily takes three weeks for Wallerian degeneration to occur and the reaction of degeneration to be definable on electrodiagnostic testing. It is only in circumstances where such an underlying and predisposing neurological lesion is suspected that immediate electrodiagnostic study is indicated.

The clinical course of recovery in patients with postanesthetic palsy is usually characterized by recovery that may begin almost immediately and is often completed by six to eight weeks. The cases summarized by Kwaan and Rappaport[19] varied from "a few weeks" to 11 months in their recovery. In most of the cases reported in the literature, as well as in my personal experience, the degree of recovery has been complete. However, I have had the opportunity to observe a 54-year-old man who incurred bilateral brachial plexus palsies following a 10-hour abdominoaortic replacement with his arms in the "hands-up" position. After five years of follow-up, his only deficit was a slight atrophy and weakness of the anterior deltoid on one side. However, his neurological status improved to its maximum by the end of the first year (Fig. 6.4).

Although the occurrence of a postanesthetic palsy is a distressing complication, it usually has such a good prognosis that both patient and surgeon may be reassured, unless there is a significant underlying neuropathy. Of course, it is possible to superimpose an additional peripheral nerve injury upon the plexus lesion or to injure a peripheral nerve and spare the plexus. For these lesions the prognosis may be quite variable.[25]

Following careful neurological evaluation with establishment of the diagnosis and prognosis, there is usually an urgent desire on the part of all concerned to institute some type of therapy. If weakness has resulted in a subluxation of the shoulder or inability to flex the elbow actively, then a sling should be worn. However, care must be taken to ensure that a full passive range of motion is performed several times a day to avoid the development of contractures. Particularly in elderly patients, this possibility must be anticipated. The paralyzed wrist and fingers should be supported as needed with appropriate splints and, here too, range of motion exercises are indicated. There is no hard evidence that the use of steroids in these patients has any validity, although it has been suggested. The use of electrical stimulation of paralyzed muscle is, in my opinion, not justifiable on the basis of rigorous proof, but it may contribute to the patient's confidence that something tangible is being done to aid recovery. I do not routinely employ it.

POSTANESTHETIC PALSY—BRACHIAL PLEXUS BLOCK

General and Historical Consideration

The advantages to patient, surgeon, and anesthetist that successful brachial plexus block offers have established for it a firm place in upper extremity surgery. Compared with general anesthesia, the obvious benefits of having to only anesthetize the upper limb makes its use ideal in patients with significant medical complications such as cardiac, pulmonary, or renal disease. In addition, the patient who is otherwise well but who has a full stomach, or one who simply rejects losing consciousness, may elect regional anesthesia by block. For the surgeon, muscular relaxation may be attained in the limb without the requirement for deep general anesthesia or the use of additional muscle relaxants. Certainly, under the adverse conditions of battlefront surgery, brachial plexus block has proved of inestimable value. Suffice it to say that the anesthetist or surgeon administering the block must have thorough knowledge of the pertinent anatomy, the techniques of administration, the pharmacology of the anesthetic agents, and the potential complications that may be caused by this mode of anesthesia.

The first reported brachial plexus block is ascribed to Halstead,[11] who performed an open block in 1884 with cocaine. Crile[6] performed a disarticulation of the shoulder in 1897 using this method, and 14 years later, two Germans, Hirschel[12] and Kulenkampff[18] each independently described percutaneous block of the brachial plexus.

As with the documentation of complications affecting the brachial plexus following general anesthesia, the exact incidence has been difficult to determine. Furthermore, the possibility of direct damage to peripheral nerves in the operative field, either by fracture fragments or surgical manipulation, may be a very real and confusing factor. Added to this is the fact that many upper extremity surgical procedures are performed under the ischemia of a tourniquet. Thus, one can see the obvious difficulties in statistical analysis.

A number of clinical series dealing with the problem of complications of regional anesthesia, and specifically brachial plexus block anesthesia, are of interest generally and with reference to the relative infrequency of neural complications, as opposed to more frequent ones, such as pneumothorax. For example, Moore[23,24] quotes an incidence of pneumothorax following supraclavicular brachial plexus block, ranging from 0.5 to 6.0%, and reports that from 1965 to 1968 at his institution, there was one pneumothorax following 616 supraclavicular brachial plexus blocks (0.16%). It is of interest that he does not quote any statistics for peripheral nerve lesions following regional block, but makes the very important point that since the literature contains reports of neurologic involvement of peripheral nerves following regional block, general anesthesia, or no anesthesia, it is important to be certain that the inadvertent or unexpected postoperative palsy did result from the regional anesthetic. He has provided us with a list of causes of peripheral nerve lesions following regional block that is useful in thinking about the problem, although I am not convinced that items 6 and 11 are necessarily adverse factors.

1. Faulty positioning of the patient or of the surgical retractor
2. Neurolytic agents
3. Surgical trauma
4. Improperly applied casts, tourniquets, or both
5. Neurolytic action of local anesthetic agents
6. Intraneural injections
7. Damage from direct contact of the needle point with the nerve
8. Contamination of solution or equipment
9. Preexisting lesions
10. Metallic ions released from receptacles and syringes
11. Repetition of a specific block within 24 hours

It should be realized that, although all local anesthetic agents are neurotoxic in high concentrations, they are generally not toxic in the concentrations that are used in clinical anesthesia. Furthermore, it is not universally agreed that intraneural injections will produce clinically significant nerve lesions.[21] The damage from direct contact of the needle point with the nerve has been the subject of some interesting studies, which will be described later.

Adriani and Evangelow[1] in 1955 described 1400 blocks performed on 513 patients and reported 11 pneumothoraces due to brachial plexus block, but only one neuritic complication, which was an injury to the medial cord of the brachial plexus, not further documented.

Woolley and VanDam[37] in 1959 reviewed the literature on this subject and pointed out the difficulty of documentation of neurological sequelae of brachial plexus block. In addition to five cases that they presented, they did a brief retrospective study and made recommendations regarding this entity.

CLINICAL PRESENTATION OF BRACHIAL PALSY FOLLOWING BLOCK ANESTHESIA

The distribution, time of onset, severity, and clinical course of nerve injuries resulting from brachial plexus block anesthesia will depend upon the factor or factors that can be identified as having produced them. In general, paresthesias and hypalgesia suggest involvement of small-diameter nerve fibers and more likely injury by the local anesthetic or hematoma. Therefore, symptoms and signs are usually sensory, rather than those of motor paralysis or paresis. Gross motor loss following block anesthesia is usually the result of something other than the above mechanism. I have had the opportunity to personally review the records of two cases of total and permanent motor and sensory loss following block anesthesia in which alcohol was inadvertently substituted for local anesthetic.

The report by Bonica et al.[2] in 1949 analyzing the results of 1100 consecutive brachial plexus blocks describes four patients who had transient and minimal degrees of paresis and analgesia in the areas supplied by the ulnar nerve. These were ultimately found to have resulted from the surgeon's placing the arm on the operating table in a way that caused pressure on the ulnar nerve at the elbow. Bonica further commented that phrenic nerve block with diaphragmatic paralysis could occur, but that he had not observed any signs or symptoms related to its presence. Dhuner and coworkers[8] specifically addressed this point in 1954 and reported some degree of paresis of the ipsilateral hemidiaphragm in 27.7% of 204 cases examined fluoroscopically after brachial plexus block. However, the paresis disappeared rapidly, usually before the paresis of the arm had dissipated. Of interest was their further investigation of the effect of diaphragmatic paresis on respiratory function. In five cases so studied, there was an average decrease of the vital capacity from 3.5 liters before the block to 2.54 liters after the block (28%). The maximum decrease was 3.6 to 2.1 liters (41%). Tidal air and minute volume were unaffected. They did not believe that a healthy person would be affected by a decrease of 40% of the vital capacity. However, in patients with poor lung function on the opposite side, this could be significant. I have examined a patient with diaphragmatic paralysis due to a block done for an elbow operation 1 1/2 years previously. He is otherwise healthy but now experiences dyspnea when running, whereas he had none preoperatively.

The duration of neurological sequelae of brachial plexus nerve block have varied from case to case but in general have been of short duration. Woolley and VanDam[37] stated that they have not been severe or permanently incapacitating. Moberg and Dhuner[22] published a series of 400 consecutive brachial plexus blocks comparing the effects of procaine and xylocaine. Radiating paresthesias occurred postoperatively in ten of the procaine cases and in seven of the xylocaine group. This symptom persisted for less than three weeks in seven of the procaine group and in three of the xylocaine group. Paresthesias persisted for more than three weeks in three of the procaine and four of the xylocaine group. They commented that, in the few cases where paresthesias of two to three months duration followed plexus block, the cause was probably a small intraneural hematoma. In this regard, there was no difference between xylocaine and procaine.

MECHANISM AND PATHOLOGY

Reference has already been made to the multiplicity of factors that might conceivably be responsible for postanesthetic brachial plexus neuropathy following regional anesthesia. They may be summarized as follows:

1. Local trauma from needles
2. Toxicity of anesthetic agents

3. Contaminants
   a. Infections
   b. Ionic contaminants
   c. Preservatives
4. Effect of underlying neuropathy

The question of local needle trauma has been extensively studied by Selander, Dhuner, and Lundborg.[30] They quoted Bonica[2] as follows: "While it is true that promiscuous, repeated and rough probing of nerves may cause neurological sequelae, gently touching the nerve with the needle point does not cause any clinically apparent damage." They experimentally studied the damage to nerve fascicles and fibers caused by piercing or injecting a nerve with two different needles used for regional block of the rabbit sciatic nerve. In their study, two different bevels, one long (14-degree bevel angle) and one short (45 degrees) were evaluated. The risk of fascicle injury was shown to be significantly reduced when a short-beveled needle was used. They felt that this difference was due to the fascicle's sliding or rolling away more easily from the short-beveled needle. They quoted the observation that others had made of endoneurial herniations with hemorrhage, degeneration, congestion, and edema resulting in functional impairment. They cited the importance of the perineurial sheath, indicating that damage to it might change the endoneurial milieu and thereby interfere with nerve fiber function, as might lesions of the endoneurial blood vessels. They also correlated the degree of fascicular injury with the orientation of the long bevel, so that fewer fibers were cut when the bevel was parallel to the nerve than when it was transversely oriented. Such differences were less evident in fascicular injuries due to the short-beveled needle.

A follow-up clinical study by Selander and colleagues[31] describes symptoms varying from light paresthesias lasting a few weeks to serious paresthesias, ache, and sensory disturbances and weakness lasting more than a year. The motor weakness was minimal. They stated that symptoms arising within the first day generally indicate extra- or intraneural hematoma and/or intraneural edema or a lesion of nerve fibers. Symptoms appearing within three weeks of the block may indicate the secondary effects of the initial trauma such as an expanding hematoma, edema, or constricting scar formation. They found the median and ulnar nerves were most frequently injured as a result of their superficial position in the axillary neurovascular sheath.

From these studies, the authors concluded that paresthesias should be elicited with the greatest care or, if possible, avoided in order to reduce the risk of postblock nerve lesions.

REFERENCES

1. Adriani J, Evangelow M: Complications of regional anesthesia. Curr Res Anaesth Analg 34:2 1955
2. Bonica JJ, Moore DC, Orlov M: Brachial plexus block anesthesia. Am J Surg 78:65, 1949
3. Budinger K: Ueber Lahmungen nach Chloroformnarkosen. Arch Klin Chir 47:121, 1894
4. Clausen EG: Postoperative (anesthetic) paralysis of the brachial plexus. A review of the literature and report of nine cases. Surgery 12:933, 1942
5. Cotton FJ, Allen SW: Brachial paralysis, post narcotic. Boston Med Surg J 148:499, 1903
6. Crile GW: Anesthesia of nerve roots with cocaine. Cleve Med J 2:355, 1897
7. Dhuner KG: Nerve injuries following operations: A survey of cases occurring during a six year period. Anaesthesia 11:289, 1950
8. Dhuner KG, Moberg E, Onne L: Paresis of the phrenic nerve during brachial plexus block anesthesia and its importance. Acta Chir Scand 109:53, 1955
9. Ewing MR: Postoperative paralysis in the upper extremity—Report of five cases. Lancet 1:99, 1950
10. Graham JG, Pye IF, McQueen IN: Brachial plexus injury after median sternotomy. J Neurol Neurosurg Psychiatry 44:621, 1981
11. Halstead AE: Anesthesia paralysis. Surg Gynecol Obstet 6:201, 1908
12. Hirschel G: Die Anaesthesierung des Plexus Brachealis. Für die Operationen an der oberen Extremität. München Med Wochenschr, 58:1555, 1911
13. Honet JC, Raikes JA, Kantowitz A, et al: Neuropathy in the upper extremity after open-heart surgery. Arch Phys Med Rehabil 57:264, 1976
14. Jackson L, Keats AS: Mechanism of brachial plexus palsy following anesthesia. Anaesthesia 26:190, 1965
15. Kiloh LG: Brachial plexus lesions after cholecystectomy. Lancet 1:103, 1950
16. Kirsh MM, Magee KR, Gago O, et al: Brachial plexus injury following median sternotomy incision. Ann Thorac Surg 11:315, 1971
17. Krum F: Ueber Narkosenlahmungen. Sami Klin Vortr 1894
18. Kulenkampff D: Die Analesthesierung des Plexus Brachialis. Deut Med Wochenschr 38:1878, 1912

19. Kwaan JHM, Rappaport I: Postoperative brachial plexus palsy. Arch Surg 101:612, 1970
20. Lincoln JR, Sawyer HP: Complications related to body positions during surgical procedures. Anaesthesia 22:800, 1961
21. Mannerfelt L: Studies on the hand in ulnar nerve paralysis. A clinical experimental investigation in normal anomalous innervation. Acta Orthop Scand [Suppl] 87, 1966
22. Moberg E, Dhuner KG: Brachial plexus analgesia with Xylocaine. J Bone Joint Surg 33A:884, 1951
23. Moore DC, Bridenbaugh LD: Pneumothorax: Its incidence following brachial plexus block analgesia. Anaesthesia 15:475, 1954
24. Moore DC: Complication of regional block. Charles C Thomas, Springfield, IL, 1955
25. Nicholson MJ, Eversole UH: Nerve injuries incident to anesthesia and operation. Anaesth Analg 36:19, 1957
26. Parks BJ: Postoperative peripheral neuropathies. Surgery 74:348, 1973
27. Petrick EU: Paralysis of the brachial plexus following elective surgical procedures. Curr Res Anaesth Analg 34:119, 1955
28. Po BT, Hansen HR: Iatrogenic brachial plexus injury: A survey of the literature and of pertinent cases. Anaesth Analg 48:915, 1969
29. Raffan AW: Postoperative paralysis of the brachial plexus. Br Med J 2:149, 1950
30. Selander D, Dhuner KG, Lundborg G: Peripheral nerve injury due to injection needles used for regional anesthesia. Acta Anaesth Scand 21:182, 1977
31. Selander D, Edshage S, Wolff T: Paresthesiae or no paresthesiae? Nerve lesions after axillary blocks. Acta Anaesth Scand 23:27, 1979
32. Slocum HC, O'Neal KC, Allen CR: Neurovascular complications from malposition on the operating table. Surg Gynecol Obstet 86:729, 1948
33. Stephens JW: Neurological sequelae of congenital heart surgery. Arch Neurol 7:450, 1962
34. Wall W: Unilateral brachial paralysis after anesthesia with thiopentone, "Flaxedil" and nitrous oxide. Med J Aust 2:674, 1954
35. Westin B: Prevention of upper limb nerve injuries in Trendelenburg position. Acta Chir Scand 108:61, 1954
36. Wood-Smith FG: Postoperative brachial plexus paralysis. Br Med J 1:1115, 1952
37. Woolley EJ, VanDam LD: Neurological sequelae of brachial plexus nerve block. Ann Surg 149:53, 1959

7

Open Wounds of the Brachial Plexus

Open wounds of the brachial plexus differ considerably in mechanism, pathology, and management from closed injuries. In addition, they constitute a significantly smaller group of patients. The large database that is available from military sources indicates that even under wartime circumstances, they represent a fraction of nerve injuries treated. For example, the United States Surgeon General's Report,[4] which describes the activities of World War II, indicated that in one neurosurgical center 5% of all nerve sutures performed were for injuries of the brachial plexus. Of the peripheral nerve injuries treated at the Wingfield-Morris Orthopaedic Hospital in Oxford, England between 1940 and 1945, 52% of the first 1600 cases were due to penetrating wounds. The brachial plexus was damaged in 42 (6%) of these 820 cases. Similar proportions were reported for World War I, according to Brooks.[2] Gunshot wounds and lacerations by shrapnel account for most of the wartime injuries.

In civilian circumstances, bullets and sharp instruments such as knives and pieces of glass account for most of the injuries, although the widespread use of chainsaws, often by those unskilled in their operation, has created a new category of particularly pernicious open injury. Falls through glass windows (outside the sets of Western movies where no one ever seems to be injured) can cause extensive damage with complete transection of all the nerves and vessels in the axilla or neck. Unfortunately, iatrogenic open injury to the brachial plexus may occur during the performance of angiography with axillary artery puncture,[3] in the course of regional surgery (first rib resection for thoracic outlet syndrome), or during the course of the placement of invasive lines for diagnosis or treatment.

ANATOMICAL RELATIONSHIPS AS A DETERMINANT OF SURVIVAL AND THE OBSERVED SPECTRUM OF NEUROLOGICAL DEFICIT

The anatomical relationships between the components of the brachial plexus, the external configuration of the overlying neck, thorax, and axilla and the associated major vessels and pleura will determine not only what is injured in a particular situation, but how life-threatening the combined injury will be (Fig. 7.1). It is not at all uncommon for spectacular bleeding or a major intrathoracic wound to obscure the recognition and treatment of a significant injury to the brachial plexus. In a series of nine patients at the Valley Forge General Hospital who, during the Vietnam war, sustained wounds of the chest with associated injury to the brachial plexus, prompt treatment of the chest wounds resulted in rapid recovery, but recognition of the brachial plexus injury was frequently delayed.

Some less fortunate individuals may die of massive hemorrhage or intrathoracic pathology before they can be treated, in which case the brachial plexus injury is of no consequence. Particularly in emergency room settings, patients may actually incur significant damage to the brachial plexus during attempts to arrest severe bleeding from the subclavian vessels. Since the upper and intermediate trunks are not intimately associated with these large vessels and do not have the protection afforded by the clavicle and first rib, they tend to be injured more often, and the patients are more likely to survive than are those who sustain wounds of the lower trunk. In the latter situation, not only may either the subclavian artery and/or vein be injured, but the pleura and underlying

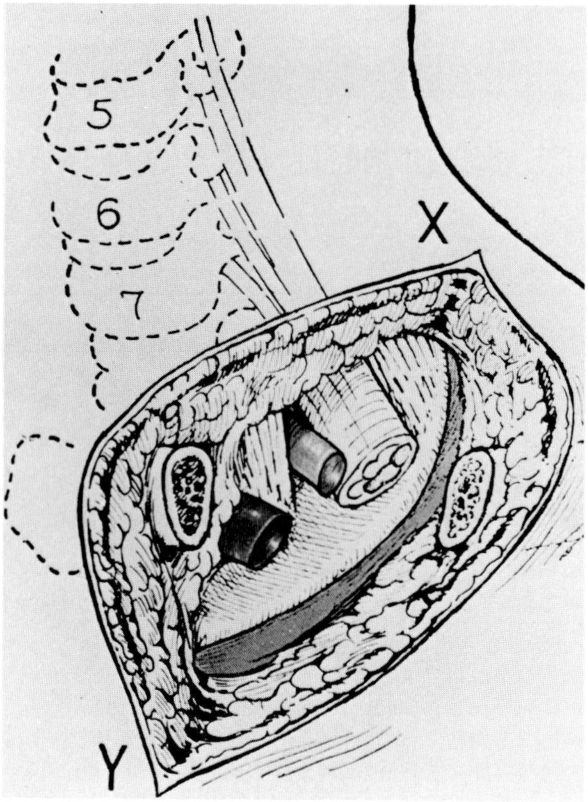

Fig. 7.1. Note the close relationship between the subclavian artery and the lower trunk of the brachial plexus.

lung may also be lacerated. Most authors have commented on the higher frequency of upper and intermediate trunk lesions as clinically observed.[2,4,7,8]

THE NATURE OF THE WOUNDING AGENT AND THE PATHOLOGY PRODUCED

It is most important to realize that all open wounds are not the same and that the nature of the pathology that they produce can vary tremendously. The simplest situation, that of a sharp laceration by a knife or shard of glass, involves a clean transection of nerve with virtually no traction element, and unless the injury is of a skiving type, there will be a relatively clean cut. The advantage of this situation is that little or no nerve substance will be destroyed beyond the relatively small area of the laceration. Little resection will be required, thus making direct suture possible. If, on the other hand, the laceration is produced by the kickback of a chainsaw, the damage will be considerably more extensive. Assuming the patient survives and can get to a hospital, the first priority will be that of resuscitation with treatment of the hemorrhage and the pulmonary problem that is often present. I have seen three such patients in the last two years and have explored two of them late, while my colleagues in the Department of Neurosurgery verified the pathology in the third patient at the time of his initial trauma and vascular reconstruction. In all three cases, there was extensive damage to the plexus over a wide area, and in one, actual nerve root avulsion at two levels was demonstrable. The possibility of reconstruction in such patients is considerably more limited than those in whom a sharp transection of the nerves has occurred, and in one of my cases there were no remnants of the brachial plexus to be found above the clavicle.

Gunshot wounds of the plexus are rarely complete in terms of their neurological deficit and may or may not be accompanied by significant vascular or pulmonary problems. If they are complete, they very often become partial over the first few weeks after injury.[2,8] This phenomenon results from the fact that the nerves may be either partially injured by a direct hit, or they may be concussed by the near miss of a bullet that produces significant shock wave distortion of the soft tissues surounding its path. Such lesions are often temporary and represent either neurapraxias or axonotmesis. The further implications of these phenomena will be discussed in subsequent parts of this chapter.

EXPERIENCE AND TREATMENT OF OPEN WOUNDS OF THE BRACHIAL PLEXUS

As has already been stated, the number of patients who sustain and are treated for open wounds of the brachial plexus is relatively small, and reports are sparse. The most extensively documented experience in the literature is that of Brooks[2] working at the Oxford Peripheral Nerve Injury Center during World War II. There were 42 patients. Twenty-two operative explorations were undertaken because there was either a severe lesion involving the whole plexus, a complete lesion of a localized part of the plexus, or persistent pain in the limb. In only four cases were the nerves found to be divided, with repair being possible in three. Brooks commented that, in general, scarring was severe and it was not always possible to expose the entire plexus. In addition, he found no evidence to suggest that neurolysis would influence motor or sensory recovery, although on one occasion it relieved persistent pain in the limb. It was exceedingly difficult to correlate the operative findings with prognosis.

In relating the eventual outcome to the location of the lesion, Brooks grouped his cases as follows:

Group 1: lesions of the roots and trunk of C5, C6
Group 2: lesions of the posterior cord
Group 3: lesions of C8-T1 or the medial cord

The recovery of cases in Group 1 was good, in Group 2 fair, and in Group 3 poor. With one exception, no recovery took place in the small muscles of the hand after a lesion in continuity was found. The good spontaneous recovery that occurred in Groups 1 and 2, the poor recovery in Group 3, and the rarity with which division of nerves was found in operation, as well as the discouraging results of repair in the three cases, forced Brooks to conclude that routine exploration of open wounds of the brachial plexus was neither profitable nor justifiable.

Nelson, Jolly, and Thomas,[8] who reported the nine cases from Vietnam associated with missile wounds of the chest, found the fifth cervical root to be the most vulnerable, and it was involved in each of the patients in their series. They recommended against surgical exploration and suggested that the rapidity and the magnitude of recovery of nerve function observed in their nine patients suggested that conservative management with physical therapy after reestabishment of cardiorespiratory stability was as effective as surgery in treatment of the neurological lesion.

In 1977 Millesi[6] stated that there were few indications for emergency surgery in cases of brachial plexus lesions, but he wrote that if there was an open injury by sharp instrument, the wound should be treated surgically. He also indicated that a missile injury with involvement of the plexus usually results in a partial lesion and that the chances of recovery are good, so that it should be treated conservatively, unless spontaneous recovery does not occur or is incomplete.

Narakas[7] reported having operated upon four of 12 patients seen with open injuries and repaired three of the lesions with grafts five to 10 days after the injury. In two, a good result was obtained. He also commented that it was difficult to judge the extent of the injury without inflicting additional trauma.

RECOMMENDATIONS FOR THE MANAGEMENT OF PATIENTS WITH OPEN WOUNDS OF THE BRACHIAL PLEXUS

The most pressing question in patients with open wounds of the brachial plexus is whether, in addition to the injury to the brachial plexus, there has also been damage to the vessels, pleura, or intrathoracic contents. Since these injuries are life-threatening, they must be dealt with immediately. During the resuscitation efforts, all care must be taken to avoid further neurological trauma. Many of these patients are in extremis when first seen. They are not good candidates for the prolonged additional operating time that would be necessary to repair their nerves, and such procedures should be done secondarily. In order to facilitate later reconstruction, however, the nerves should be identified and tagged with nonabsorbable sutures of different colors for later identification. If the length of nerve will permit it, a sling suture between the proximal and distal ends can prevent later retraction of the nerve ends, malrotation, or even gross mismatch.[1]

Sharp Cuts

Sharp cuts are produced by knife wounds or glass and invariably produce a neurotmesis. If there has been no significant vascular or pulmonary damage, if the patient's general condition is stable, and if the optimal facilities in terms of equipment and personnel are available, these lesions can be repaired primarily, although there is no evidence to suggest that a delayed primary or even secondary repair will produce inferior results. Obviously, if the neurological deficit is trivial, one must weigh the potential benefits of an extensive operative exploration against risks, including those of worsening the defect (Fig. 7.2). The upper and intermediate trunks in adults might be repaired with reasonably good prognosis for recovery, assuming that anatomical continuity can be restored and a large resection or extensive grafting is not necessary. With limited sharp

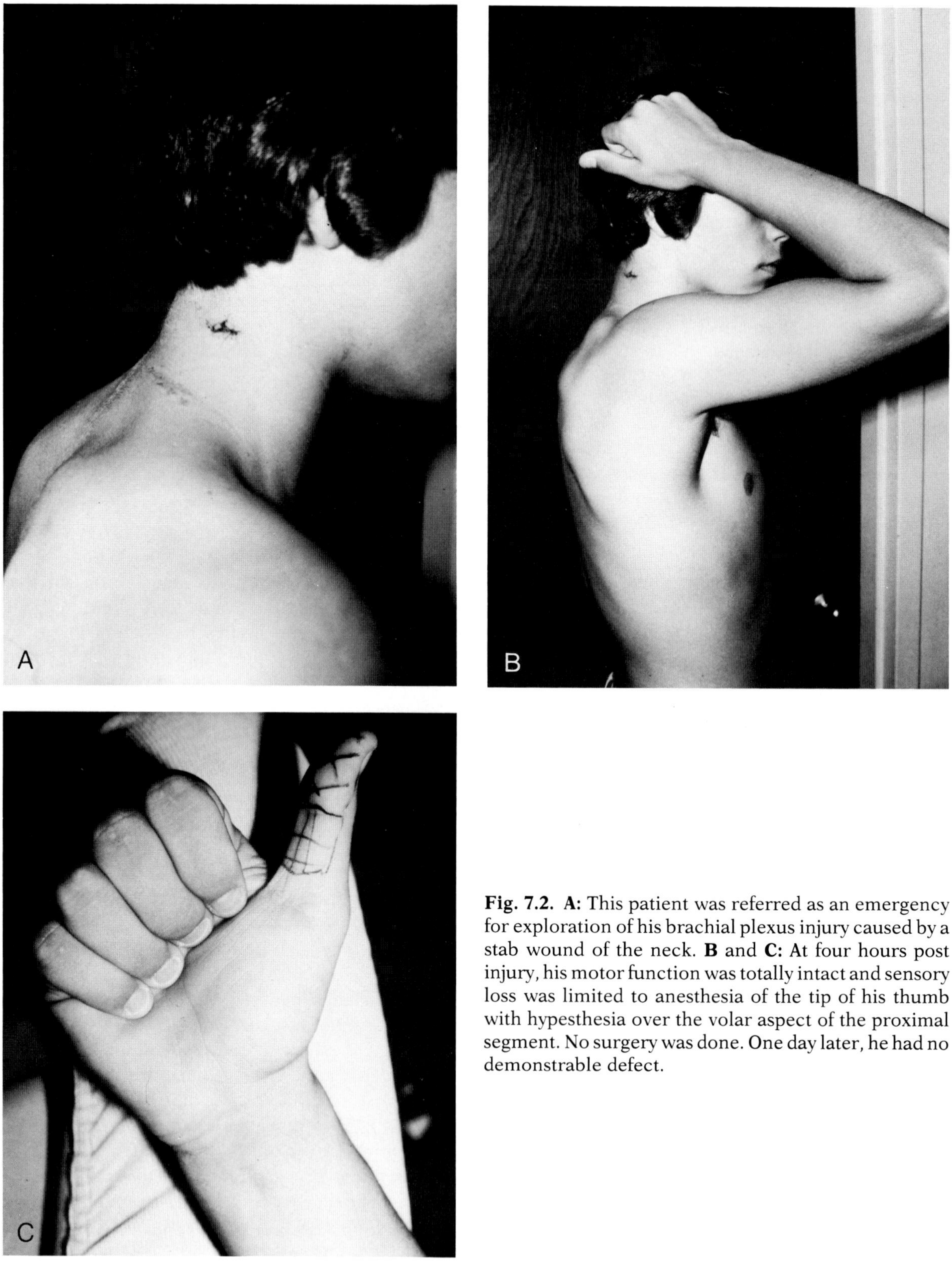

Fig. 7.2. **A:** This patient was referred as an emergency for exploration of his brachial plexus injury caused by a stab wound of the neck. **B** and **C:** At four hours post injury, his motor function was totally intact and sensory loss was limited to anesthesia of the tip of his thumb with hypesthesia over the volar aspect of the proximal segment. No surgery was done. One day later, he had no demonstrable defect.

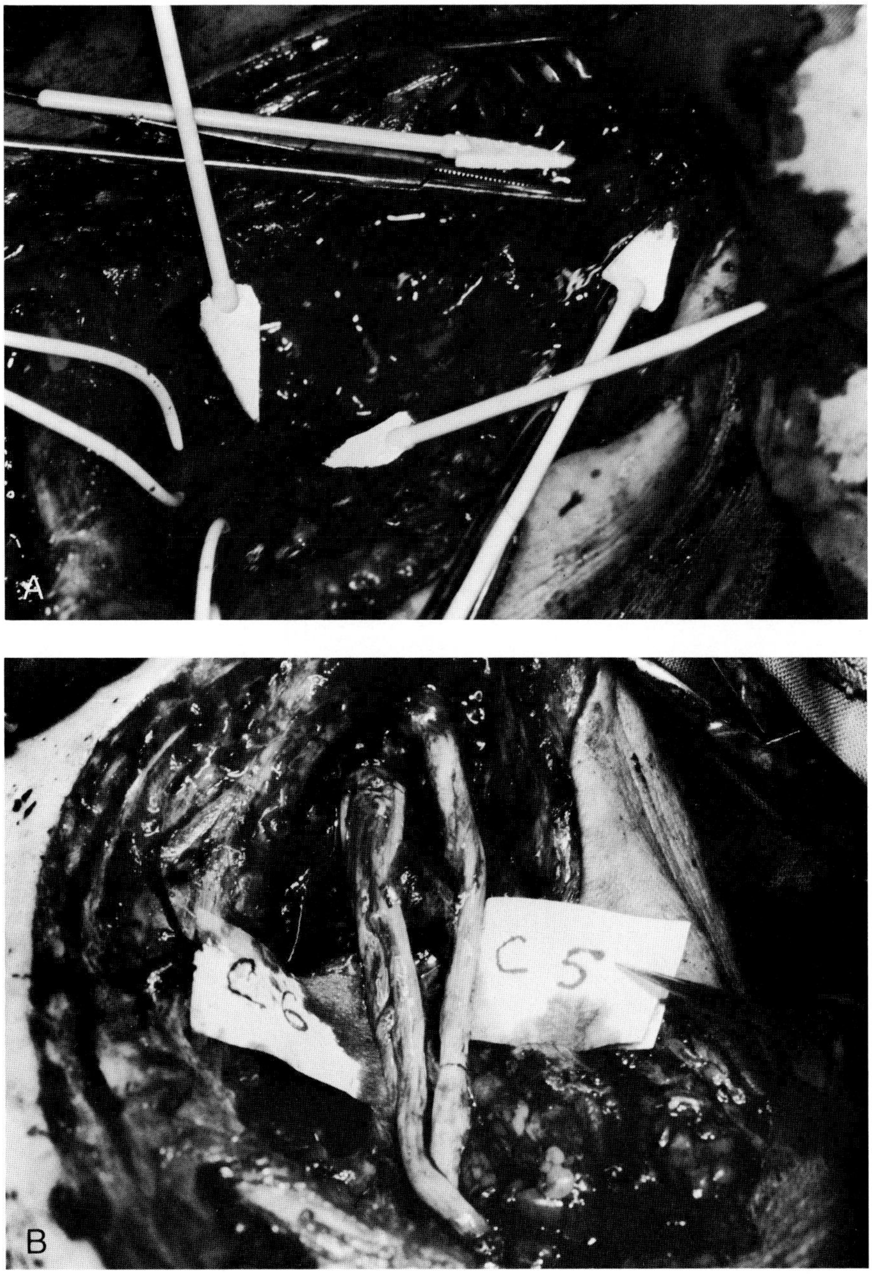

Fig. 7.3. A: Operative photograph of the posterior triangle of the neck of a 25-year-old patient who was explored 3 months following a chainsaw injury to his neck that resulted in a flail-anesthetic arm. Detail between the upper arrows (indicating upper trunk) and lower arrows (divisions of the plexus) is essentially unrecognizable. **B:** Following extensive dissection only C5 and C6 were found to be available for grafting. The ipsilateral ulnar nerve was removed from the forearm, thinned by removal of the dorsal sensory branch, and used as a graft between the roots and corresponding divisions.

cuts, this will usually be the case. In children, everything that can be repaired should be repaired, since, as differs from the adults, even the lower trunk and its terminal branches may be repaired with benefit. In adults, I do not believe that it is worthwhile to attempt repair of the lower trunk.

Chainsaw Injuries

Patients who have chainsaw injuries are often moribund or close to it when they are initially treated. There is extensive damage which involves not only laceration, but traction and chewing-up of nerve so that long segments may actually be absent

(Text continues on p. 138.)

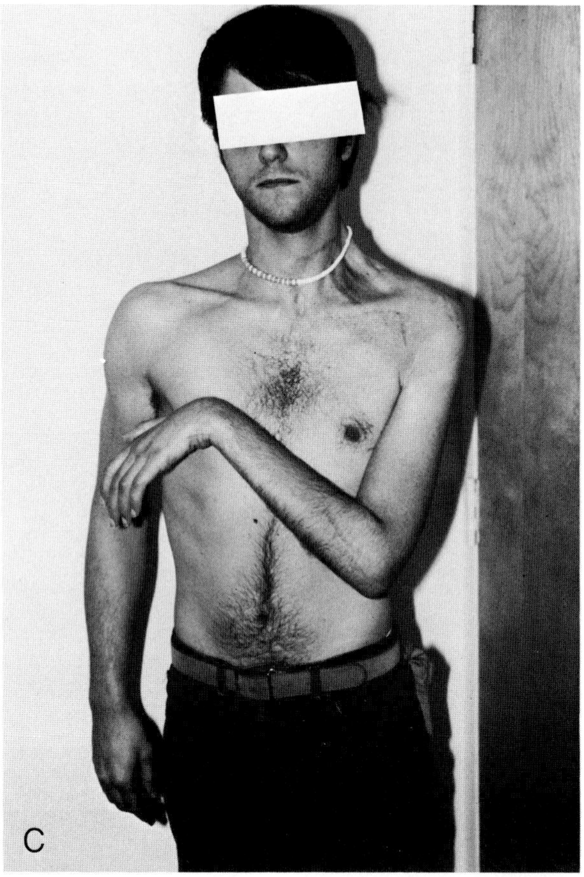

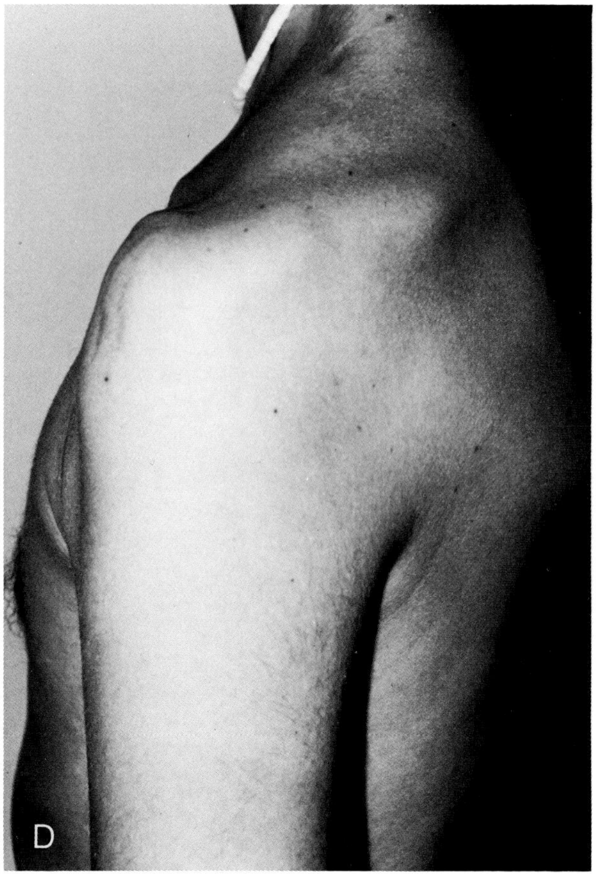

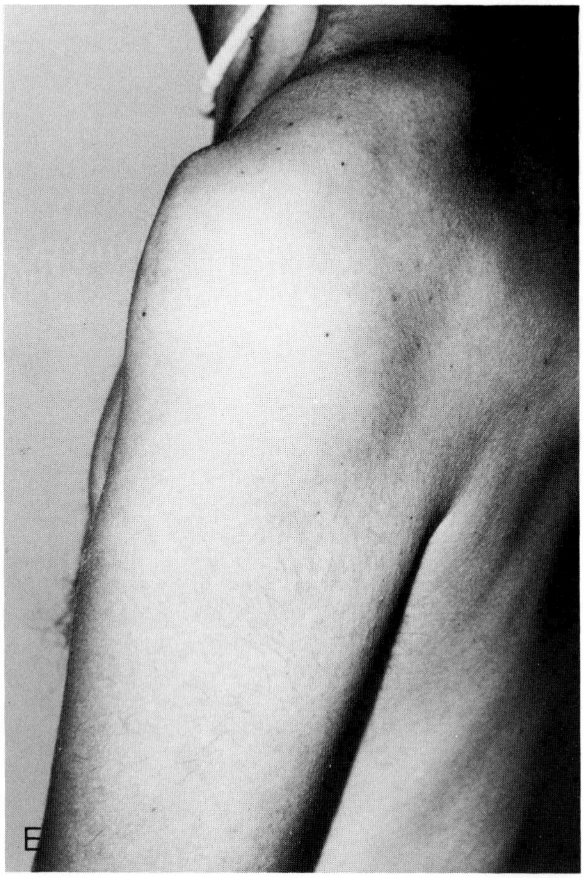

Fig. 7.3. *(continued)* **C:** Same patient one year later. Elbow flexion against gravity. **D:** Inferior subluxation of paretic glenohumeral joint. **E:** Demonstrating active contraction of deltoid to overcome subluxation.

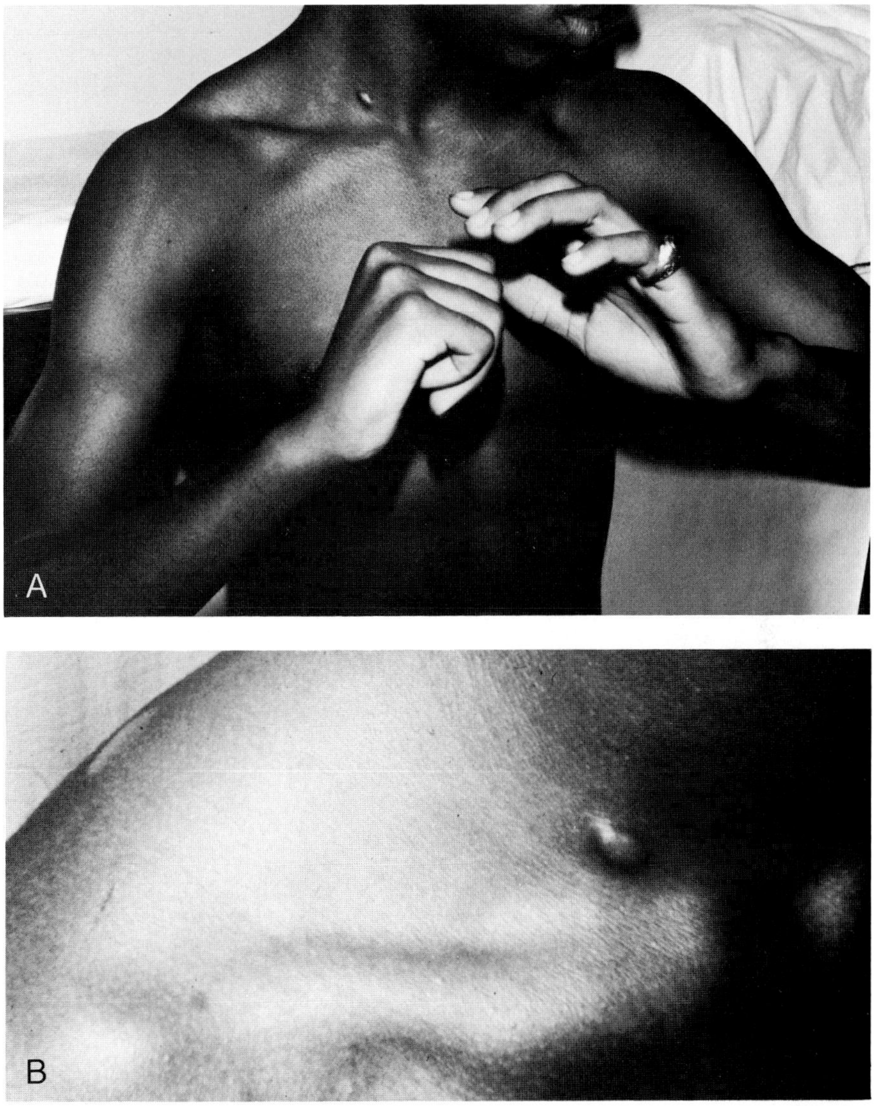

Fig. 7.4. A: A 17-year-old patient with small caliber gunshot wound of the right brachial plexus. Remaining motor deficit of finger extension. **B:** Closeup of same patient's neck showing wounds of entrance and exit. **C** and **D:** Active range of motion of fingers following tendon transfer of flexor carpi ulnaris to finger extensors.

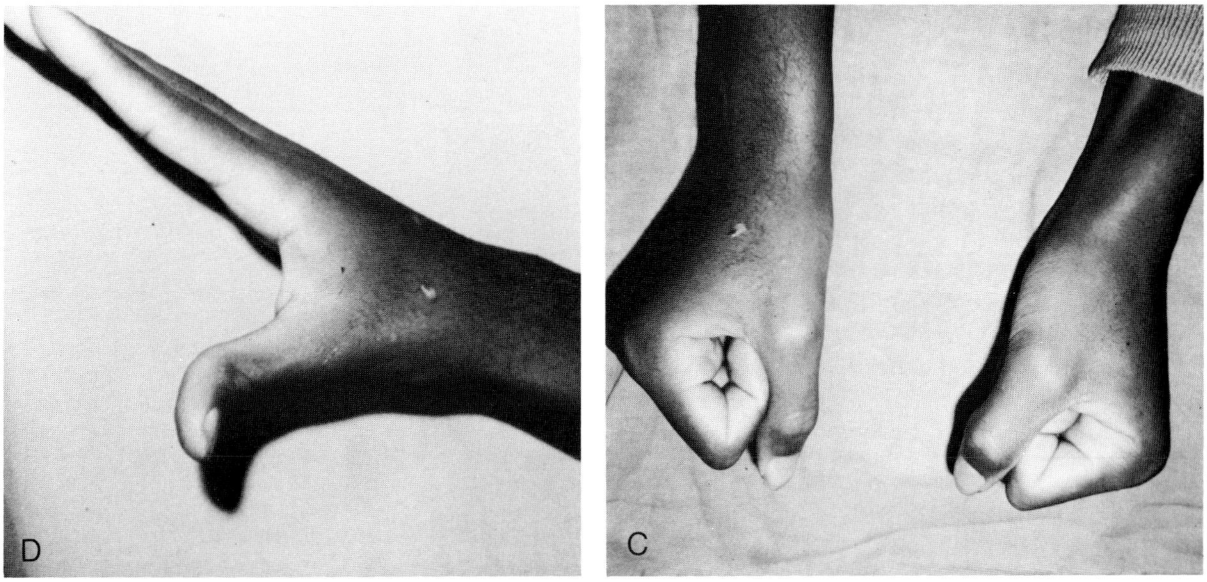

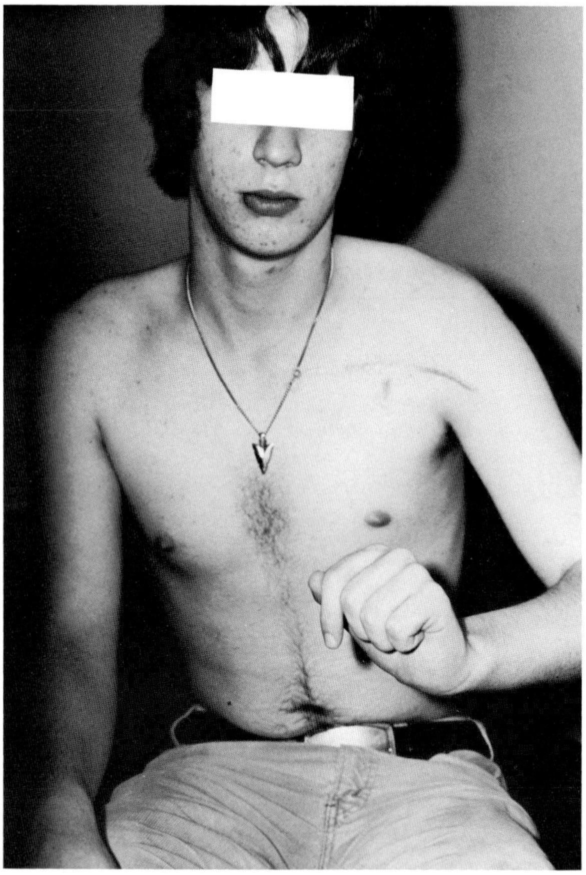

Fig. 7.5. Gunshot wound of infraclavicular brachial plexus that required arterial graft. In addition to partial median neuropathy which was residual at seven months when we saw him, he had severe pain successfully treated with continuous sympathetic blockade.

and require later grafting. Avulsion of nerve roots may occur. In these patients, the nerves should be identified and tagged. Myelography may be required prior to secondary exploration for clarification of their lesions. At neurological reconstruction (Fig. 7.3), which should be done as early as possible, before scarring is established but after the patient has convalesced from the initial trauma, it will be most important to avoid damaging the vascular reconstruction. Often arteriography and venography are of benefit in this situation. These patients invariably need grafting because of the long segments of nerve that have been lost.

Bullet or Shrapnel Wounds

Assuming there is no vascular or pulmonary problem, patients with bullet or shrapnel wounds should be treated conservatively with local wound care and physical therapy, as indicated. It is unusual for them to have complete lesions. Those cases that are complete usually become partial within weeks. If there is no recovery at all in three months, or it is incomplete with a major area of neurological deficit, then they should be explored secondarily. Peripheral reconstruction in the limb may, in some cases, be indicated (Fig. 7.4). Also, some patients may be left with chronic pain that may be extremely difficult to treat (Figs. 7.5, 7.6).

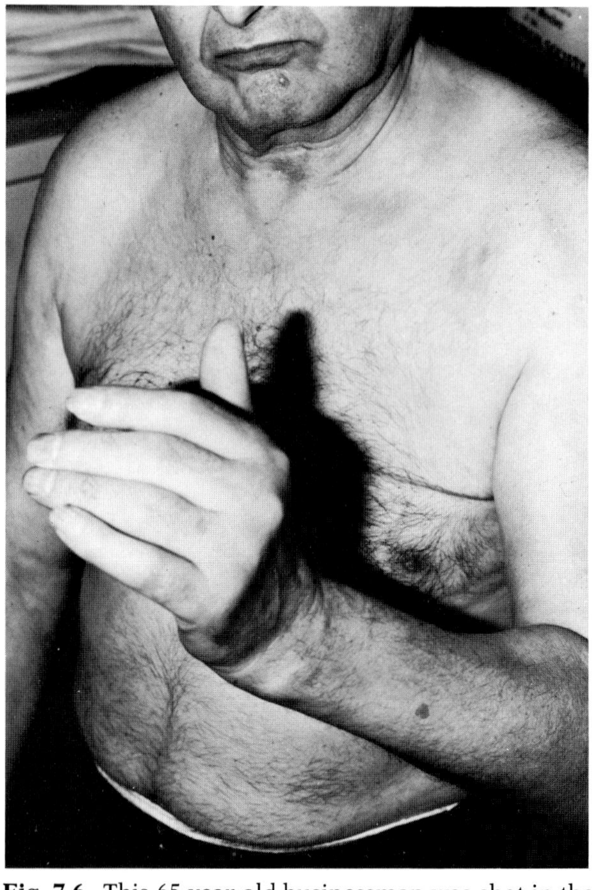

Fig. 7.6. This 65-year-old businessman was shot in the chest during a holdup three years prior to this picture. In addition to a massive hemopneumothorax, he sustained a total loss of lower trunk function. His chronic pain syndrome did not respond to therapy.

Brachial Plexus Injury with Arteriography or as a Result of Placement of Invasive Lines or Arteriography

Patients who have received brachial plexus injury through arteriography[3] should be forewarned about the possibility of neurological damage and informed of the symptoms that they might experience. As soon as neurological loss is appreciated along with increasing local and referred pain, they should be explored.

Operative Injury

If brachial plexus injury occurs at the time of surgery done in the region of the nerves and it is not deemed due to positioning on the operating table or the effect of rib spreaders in a median sternotomy incision, subsequent operative decisions must relate to the mechanism of injury and the part of the plexus that has been injured, as well as its individual prognosis for recovery following reconstruction. For example, a laceration of the upper trunk of the plexus incurred intraoperatively should be primarily repaired if possible. The prognosis for patients who sustain injury to the lower trunk of the brachial plexus during the performance of transaxillary first rib resection is generally poor. The injury may be sustained as an inadvertent laceration with the rib cutters, or as a traction lesion by placing a retractor on the nerves during the course of the dissection along the inner and superior aspects of the first rib. Some patients may actually sustain traction injury to the brachial plexus because of unrelenting pull on the arm during the course of the procedure. In these patients, the intrinsic muscles that have been completely paralyzed usually do not recover, even if partially paralyzed long flexors do. In such cases, the degree of clawing of the fingers will actually increase as the long flexors recover because of the increased disparity in muscle balance. I do not believe that surgery is of any benefit on the nerves but have found that peripheral reconstruction of the hand can help to restore function.

REFERENCES

1. Armine ARC, Sugar O: Repair of severed brachial plexus. JAMA 235(10):1039, 1976
2. Brooks DM: Open wounds of the brachial plexus. J Bone Joint Surg 31B(1):17, 1949
3. Carroll SE, Wilkins WW: Two cases of brachial plexus injury following percutaneous arteriograms. Can Med Assoc J 102:862, 1970
4. Coates JB Jr (ed): Surgery in World War II. Vol. 2: Neurosurgery. Published by the Office of the Surgeon General, Department of the Army, 1959
5. Lusskin R, Campbell JB, Thompson WAL: Post-traumatic lesions of the brachial plexus. Treatment by transclavicular exploration and neurolysis or autograft reconstruction. J Bone Joint Surg 55:1159, 1973
6. Millesi H: Surgical management of brachial plexus injuries. J Hand Surg 2(5):367, 1977
7. Narakas A: Brachial plexus surgery in symposium on peripheral nerve injuries. Orthop Clin North Am 12(2):303, 1981
8. Nelson KG, Jolly PC, Thomas PA: Brachial plexus injuries associated with missile wounds of the chest. J Trauma 8(2):268, 1968
9. Stevens JC, Davis DH, McCarthy CS: A 32-year experience with the surgical treatment of selected brachial plexus lesions with emphasis on its reconstruction. Surg Neurol 19:334, 1983

8

Radiation Neuropathy of the Brachial Plexus

GENERAL STATEMENT OF THE PROBLEM

Although the use of therapeutic radiation for nonmalignant conditions has greatly declined, radiotherapy for cancer remains an important and even increasing modality of treatment. Analysis of end results following radical mastectomy for treatment of early breast cancer, as opposed to therapy with limited surgery and radiation have shown the latter to have comparable survival rates. The evolution of radiotherapy technique from kilovoltage to small-field, high-dose megavoltage radiation has virtually eliminated the all-too-common and sometimes utterly disastrous skin changes that were seen with the earlier techniques (Fig. 8.1). However, because the peak dosage of the newer megavoltage radiation is several centimeters below the skin level, the superficial skin erythema is eliminated and the risk of damage to the deeper structures is significant.[16] For many years it was considered that nerve tissue, particularly that of adult animals, was remarkably radioresistant.[4] With more careful scrutiny of the experimental conditions from which such conclusions regarding animals, and by extrapolation, humans, were derived, it became apparent that these assumptions were unwarranted.[6,9] Clinical studies of patients who have developed neuropathy of the brachial plexus following radiotherapy have made moot any further debate, since there is little question that radiation-induced brachial plexopathy does exist.[8,10,16,18]

The effects of radiation on peripheral nerve function and structure are not only complicated, but must be assessed over a sufficiently long time to appreciate the widespread nature of the changes that are produced. Thus, earlier investigators failed to recognize the delayed effects and considered peripheral nerves to be relatively resistant to radiation.[4]

The early axonal response to radiation is an increase in the conduction velocity of peripheral nerves, which then gradually declines with time.[17] The late effects, in addition to those on the axon, are also angiomesenchymal. They result in changes in the vasa nervorum that obliterate the blood vessels and result in progressive fibrosis and ultimate disappearance of the neural elements.[9] Finally, the fibrosis induced in the supraclavicular and axillary tissues by radiation can result in edema, which may well further compound the problem of nerve compression and ischemia by producing more scarring.

From the point of view of the clinician having to evaluate a patient with brachial plexopathy presumed to be radiation-induced, it is, unfortunately, not always possible to obtain clear information as to the time and dosage schedules, as well as the size of the fields that were employed.

A number of studies exist to provide us with information regarding the incidence of this entity. Stoll and Andrews[16] in 1966 reported on several groups of patients. They stated that if it is assumed that the affected portion of the brachial plexus lies at a depth of 2–4 cm below the skin, a megavoltage dose of 6300 rads peak delivers a minimum dose of 5500 rads at the plexus, and a dose of 5775 rads delivers a minimum dose of 5100 rads at the same depth. In their series, both doses were given in 11 or 12 increments in 25 to 28 days. The incidence of neuropathy was 73% with the higher dose and 15% with the lower dose. They also reported two other series, the first a group of 25 patients who were treated by 4 MeV x-rays to a large supraclavicular

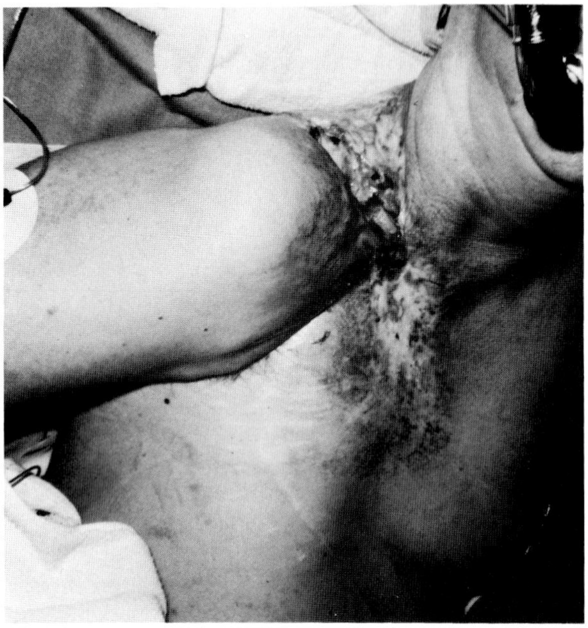

Fig. 8.1. Radiation necrosis of the skin, clavicle, and brachial plexus in a patient who was irradiated following radical mastectomy for breast cancer.

field to a peak dose of 4650–5550 rads in 18 to 20 days. About 16% of these patients became symptomatic. Westling, Nordin, and Hele[21] reported plexus complications in 35% of 80 patients receiving 4500 rads over a period of three to four weeks, while Notter et al.[13] reported an incidence of 17% at calculated dosages between 4500 rads in 27 days and 8100 rads in 21 days.

THE CLINICAL PICTURE OF RADIATION NEUROPATHY

As the reader may deduce from consideration of the data that has been cited above, there are still basic uncertainties in the understanding of the entity of radiation neuropathy. These are paralleled by problems in diagnosis, differential diagnosis, and, ultimately, in therapy. Most of the patients seen on a clinical basis will have received their radiation in the course of treatment for malignancies of the breast, although radiation neuropathy may be seen in patients radiated for other neoplasms and even nonmalignant conditions. However, because infiltration of the nerves of the plexus by malignant processes can cause similar if not identical signs and symptoms to those resulting from irradiation, the differential diagnosis may be quite difficult. Since most of the clinical studies that have been done in an attempt to further define the nature of radiation neuropathy have been retrospective, it has been necessary to evolve reliable criteria for assuring that patients who are labeled as having radiation neuropathy did not have local malignant disease. Although that would seem to be a relatively simple task, in practice it is not because of the similarity of clinical presentations of the two entities. There has been no absolute uniformity of criteria for assigning a particular patient to either the neoplastic brachial plexopathy group or the radiation neuropathy group.

In 1983 Lederman and Wilbourn[8] designated patients as belonging to the neoplastic brachial plexopathy group if

1. there was pathological confirmation of malignancy involving the affected brachial plexus or its immediate environs;
2. there was no history of irradiation to the region of the brachial plexus at the time of onset of the upper limb symptoms;
3. there were multiple metastases identified at the time of evaluation but no histological confirmation of brachial plexus involvement.

Thomas and Colby[18] in 1972 adopted a presumptive diagnosis of radiation damage when (1) surgical exploration of the plexus failed to identify a neoplasm but showed extensive scarring; (2) an observation period of more than three years from the onset of plexus involvement failed to demonstrate distant metastases; or (3) the radiation treatment had been given for a nonmalignant lesion.

A carcinomatous origin was suggested when (1) surgical exploration, biopsy or autopsy revealed evidence of malignancy in the plexus; (2) in the absence of direct tissue diagnosis, multiple distant metastases were found; or (3) plexus symptoms preceded radiation.

Despite the difficulties inherent in excluding patients with neoplastic involvement of the brachial plexus from the radiation neuropathy group, such determinations must be made on a practical clinical basis. The following factors must be considered.

Onset of Delay of Symptoms

In both groups of patients, there may be considerable delay in the onset of symptoms following either the administration of radiation or the discovery of the neoplasm. In Stoll and Andrews'[16] group of 117 patients treated with megavoltage x-ray therapy after radical mastectomy, initial symptoms were not noted earlier than five months or later than 30 months after irradiation. Match's[10] 15 patients radiated for neoplasms (13 women for breast cancer and two men for lung cancer) were reported as having had peripheral neurological symptoms and signs "at least 1–3 years after their radiation therapy." Thomas and Colby,[18] in a group of 25 patients, found a symptom-free period that was similar in both groups, with radiation plexopathy ranging from 5 months to 20 years, mean 6 years 1 month; metastatic plexopathy, range 2 months to 16 years, mean 6 years 7 months.

Dosage

The question of dosage has already been commented upon. The range has been great and not always definable in an individual case. Stoll and Andrews[16] have recorded neurological symptoms even after radiation doses in the order of 3500 to 3700 rads in 20 increments in 25 to 27 days, given by 200 kV x-rays. They also reported an incidence of neuropathy in 10–20% of cases noted for three dose levels: minimum 5100 rads in four weeks with 4 MeV x-rays; minimum 4100 rads in three weeks with 4 MeV x-rays; minimum 4350 rads in four weeks with 200 kV x-rays. Clearly, however, the incidence would appear to be related to the level of dosage and the higher dose group tends to develop symptoms before the lower dose group.

Clinical Presentation

Paresthesias in the upper extremity are commonly the first symptom of both radiation neuropathy and neoplastic infiltration. Although Mumenthaler[11] in 1969 reported that pain was usually the first symptom in the radiation group, the majority of the other authors have concluded that pain as a presenting or predominant complaint was considerably more characteristic of the neoplastic infiltration group and usually began early in the course of the disease. In the series of Thomas and Colby,[18] two of eight patients with radiation-induced plexopathy in whom pain was a predominant complaint had their pain begin relatively late in the course of the disease. Even in patients who had no pain, other sensory symptoms, such as numbness or paresthesias, were usually present. In both groups of patients, the sensory symptoms were more prominent than motor symptoms, although there were some in both groups in whom muscle weakness appeared first. Obviously, the distribution of the weakness and of the sensory symptoms depended on which parts of the plexus were affected. Here again there was no uniformity of agreement, although the outflow of the lower trunk of the brachial plexus appeared to be more commonly affected in most patients with either neoplastic or radiation-induced plexopathy. This has also been my experience (Figs. 8.2, 8.3). However, Kori

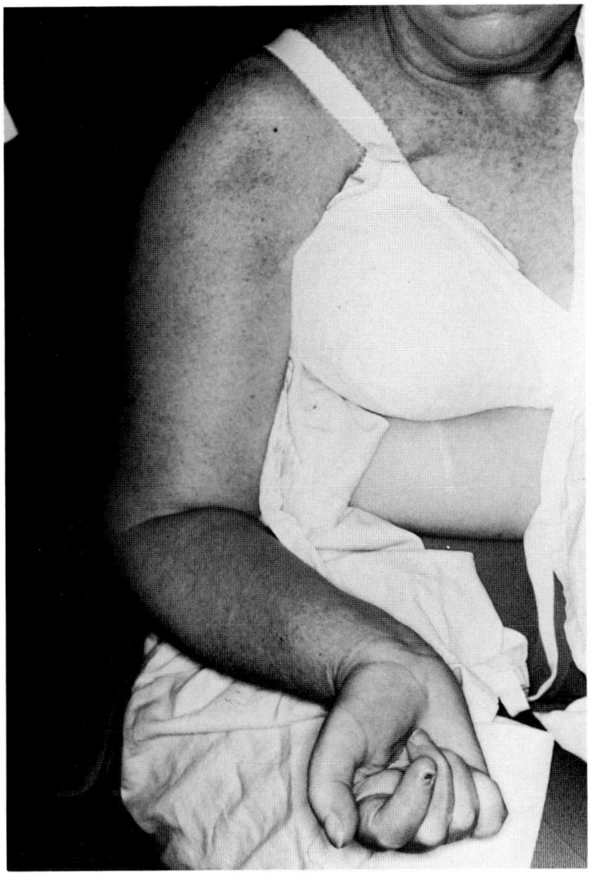

Fig. 8.2. Three years following mastectomy and radiation, this patient has predominantly lower trunk palsy with diffuse edema of her arm.

Fig. 8.3. Radiation neuropathy following treatment for lymphoma. **A:** Irradiated sites on both sides of the neck. **B** and **C:** The neuropathy was unilateral and spared the distribution of the upper trunk of the plexus.

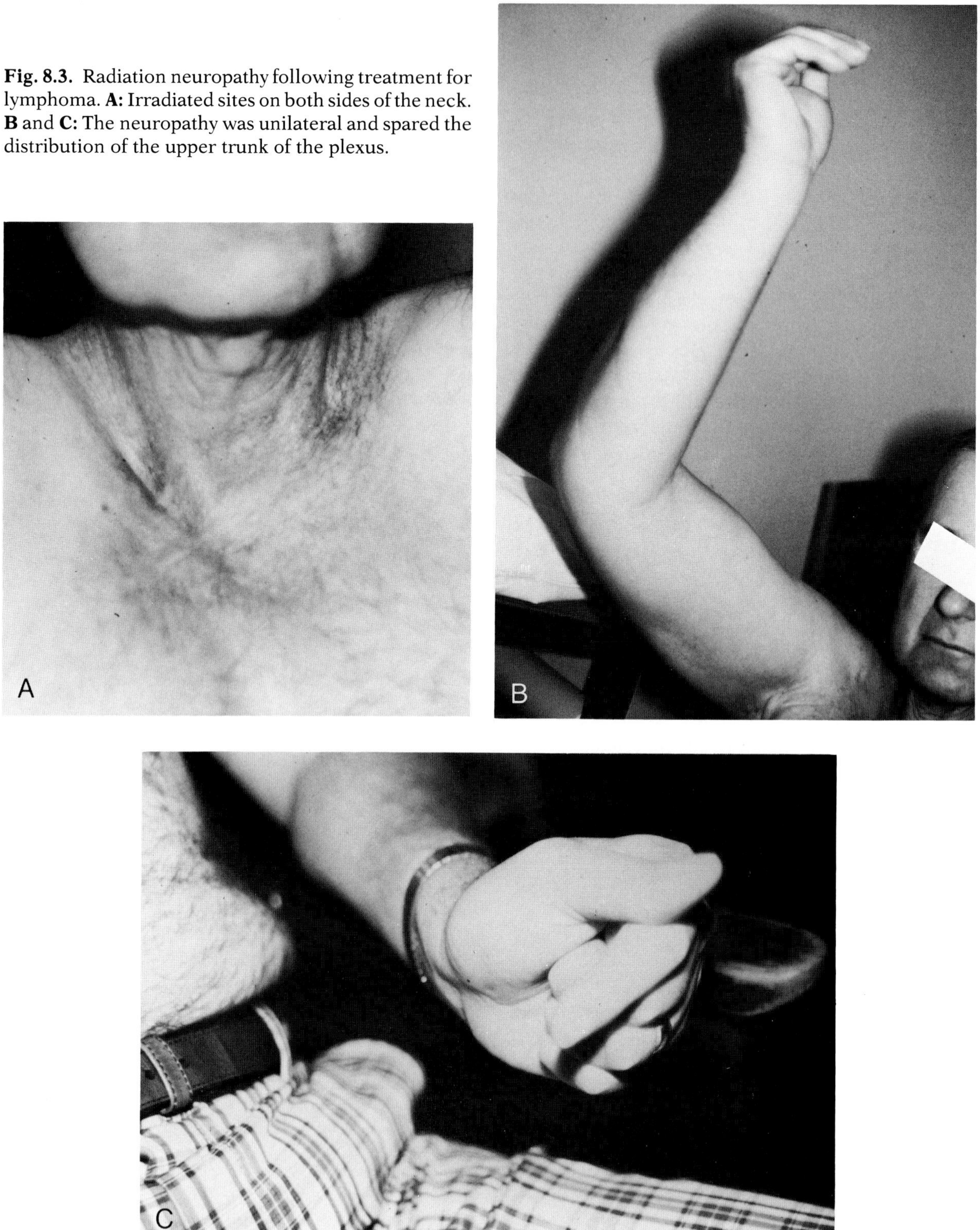

and coworkers[7] found 78% of the radiation injuries affecting the upper plexus (C5–6). The presence of Horner's syndrome was more consistent with neoplastic infiltration than radiation-induced neuropathy.[7,8]

Clinical Course

The natural history of both radiation neuropathy and neoplastic brachial plexopathy is of progressive loss of neurological function in most cases. Although there have been occasional reports of spontaneous halting of this progression,[18] there is only one study reported in the literature that documents actual regression of symptoms without treatment. This paper, by Salner, Botnick, et al.[14] reported on 565 patients treated between January 1968 and December 1979 with moderate doses of supervoltage radiation therapy (average axillary dose of 5000 rads in five weeks), of whom eight patients (1.4%) developed characteristic symptoms at a median time of 4.5 months after radiation therapy. All patients had paresthesias with weakness and, less commonly, pain. What distinguishes this group is that they underwent resolution of their neurological deficits. The factors responsible for the atypical behavior of these patients were not clearly defined, although they did demonstrate temporal clustering and a possible relationship to adjuvant chemotherapy.

EVALUATION AND TREATMENT OF RADIATION-INDUCED BRACHIAL PLEXOPATHY

Despite the difficulties of evaluation of patients with presumed radiation neuropathy, the clinician should avoid adopting an attitude of diagnostic and therapeutic nihilism and must perform a thorough examination with full knowledge of the limitations inherent in it. A search for distant metastases, including plane x-rays as well as bone scans (usually low yield), will define those patients in whom peripheral lesions are present, but if negative, it will convey no assurance of freedom from neoplastic infiltration of the plexus. Although one might assume that the absence of peripheral metastases could be assured after an interval of three years of plexopathy, there have been patients reported who have had malignant disease confined to the plexus for as long as four years without metastases.[18] Although the presence of edema in the upper extremity and local fibrosis are more consistent with radiation change, the diagnosis is certainly not assured by their presence.

Electrodiagnostic studies can be of benefit, particularly in ruling out patients with peripheral nerve compression lesions such as median neuropathy within the carpal canal or ulnar neuropathy at the elbow. The differentiation of radiation neuropathy from neoplastic involvement of the plexus in and of itself may be quite difficult. Recent experience at the Cleveland Clinic reported by Lederman and Wilbourn[8] is that the findings of fasciculations and/or myokymia in the radiation plexopathy group is extremely helpful in defining this group from the neoplastic patients. In their experience, it was the single most useful differential point in the electrodiagnostic studies, as had previously been reported by Albers and coworkers.[1] The Cleveland group also suggested that the CT scan or nuclear magnetic resonance (NMR) may also provide a more accurate and less invasive means of differentiating the two entities.

The question of surgical exploration must be considered from the perspectives of both diagnosis and treatment. There are no simple indications. However, when the factors that have been described above point considerably more toward a neoplastic etiology rather than radiation injury, surgical exploration must be considered. Since the pain of neoplastic infiltration can be palliated by additional radiation whereas that accompanying radiation neuropathy will not only not be helped but can be worsened, the differential diagnosis is more than academic. Such surgery must be meticulously performed with visualization of all neural elements of the plexus potentially responsible for production of symptoms, else a false-negative conclusion will be reached or, even worse, additional damage inflicted on the plexus. Limited "keyhole" explorations are not only likely to miss existing lesions, but are actually dangerous in an area where there is an increased risk of hemorrhage from vessels already damaged by radiation.

Surgical Exploration

Surgical exploration for treatment of patients presumed to have radiation neuropathy and who are experiencing progression of their symptoms remains a question that must be addressed on an individual basis. Unfortunately, the clinical data available upon which to make an informed decision are scanty. The questions that must be addressed are as follows:

1. Will decompression be helpful?
2. Should neurolysis be done, and if so, when?
3. Should neurolysis be accompanied by an attempt at neovascularization?

In 1962 Bateman[2] stated: "Release of the constricting scar by careful neurolysis markedly improves these problems." No supporting data was given. In 1966 Stoll and Andrews[16] discussed two patients who had severe sensory symptoms and underwent exploration of the brachial plexus above the clavicle. They were reported as having "derived some relief of their symptoms from this procedure, though motor and sensory changes persisted." Thomas and Colby[19] had four patients who did not improve after surgical treatment, which was attributed to the fact that these patients were operated on late in the course of their disease. Thomas and Colby tentatively advocated surgical exploration of the brachial plexus in every case in which there was a doubt as to whether radiation or metastasis was causing the symptoms, and suggested that early surgery in patients with presumed radiation damage might prevent some of the strangulating effects of fibrous tissue. In 1975 Match[10] described 12 patients who had undergone surgery on the plexus and who failed to improve in their pain or motor paralysis. Two of those patients demonstrated delayed wound healing of the irradiated tissues with substantial infection over the plexus. In one patient tissue necrosis developed with erosion of the axillary artery, which resulted in massive hemorrhage, amputation of the extremity, and death.

Recent reports from Brunelli[3] in Brescia, Italy and Uhlschmid and Clodius[19] in Germany describe neurolysis accompanied by transplantation of omentum in an attempt to revascularize the plexus damaged by radiation fibrosis. The reported results are favorable, particularly with reference to pain, but I believe that these procedures should presently be regarded as experimental and that they should be done only by those who are well acquainted with surgery of the brachial plexus and microsurgical technique. No patient should be subjected to such surgery without a thorough explanation of the nature of the surgery and the significant risks of making the neurological deficit worse.

The use of medical therapy to attempt to prevent some of the strangulating effects of fibrous tissue has been reported by several workers. Von Albert and Mackard[20] have been quoted by Thomas and Colby[18] as having used protein-free extract of blood, Actihaemyl, in eight patients with radiation-induced plexopathy and claim to have achieved arrested progression of the disease in all cases, with partial improvement of arm function. They also cite the work of Glicksman et al.[5] in the use of triiodothyronine, which has been advocated for radiation damage.

In a number of cases of radiation neuropathy that I have seen, the use of steroids has been suggested and tried. In my experience, neither this mode of therapy nor any other medical regimen has been proven to be effective. I have only explored three patients with radiation plexopathy. Pain relief was temporary and the neurological deficit was not improved. However, within the past six months, I have seen two patients who presented with the differential diagnosis of radiation neuropathy versus carcinomatous neuropathy from recurrent breast cancer without other evidence of metastases. In both patients the major complaint was pain, and both were proved, on biopsy, to have tumor. In one, a preoperative CT scan was diagnostic.

Thus, the problem of radiation-induced plexopathy remains unsolved. Only by accurate and long-term documentation of clinical data, and particularly operative results, will true progress in treatment be made as long as radiation is required for the treatment of neoplasms in the vicinity of the brachial plexus. It is hoped that, with advances in the treatment of cancer, the entity will eventually be eliminated.

REFERENCES

1. Albers JW, Allen AA, Bastion JA, Daube JR: Limb myokymia. Muscle Nerve 4:494, 1981
2. Bateman JE: Trauma to Nerves and Limbs. Saunders, Philadelphia, 1962
3. Brunelli G: Neurolysis and free microvascular omentum transfer in the treatment of postactinic palsies of the brachial plexus. Int Surg 65:6, 1980
4. Clemedson CJ, Nelson A: In Errera M, Fossberg A (eds): Mechanisms in Radiobiology. Vol 2. Academic Press, New York, 1960

5. Glicksman AS, Kitagawa T, Fillmore RR, et al: Effect of L-triiodothyronine on post-irradiation fibrosis. Radiology 77:799, 1961
6. Haymaker W, Lindgren M: Nerve disturbances following exposure to ionizing radiation. In Vinker DJ, Bruyn GW (eds): Handbook of Clinical Neurology. Vol 7: Diseases of Nerves. Part II. North-Holland Publishing, Amsterdam, 1970
7. Kori SH, Foley KM, Posner JB: Brachial plexus lesions in patients with cancer. Neurology (NY) 31(1):45, 1981
8. Lederman RJ, Wilbourn AJ: Brachial plexopathy: Recurrent cancer or radiation? Presented at the American Academy of Neurology Meeting, San Diego, CA, April, 1983
9. Linder E: Über das funktionelle und morphologische Verhalten peripherer Nerven längere. Z Nachbestrahl Fortschr Röntgenstr 90:618, 1959
10. Match RM: Radiation-induced brachial plexus paralysis. Arch Surg 110:384, 1975
11. Mumenthaler M: Armplexusparesen in Anschluss an Röntgenbestrahlung: Mitteilung von 8 eigenen Beobachtungen. Schweiz Med Wochenschr 94:1069, 1964
12. Nisce LZ, Chu F: Radiation therapy of brachial plexus syndrome from breast cancer radiation 91:1022, 1968
13. Notter G, Hallberg O, Vikterlof KJ: Strahlenschaden am Plexus brachialis bei Patienten mit Mammakarzinom. Strahlentherapie 139:538, 1970
14. Salner AL, Botnick LE, Herzog AG, et al: Reversible brachial plexopathy following primary radiation therapy for breast cancer. Cancer Treat Rep 65(9–10):797, 1981
15. Spiess H: Schädigungen am peripheren nervensystem durch ionisierende Strahlen. Springer-Verlag, Berlin, 1972
16. Stoll BA, Andrews JT: Radiation-induced peripheral neuropathy. Br Med J 1:834, 1966
17. Sunderland S: Nerves and Nerve Injuries, 2nd Ed. Churchill Livingstone, Edinburgh, London, and New York, 1977
18. Thomas JE, Colby MY: Radiation-induced or metastatic brachial plexopathy? JAMA 222, 1972
19. Uhlschmid G, Clodius L: A new use for the freely transplanted omentum. Management of a late radiation injury of the brachial plexus using freely transplated omentum and neurolysis. Chirurgie, 49(11):714, 1978
20. Von Albert HH, Mackert B: Eine neue Behandlungsmöglichkeit strahlenbedingter Armplexusparesen nach Mammakarzinomoperation. Dtsch Med Wochenschr 95:2119, 1970
21. Westling P, Nordin G, Hele P: Cervikalplexuslasioner efter postoperativ stralterapi vid cancer mammae. Nord Med 80:1636, 1968

9

Conservative Management of Patients with Brachial Plexus Injury

In many cases, long periods of time may elapse in the treatment of patients with brachial plexus injury where no overt or dramatic evidence of recovery appears to be occurring. A general philosophy of vigilant, active care-taking and guidance must therefore be adopted by the responsible physician or surgeon. Only the uninitiated or those without knowledge of the complexity of the problem would fall into the trap of regarding the situation as necessitating only "benign neglect."

Once the therapeutic relationship has been established, it is the doctor's responsibility to have reviewed all facets of the diagnostic workup, including the initial history and physical examination and radiographs. Rarely are complete or formal manual muscle testing charts available, but sometimes they may be reconstructed from narrative summaries. It is useful to ask the patient to describe in his own words the initial extent of motor loss or sensory deficit and what has changed with the passage of time, assuming that someone else has cared for him previously. If electrodiagnostic studies have been performed, then the details must be reviewed to avoid merely accepting the diagnostic impression at the end of the report, since it may be neither pertinent nor correct. Particular attention should be paid to the time between injury and the first electrodiagnostic studies, since those done before three weeks post injury will rarely accurately reflect the degree of damage unless it was preexistent.

If myelography has been performed, it is absolutely vital to obtain the actual films or good copies of them, rather than the reports. I have had the startling experience of referral of a patient who reportedly had myelographic indication of avulsion of all his roots, only to find on reviewing the actual films that his myelogram was normal! Rather than an amputation of his arm he underwent a partial reconstruction of his brachial plexus along with a neurolysis and obtained useful function in the limb.

It is unfortunate, but true, that patients who sustain injury to the brachial plexus, particularly in motorcycle accidents, often suffer from multisystem trauma. They may have incurred a variety of injuries, any or all of which may seriously and adversely affect the ultimate functional result in the limb. Because of the overwhelming menace of the brachial plexus injury, fractures and joint injuries may have been treated inadequately, or, as in the case of the immobilization that is required for their treatment, the result may be incapacitating stiffness. Skin coverage problems may produce a similar result or such fragile or painful soft tissue that function may be further compromised.

Infections anywhere in the body, and particularly in the paretic limb, must be noted and controlled. Obviously, all considerations of surgical reconstruction must be delayed until sepsis has resolved. This prohibition should extend even to considerations of myelography, although with care it is possible to perform needle electromyography if the infection is not particularly virulent and is sufficiently far removed from the site being examined.

Vascular injury in the upper limb often accompanies neural injury and may, to a large degree, serve as a prognostic factor. Where sufficient traction has been produced on a limb to rupture the subclavian artery and vein, the outlook for the neural structures is extremely poor. Furthermore, with vascular insufficiency, the quality of the neural recovery will be adversely affected as well. It should be noted, however, that virtually all patients with significant nerve injury will be cold-sensitive, and their limbs may appear dysvascular, despite the absence of a discrete arterial or venous lesion.

The presence of a brachial plexus injury does not confer immunity against peripheral nerve injury further distally in the same limb. It can be very difficult to make such a diagnosis with certainty in some cases, although in the presence of open wounds and with some closed fractures where there is sufficient anatomical disruption that such nerve injury would be likely under ordinary circumstances, there should be a high index of suspicion. The combination of a brachial plexus injury and injury to ipsilateral peripheral nerves further distally may constitute a most difficult problem in treatment.

Not uncommonly, and particularly where a motorcyclist was not wearing a helmet at the time of impact, a head injury may either mask the presence of the brachial plexus injury or complicate its management.

The social and emotional problems of patients with brachial plexus injury are many and varied. Not only is the fact of suddenly losing all or part of the function of a limb emotionally and economically catastrophic, but some of these patients have already had premorbid difficulties that may have directly contributed to the circumstances of the brachial plexus injury. Since the largest single group of patients have been motorcyclists, and since they tend to be people who work with their hands, the alteration in their potential for making a living or even taking care of themselves is very dramatic indeed. The social and economic problems stemming from the brachial plexus injury may generate reams of paperwork from governmental agencies and insurance companies that may plague the physician and ultimately so annoy him that he may simply begin ignoring them. Unfortunately, they may constitute the sole source of support of the patient, and failure to process them promptly may literally cost him a great deal.

PROBLEMS STEMMING FROM BRACHIAL PLEXUS INJURIES

Paralysis

The degree of paralysis may be complete, in which case the result is a flail arm, or it may be incomplete and some function may be preserved. For the patient with a totally paralyzed upper extremity, the management of that paralysis may have been solved by the patient who elects to keep his hand in his pocket, usually not a very satisfactory solution. Most patients use some type of a sling that will support the paralyzed limb and keep it out of the way, and prevent further traction on the neurovascular structures, particularly if the shoulder is subluxated. Although the concept of a sling is very simple and generally appreciated, it should be remembered that its unremitting use can result in a medial rotation and adduction contracture at the shoulder, a flexion contracture at the elbow, and a wrist that is maintained in flexion, the thumb in the plane of the palm and the fingers stiff in full extension at all joints. In effect, the hand conforms to the abdomen against which it is held unless measures are taken to preserve its functional posture.

For the patient with a totally paralyzed arm, there is usually sensory loss as well, so that functional bracing must not only enhance use but also protect the limb from injury. Regardless of whether it was the dominant or the nondominant hand, it is obvious that the patient will now be a one-handed individual, and, in addition to whatever adaptations and techniques he learns on his own, it will be helpful to instruct him in one-handed activities, particularly if recovery is not expected. The occupational therapist can be particularly helpful in this regard and can suggest a number of printed references that are available to instruct patients in one-handed activities.

For those patients who have incomplete loss of motor power in the limb, the options as well as the outlook for continued or restored function is significantly better. Although one cannot consider motor paralysis in the absence of sensory loss, our discussion for this section will pertain to the former. Many of the same considerations of protection and keeping the partially paralyzed limb in a comfortable position will be identical to those of the patient with complete paralysis. No matter what the specifics of muscle weakness are, the most important consideration is that of preserving or enhancing function, if that is possible. All modalities that are brought to bear in the treatment of the patient must be simply equated in terms of whether they have this potential or whether they may actually hinder the use of the limb. Complicated braces may actually negate any benefit they could have because they are too heavy, difficult to don, or they may interfere with the use of the hand, if it can be used safely. Simple orthoses that can be custom-made by the occupational therapist for the individual patient are desirable. If they prove to be successful by a trial of use, they may be made in more permanent or durable form by the orthotist if desired. Often the commercially available splints that are advertised as "one size fits all," fit none properly. In addition to the various types of slings, of which there are many, orthoses may serve the function of static support of flail joints or, in a dynamic mode, they may actually be assistive and enhance active function. For the partially paralyzed patients, because they have more motor power and usually more sensibility, the use of functional braces may be quite beneficial. Even in patients who do not have function in the hand, but who wish to retain that hand, a functional brace in the form of a cable-activated exoprosthesis may be much appreciated by the patient (Figs. 9.1, 9.2, 9.3, 9.4).

It cannot be overemphasized that all joints in the paretic limb must be put through a passive range of motion where active motion is impossible, and that this must be done regularly and gently lest contractures or joint injury occur. It is unfortunate to see a patient who has developed the opposite deformity from what would be expected due to the nerve injury when a splint has been improperly and uninterruptedly used. Most patients can be taught to conscientiously perform a self-ranging program to maintain the mobility of their paralyzed joints. Some patients require more and some less supervision. Supervision should be done by both the therapist and the responsible physician, so that the constant monitoring of the patient helps to avoid the problem of joint stiffness.

The cornerstone of the treatment of the weakness due to brachial plexus injury is, of course, active exercise for those muscles that are capable of voluntary contraction. The best way of performing that function is by active use of the hand and the upper limb, but it may be quite beneficial to have the patient exercise to strengthen specific muscles. After reviewing the available literature on the subject of galvanic stimulation of paralyzed muscle, I am not sufficiently convinced that it offers significant benefit to advise or encourage my patients to use it, even though relatively inexpensive home stimulators are now available.

Sensory Loss

The major factor that makes the prognosis for function in patients with brachial plexus injury whose motor deficit may be identical to those with polio much worse than the polios is their loss of sensibility (Fig. 9.5). Not only is discrete function ad-

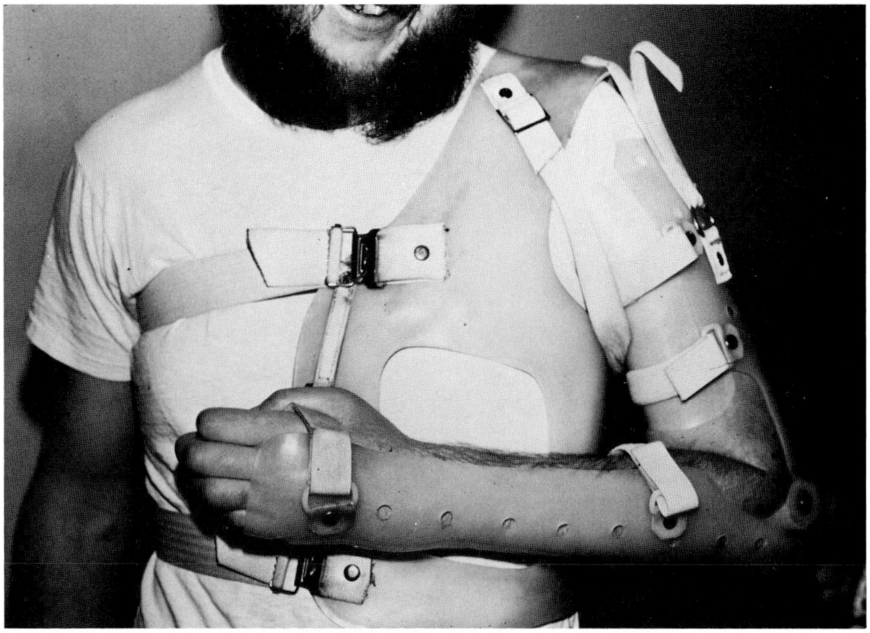

Fig. 9.1. A landscape gardener with a flail-anesthetic arm. The orthosis relieved his shoulder subluxation and protected his hand and arm while he worked.

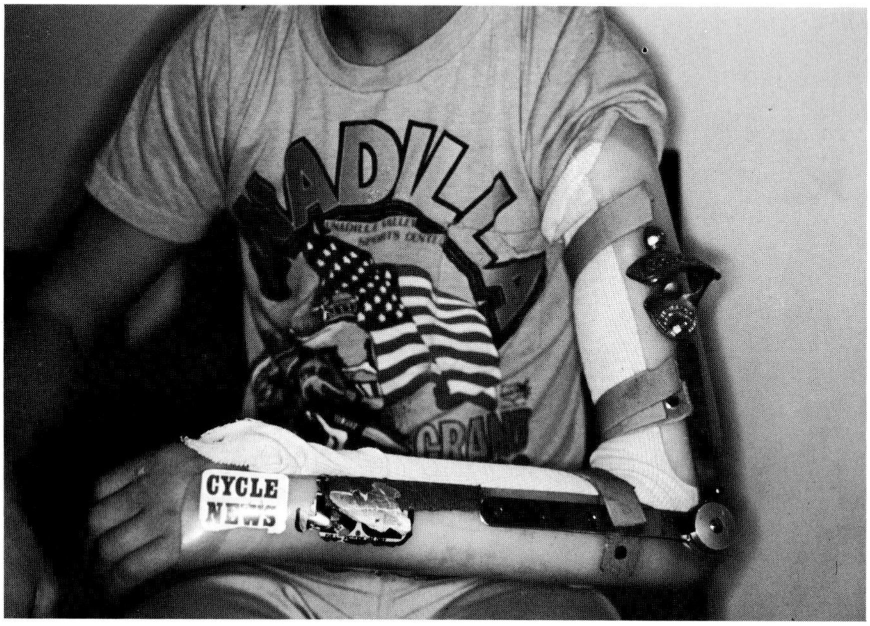

Fig. 9.2. This patient had minimal requirements from his flail-arm orthosis.

versely affected, but even the application of voluntary muscle contraction to gross tasks will be prejudiced. Those patients with C5 or C6 root lesions will have good grasp and release as well as intrinsics, but their hand function will be prejudiced because of loss of sensibility in the thumb and index fingers. For those with lower trunk or C8–T1 lesions, although the thumb and index finger sensibility will be spared, they will lack the motor power for grasp and, in addition, will have the vulnerability of anesthesia of the little finger even when that grasp is restored by means of tendon transfer. The problem of skin vul-

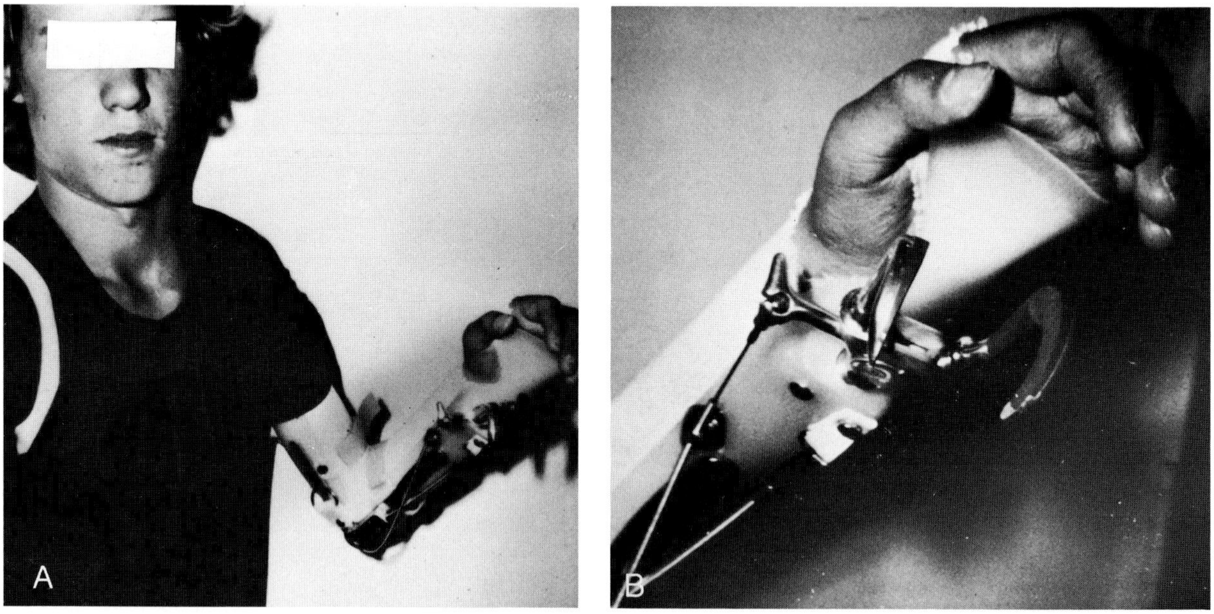

Fig. 9.3. A: This patient had shoulder and elbow control but no hand function. **B**: Closeup of the cable-activated voluntary-opening hook that allowed him some function in the limb without endangering his insensate hand.

Fig. 9.4. Types of orthoses for patients with partial function using spring assists and cables.

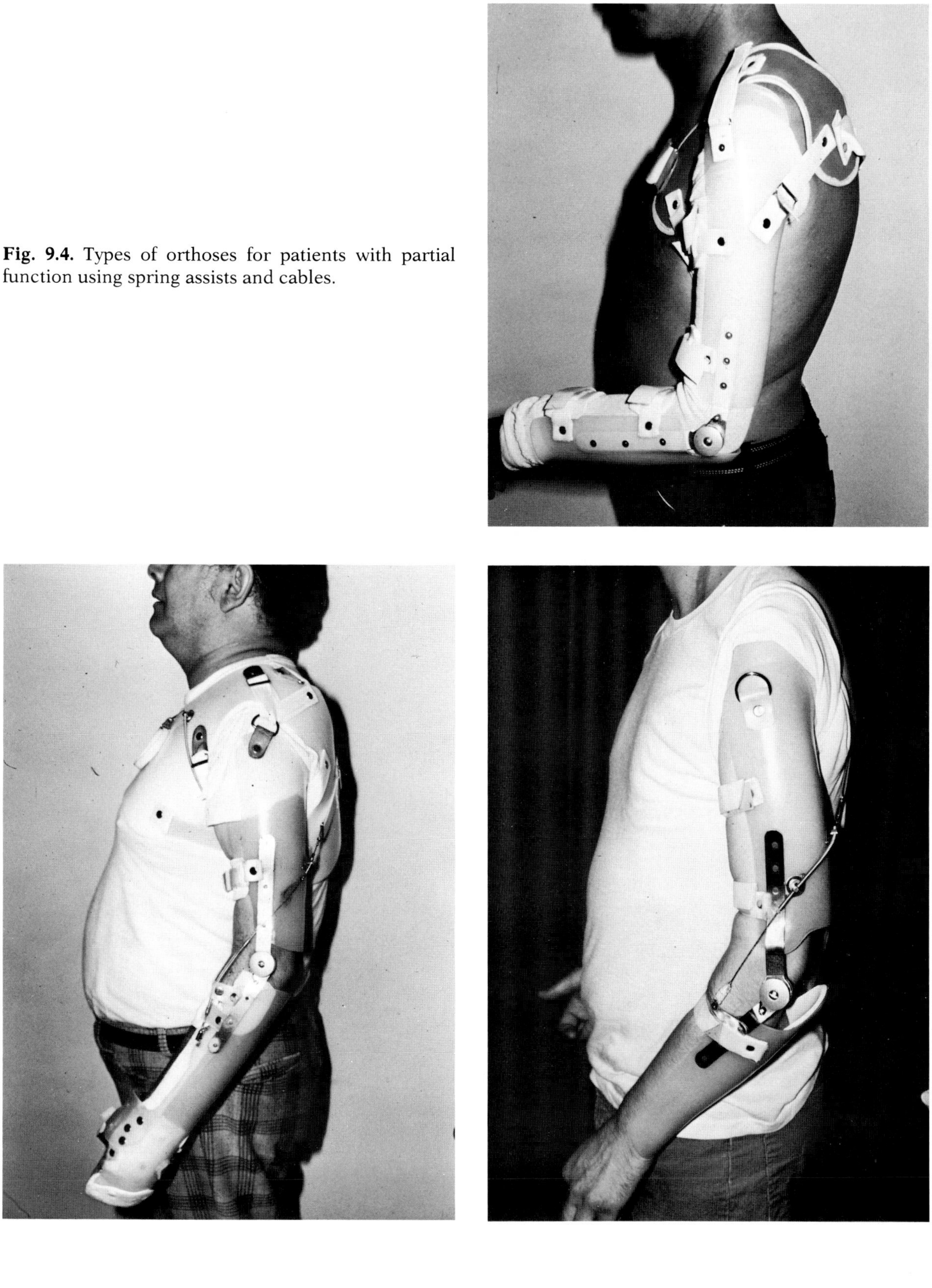

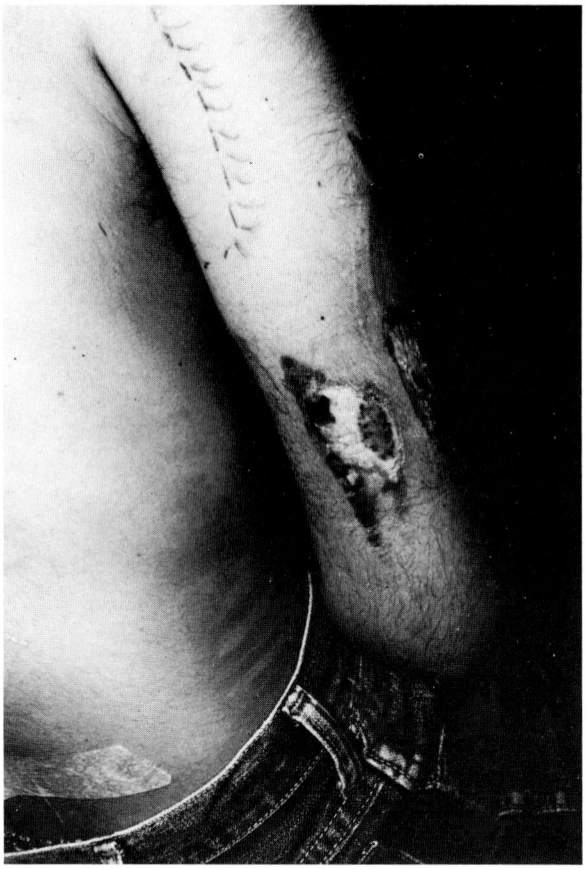

Fig. 9.5. Severe skin burns in the insensate arm of a patient with brachial plexus injury.

nerability requires that the patient be educated early in the necessity for protection, and this is particularly true for motorcyclists who tinker with engines. Even in patients who have undergone extensive reconstructions of their hands and who are able to use them for mechanical tasks, the anesthetic little finger is often the site of a burn. In some patients, because of infections around the fingernails due to habitual nail-biting, the trophic changes may be accelerated, and osteomyelitis of the terminal phalanges may eventuate in digital loss (Figs. 9.6, 9.7). In some cases, particularly in those with major sensory loss, the only alternative available may be amputation. Even more proximally in the limb, and particularly in areas where the patient may not be able to easily see the part without a mirror, the liability of burns on steam pipes or stoves is very real. Patients must be aggressively educated in the prophylaxis of skin problems and their early recognition and treatment. The experience with such prophylactic programs in leprosy patients has resulted in a very high limb salvage rate despite major sensory loss.

Ordinarily patients do not need to be told that if there is any significant loss of dominant hand function they will almost automatically shift to the well side. Nevertheless, such patients can obtain significant benefit from discussion of the problem with the occupational therapist.

Joint Stiffness and Muscle Contracture

The effect on upper extremity function of sensory and motor loss is considerably more than the sum of these two factors. In an adult, untreated muscle imbalance will ultimately produce contracture of the stronger muscles and overstretch, additional weakness, and local tendinitis of the weaker muscles. For the joints that these muscles cross and normally

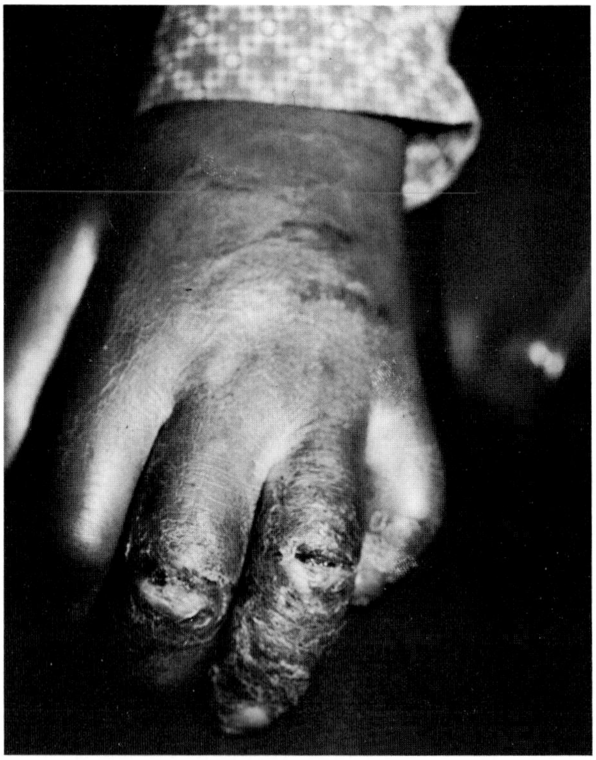

Fig. 9.6. This boy's anesthetic hand shows chronic infection due to nail-biting and lack of protection.

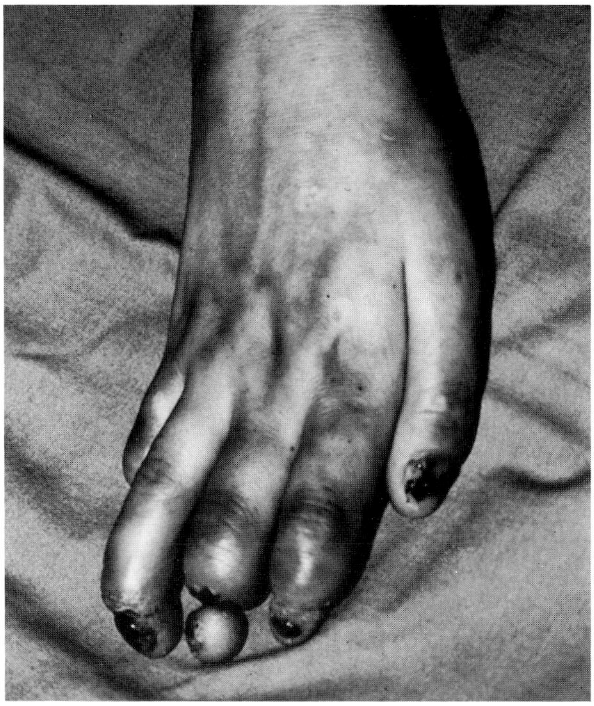

Fig. 9.7. Trophic changes and autoamputation of the fingers following brachial plexus injury.

activate, with time, articular contractures will supervene and make even therapeutic passive manipulation either difficult or impossible. Although myostatic contracture does not occur in sensory-denervated muscles with intact motor innervation, it is precisely the muscles that have been spared that will undergo myostatic contracture if their antagonists are paralyzed. If one superimposes edema or joint injury on this situation, then the propensity for permanent joint stiffness and loss of function is great. Although most motorcyclists are young and presumably vigorous and healthy, brachial plexus injuries may occur in all age groups, including the elderly, whose liability to joint stiffness is very well known.

Edema

Edema in the limb of a patient with a brachial plexus injury may be caused by a number of factors, some of which may be controlled. For those who have had root avulsion, particularly in the lower plexus, a functional sympathectomy has been achieved because of loss of the white rami communicantes. This may result in a loss of tone in the sympathectomized vessles and a diminished capacity to adapt to changing conditions. The loss of the massaging action of muscles and the movements of joints deprives the limb of an important mechanism of preventing and dispelling edema, particularly in the hand. Without support, the effect of gravity and the dependent position will materially aggravate the edema. Finally, vascular insufficiency and the residua of local trauma to the soft tissues as well as infection may perpetuate edema or make it difficult to treat.

The easiest way of dealing with edema is to prevent it. Then one must educate the patient and those caring for him about the importance of early recognition and immediate steps to alleviate the condition. Tight casts, bandages, and splints can be particularly pernicious on an insensate limb. The patient must be taught about passive positioning of the limb above the level of the heart whenever possible, or at least in a position that will encourage dependent drainage. For those with arterial insufficiency, in the absence of vascular reconstruction, appropriate positioning is necessary to allow adequate tissue perfusion. The patient with a stiff or fused shoulder is particularly vulnerable to edema of the distal portions of the limb, particularly if the elbow flexors are weak or paralyzed. These circumstances also suggest planning staged reconstructions to begin distally with the hand. Simple measures, such as the use of pillows when the patient is in bed or seated, may be of very substantial benefit. For those patients in whom edema has become established, it is mandatory to free the limb of excess fluid before it produces fibrosis and a stiff hand. Such patients are to be treated as semiemergencies. Their ambulatory status can be preserved by fitting them with a "statue of liberty brace" that is either commercially available or that can be made by the occupational therapist (Fig. 9.8). Many patients will balk at the prospect of having to wear such a clumsy-appearing device, but reassurance and a day or two of therapy will usually convince them of its efficacy. Although it is rare to have to proceed further, some patients who either have low-grade infections or are simply recalcitrant and less cooperative, may benefit from a short but well-supervised period of hospitalization, during which time the edema can be reduced. This final measure should usually not be necessary. All patients who are mentally competent can be taught the importance of

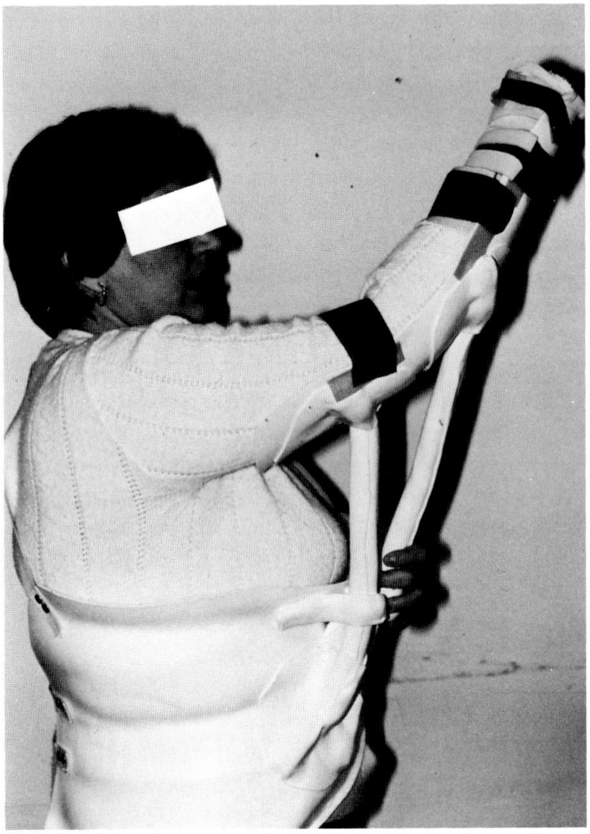

Fig. 9.8. The orthosis used for treating intractable edema of the hand.

a self-ranging program for those joints not affected by unhealed fractures, and they must thoroughly understand the importance of active use of the part in the treatment of edema. Sometimes they are afraid to use the limb, even when there is minimal sensory loss. They must be specifically instructed by the therapists with proper cautions of skin protection.

Elastic supports of various types are useful adjuncts in the treatment of edema, but like all modalities, they must be applied properly and with care to avoid distal edema due to a tourniquet effect or pressure necrosis of anesthetic skin. The various types of elastic cloth bandages can be safely applied one-handed by most patients, and the newer types of paper elastic can even be used on fingers. Elastic gloves usually require that the patient be premeasured so that the appliance will conform in a uniform manner. However, because they often take four to six weeks to be delivered from the manufacturer, the limb may change shape or size by the time they arrive, so they no longer fit.

In some situations, the use of "air splints," such as are employed in transportation of accident victims and in emergency rooms, can be quite beneficial in the temporary treatment of edema. It should be recognized, however, that there is at least a theoretical possibility of the production of a compartment syndrome in such limbs by means of external compression, although I have not yet observed it. In the setting of a physical therapy department, treatment with a compression pump apparatus as an adjunct to range of motion exercises and massage is of definite value. Finally, as has been emphasized previously, it is necessary to promptly and aggressively treat all local infections anywhere in the limb, since they tend to become indolent and progressively more difficult to eradicate with the passage of time.

Pain

The problem of the treatment of pain accompanying brachial plexus injury has remained difficult and largely unsolved, despite many and varied attempts to defeat it. Although not all patients with brachial plexus injuries have pain, a substantial number of them experience pain after the initial trauma. Most patients are able to describe painful sensations that are the sequelae of brachial plexus injury. They are generally present to some degree even if they become less severe, less incapacitating, or the patients simply learn to live with them. It is difficult to predict in an individual case whether a patient with a plexus injury will have pain, although the mechanism of injury may be a significant factor in the determination of whether or not the patient will have pain. For example, whereas not all patients with traction injuries, even avulsions, have severe pain, those with extensive avulsions, particularly involving the lower trunk, will be more likely to have significant pain. Often it is characterized as a burning type of discomfort and sometimes it has a phantom-like quality. Most patients with sharp lacerations of the plexus do not usually complain of severe pain, but those who are the victim of gunshot wounds almost invariably have pains, and in them the presentation is usually that of a classic causalgia. Possibly the type of injury inflicted by a gunshot wound predisposes to an irritative afferent barrage to the central nervous system. It would also appear that total plexus lesions cause more pain than partial injuries, and this may be a consequence of sensory deprivation. Some clinical investigators have, in fact, reported a significant improvement in pain after plexus reconstruction or neurotization.

Added to whatever neural mechanisms may be invoked to explain these painful stimuli are the effects of anxiety and depression, either or both of which may be a serious problem in the patient with a brachial plexus injury. They may considerably and adversely affect the patient's response to pain. The natural history of the severe pain accompanying traction injuries to the brachial plexus tends to be that of gradual subsidance with the passage of time. I shall discuss drug therapy later in this chapter. Suffice it to say now that it is not uncommon for patients I have seen to have spontaneously stopped taking narcotics that were prescribed by their doctors because they simply concluded that the drugs did not help the pain. In most cases, by the end of a year from the time of injury, most of the traction injury patients have occasional discomfort but do not find their pain incapacitating.

In addition to pain directly attributable to the neurological lesion, there may be significant discomfort that can be attributed to the derangements in the musculoskeletal system itself. Specifically, joints that become subluxated or dislocated because their muscles are weak or paralyzed and the limb unsupported may become significant sources of pain. The stretch of the capsular and ligamentous structures, which are well innervated, is a preventable and treatable entity. Particularly in the paralyzed and unsupported glenohumeral joint, the use of a sling can materially decrease the pain, which comes not only from the articular structures, but also from additional traction on the vessels and nerves which are not subjected to undue elongation in the normal state. Furthermore, secondary vascular compromise can occur for the same reason.

The presence of an unstable fracture in a partially denervated limb can be a continued source of pain, as can easily overlooked derangements of the sternoclavicular and acromicoclavicular joints. Finally, even in those limbs that are not frankly ischemic, cold intolerance is a virtually assured consequence of denervation, and it can be very painful. From what has already been said, it might well be deduced that the treatment of the pain of brachial plexus injury is essentially an empirical matter. Lest one become too convinced of the success of a particular modality of therapy, it is well to remember the capricious nature of the pain and the tendency to spontaneous resolution. It has been my experience that there can be very positive benefit from taking the time to listen to the patient talk about his pain, to try to identify some of the causative factors, and to provide reassurance that, in most cases, it does get better. The reader should not infer that one ought or could "talk the patient out of it," since I believe that this approach is simplistic. Furthermore, I have not had positive results from hypnosis in an attempt to accomplish the same thing.

Particularly for patients who up to the time of their injury have been physically very active, and even for those who are not, the positive effects of a generalized exercise and conditioning program should not be underestimated. It does not really matter whether you believe that the positive effects come from endorphins generated by the vigorous exercise or the psychological benefits from realizing that despite their injuries, they can still remain physically active, the end result is one that should be encouraged. Patients who have been avid joggers, swimmers, and even skiers, have been encouraged to and have continued to participate in their sports. The use of a nylon sling to hold the arm close to the body has been very useful, although some swimmers have preferred to simply let the arm float. Even for those patients who have not been exercisers, it has been my practice to try and get them to at least become avid walkers in an attempt to improve their level of conditioning. The one sport that I have consistently, but not always successfully, attempted to discourage has been motorcycle riding.

The pharmacologic approach has, like the surgical approach to the pain of brachial plexus injury, been marked by inconsistency of positive results. It is important for the physician to have taken a detailed premorbid drug and alcohol history, since failure to appreciate these details may make it impossible to properly interpret the patient's complaints of pain and to respond to them appropriately. Anxiety and depression have already been commented upon in terms of their effects on the patient's reaction to pain. Depending on how knowledgeable the individual physician is in diagnosis and treatment of these entities with drugs, there may or may not be need for additional consultation from a psychiatrist. Such referrals have the additional benefit of allowing the patient to ventilate the obvious feelings of anger, frustration, and anxiety or depression that often accompany brachial plexus injury.

It has been my practice in the long-term management of the pain of brachial plexus injury to avoid prescribing narcotics on an outpatient basis. Probably the most abused drug in this patient population is oxycodone (Percodan) and its analogues. Often the patients have been given the drug by well-meaning but short-sighted physicians who are anxious to relieve both the patient's discomfort and themselves of the annoyance of having to argue about the medications at each office visit and on the telephone between them. Since Percodan is readily available "on the street," at sometimes unbelievably inflated prices, some patients will manage to get it without a doctor's prescription. For those patients who use the argument that the previous doctor gave it to them and they cannot see why I would not continue the practice, I simply explain to them that, although I understand the fact of their pain and sympathize with it, I do not believe that it is medically indicated to continue to prescribe the narcotic. Although it is not feasible to insure that the patient will not obtain the drug from another source, I have generally informed the referring physician that all medications will be prescribed by me and that no further narcotics will be given. Obviously not every patient will be amenable to this arrangement, but a surprisingly high percentage of them will acquiesce if they are not frankly addicted. Sometimes the interval use of codeine will ease the transition to the nonnarcotic analgesics. The occasional patient who is recalcitrant or addicted may require consultation with a psychopharmacologist who is particularly skilled in this area, but it is usually these patients who are difficult management problems in every phase of their rehabilitation program, and their overall prognosis for a favorable result is generally poorer.

Propoxyphene (Darvon) in its various forms is a drug that is in very common use in the United States. It is a mild analgesic that is related to methadone, but less effective in pain relief. Nevertheless, it can be useful for the relief of mild to moderate pain, but since it can produce drug dependence, it should also be used with caution. Darvon can only partially suppress withdrawal symptoms of patients who are narcotic-addicted. It has a central nervous system depressant effect that may be additive with other depressants.

Usually, if pain has been a significant problem in the patient's management, some physician along the way has suggested the use of phenytoin (Dilantin). Although this drug is well known for the control of grand mal and psychomotor seizures, it has been used empirically in the treatment of the pain of diabetic peripheral neuropathy with some reported success. However, because of the capricious nature of the neuropathy of diabetes, it is difficult to be certain that it is indeed the pharmacological action of the drug that has resulted in improvement. Furthermore, since the most common adverse reactions are on the central nervous system and include slurring of speech, mental confusion, dizziness, nervousness, and headaches, I believe it is best avoided. Suffice it to say that in a 20-year experience of treating patients with pain of brachial plexus injury, I have never seen one in whom I was convinced that Dilantin was an effective agent in controlling the pain.

Carbamazepine (Tegretol), in addition to its use as an anticonvulsant, has had successful use in the control of chronic pain, particularly that of trigeminal neuralgia. It cannot be stated too strongly that the drug is a very powerful one with serious and potentially fatal side effects. Interference with hematopoiesis is the most common one, for which the patients must be screened weekly during the first three months of therapy and monthly thereafter. Since liver damage may also occur, baseline evaluations of liver function should be obtained and performed at regular intervals during treatment. Eye changes may also occur, as many renal dysfunction. In addition, a host of nervous system side effects may occur, as may cardiovascular problems and those of the digestive system.

The initial dosage is one-half tablet, 100 mg, twice daily on the first day. This dose may be increased by up to 200 mg a day using increments of one-half tablet every 12 hours, only as needed to achieve pain relief. If the drug proves to be effective, maintenance doses of 400–800 mg a day can be achieved in most patients. Despite the very serious potential for side effects, and the necessity for the treating physician to assume the responsibility for monitoring the drug and potential side effects, I have found that in some patients it has been very effective in the treatment of pain. Obviously, it is not a commitment that can be taken lightly by the physician or without total informed consent by the patient.

The past few years have seen the proliferation of the nonsteroidal antiinflammatory agents, which are, because of their analgesic properties, being promoted by many pharmaceutical companies as useful analgesics. In my experience, they are useful but have not proved to be more so that aspirin in therapeutic doses. The significant advantage of the new group of antiinflammatory agents is that they are considerably more convenient, since they require fewer pills, and it is easier to avoid irritation of the gastrointestinal tract. Since they are relatively safe compounds, it is worth trying them for mild to moderate pain, but they are not effective against severe pain.

The perioperative management of the patient with a brachial plexus injury who requires multiple-staged surgical reconstructions can present a difficult problem. Unquestionably, sensible medical management and basic humane considerations dictate that these patients do not suffer unnecessarily. Some of them, who have had significant drug problems in the past and who have been "clean," will express considerable concern lest they become "hooked" again in the hospital. In this group of patients, I have found the use of methadone to be effective. The drug is a synthetic narcotic analgesic that has many actions similar to those of morphine and, in itself, can produce drug dependence. In addition, it must be used with great care with general anesthetics and tranquilizers, since central nervous system depression, respiratory depression, hypotension, and coma could result. The drug must be titrated in the postoperative period, and usually a 5 to 10-mg dose repeated in 4 to 8 hours will be effective. Again, it is necessary to inform the nursing staff and the anesthetist preoperatively that this drug will be used so that an appropriate dosage schedule can be worked out and the patient's needs met while he is carefully monitored. Although narcotic antagonists can counteract the physiological depression induced by methadone, their action is relatively brief, usually not more than 1 to 3 hours, while methadone is a long-acting drug that can persist for as long as 48 hours. Again, this is a useful drug but, particularly in the nontolerant individual, it must be used with great caution.

Although a detailed treatise on the management of chronic pain is well beyond the scope or intent of this monograph, I would conclude this section by saying that I do not hesitate to ask for consultation from the anesthesiologists, pain clinics, or psychopharmacologists in the management of those patients who do not seem to be doing well with the measures outlined above.

The transcutaneous nerve stimulator has had extensive use in my department for the treatment of virtually every type of chronic benign pain (the term "benign" is used to differentiate it from the pain of maligancies and does not in any way refer to its severity). Although in some brachial plexus injury patients there appears to be a beneficial effect of the TNS unit, it has always been difficult for me to be clear as to the efficacy of this modality. True, the side effects are minor and usually confined to skin irritation or financial sacrifice, so the down-side risk is acceptable. It is quite clear that one cannot simply hand the patient the device, briefly describe how to use it, and expect a positive result. That approach or lack thereof can be predicted to fail every time. It has been our experience that a time-consuming explanation, demonstration, and adequate trial of the TNS, which includes its use at home, is really necessary if success is to be obtained.

I have no personal experience with the use of acupuncture or acupressure in the treatment of patients with pain due to brachial plexus injury, and, although several of my patients have tried it, they have not reported significant success.

For those patients in whom all conservative measures have failed to alleviate long-standing and incapacitating pain from brachial plexus injury, the question of neurosurgical intervention must be raised. Many operative procedures have been tried and have failed to stand the test of time. However, I have been cautiously optimistic about the results of the dorsal root entry zone (DREZ) radiofrequency lesion that has been described by Nashold and Ostdahl.[9]

PERSONNEL CONSIDERATIONS IN THE TREATMENT OF PATIENTS WITH BRACHIAL PLEXUS INJURY

Because of the complexity of the problems engendered by brachial plexus injury and the fact that they may have a profound effect on a patient's physical, emotional, social, economic, and future life, there are multiple opportunities for lack of a cohesive program to result in suboptimal care. There is no question that not only may physicians of diverse medical specialties, nurses, therapists, social workers, orthotists and prosthetists, rehabilitation counselors, and insurance companies, as well as attorneys be called upon to assist the patient in his rehabilitation, but any or all of these may fail to communicate in a meaningful and positive way or may actually work at cross-purposes. In the final analysis, it is the patient who bears the ultimate responsibility, since he must live with the consequences. One physician or surgeon who knows the patient best, has spent the most time with him, and will ultimately help make the treatment decisions, should assume the role of the patient's primary doctor for the care of the sequelae of the brachial plexus injury. It is desirable to have as many of the participating professionals under one roof as possible, although some, by the nature of their vocations and position, will obviously be geographically and administratively removed. A successful team captain cannot "cover all the bases," and so he must be prepared to constantly communicate and to delegate responsibilities as necessary to achieve a desired result for the patient. The cooperation of the patient is the one factor without which nothing can succeed. It is vital to convey the importance of this concept to all concerned.

Where and by whom should this care be rendered? Experience in clinical practice is an irreplaceable element, particularly in complicated situations. Although it is possible to successfully treat patients with brachial plexus injury in individual offices or group practices, the ability to marshall the requisite personnel and facilities for optimal care makes referral of such patients to specialized centers desirable in most cases and, in some, a practical necessity.

REFERENCES

1. American Academy of Orthopaedic Surgeons Committee on Prosthetics and Orthotics: Atlas of Orthotics. Mosby, St. Louis, 1975
2. Bloomberg MH: Orthopedic Braces—Rationale, Classification and Prescription. Lippincott, Philadelphia, Montreal, 1964
3. Bowden REM: Factors influencing functional recovery. In Seddon HJ (ed): Peripheral Nerve Injuries. Chap 7. Her Majesty's Stationery Office, London, 1954
4. Brand PW: Management of sensory loss in the extremities. In Omer GE, Spinner M (eds): Management of Peripheral Nerve Problems. Saunders, Philadelphia, 1980
5. Brewerton DA, Daniel JW: Return to work after injury. Hand 1:125, 1969
6. Ellenberg M: Treatment of diabetic neuropathy with diphenolhydantoin. NY State J Med 68:2653, 1968
7. Hunter J, Schneider L, Mackin E, Callahan A: Rehabilitation of the Hand. 2nd Ed. Mosby, St. Louis, 1984
8. Medical Economics Co: Physicians Desk Reference. Oradell, NJ, 1985
9. Nashold BS, Jr, Ostdahl RH: Dorsal root entry zone lesions for pain relief. J Neurosurg 51:59, 1979
10. Nickel V.: Orthopaedic Rehabilitation. Churchill Livingstone, New York, Edinburgh, London, Melbourne, 1982
11. Perry J, Hsu J, Barber L, Hoffer M: Orthoses in patients with brachial plexus injuries. Arch Phys Med Rehabil 55:134, 1974
12. Richardson NK: Type with One Hand. South-Western Publishing, Cincinnati, Dallas, New York, 1950
13. Schottsteadt ER, Robinson GB: Functional bracing in the arm. J Bone Joint Surg 38A(3):477, 1956
14. Washam V: The One-Hander's Book—A Basic Guide to Activities of Daily Living. John Day-Intex, New York, 1973
15. Wynn-Parry CB: Rehabilitation of the Hand. Butterworths, London, 1981

10

Surgical Treatment of Closed Traction Injuries of the Brachial Plexus

HISTORICAL REVIEW

> Gentlemen,—The case which I propose to bring before you today presents several points of interest. It is an admirable example of the result of complete rupture of the brachial plexus, and it is also, I believe, the first case in which suture of that plexus has been effected long after the original injury. To the various minor details which it illustrates I shall refer after describing the symptoms presented.

With these words, William Thoburn, an Assistant Surgeon of the Manchester Royal Infirmary, began his paper entitled: "A Clinical Lecture on Secondary Suture of the Brachial Plexus."[40] The year was 1900, and, although modern surgery has since evolved to a state of the art that would not have seemed possible 85 years ago, a reading of this historic paper quickly imposes a humbling perspective on even the most zealous surgeon. In fact, the problems surrounding surgical repair of the damaged brachial plexus have not been solved, and remain until this day. In order to be able to understand how honest, capable, and careful workers in the field have often come to diametrically opposed conclusions, it will be necessary for us to review in detail the history of their labors.

The variety of injuries to the plexus has already been enumerated. In 1827 the first report by Flaubert[10] described the reduction of a dislocated shoulder by the combined force of eight men. All roots except the C5 were avulsed from the spinal cord and recovered below the clavicle at autopsy. Although in the past there has been controversy over where in the plexus the traction lesions occurred, this point is no longer debated. The problems of repair are, for the most part, clearly defined. Many of the solutions continue to elude us.

Let us return to Thoburn's case to continue the story. The patient was, in 1895, a 16-year-old girl who was caught up in the machinery of a mill where she worked. She was rendered unconscious, and since there were no witnesses to the accident, the exact mode of injury is unknown. The result, however, was a flail, anesthetic arm, for which Thoburn saw her, unchanged, seven months later. Using his knowledge of the anatomy, he localized the probable site of the lesion—or, to let him tell it:

> To sum up: We have here an injury of the brachial plexus situated in an accessible region of the neck, external of the scalenus medius; the motor fibers above that level are intact, those below it are paralyzed. The plexus has been torn across or hopelessly contused in the region named, but its roots have not been torn away from the spinal cord. On these grounds a plastic operation was regarded as possible. The operation of secondary suture was performed on April 13th, 1896, seven and a half months after the injury.

The plexus was explored by a transclavicular approach, and a conglomerate neuroma, beginning just below the suprascapular nerve and extending distally for two inches and involving the entire plexus, was resected. The resulting gap was closed, reportedly without tension, by mobilization and positioning of the shoulder, and the nerves were repaired with fine silk sutures. The postoperative course was benign, except for an unexplained and violent, but fortunately transient, inflammatory process of the ipsilateral elbow. The patient returned to work in the mill six months later with no change in her paralysis. About one month later, she began to experience some return of function. On examination four years postoperatively she still had marked atrophy and was not using her hand at all. But the forearm was used for carrying things with the flexed elbow, and she was able to hold objects by adducting the arm against the chest. There was sensation throughout the entire limb, but localization of touch was quite defective. Sensibility in the hand was poorest, and she could only appreciate that it had been touched somewhere. The details of the motor recovery are of great interest. She had minimal glenohumeral control with no active lateral rotation, although the deltoid was contracting. Elbow flexion was fairly powerful and functionally useful, although elbow and wrist extension were absent. There was considerable power of wrist flexion, the remaining musculature being in the "trace" range.

On the basis of this rather startling result, the surgeon posed several questions which succeeding generations have attempted to answer, and to which we must, of necessity, return anew with each patient considered for surgery. Again, to let him speak for himself:

> . . . the question may fairly be asked, Was operation really called for in this case? The uselessness of the limb was obvious: but was there no chance of recovery without operation? The question thus becomes. *[sic]* At how late a period may complete motor and sensory paralysis resulting from injury of the brachial plexus first show signs of recovery? Upon this point I can obtain no precise information.
>
> . . . A further difficulty which was raised before operation was the impossibility of attaching the torn cords correctly to their peripheral ends, and it was suggested that the spinal nuclei on regeneration be attached to muscles other than those for which they were intended, and that hopelessly confused movements might thus result. In my opinion this is a matter of little moment.
>
> . . . Lastly, we have to inquire how far the operation was justified by results, and what hope is offered to us in similar cases. That the plexus is capable of repair after complete resection and secondary suture is clearly proved. The extent of recovery is disappointing, but its promise for other cases is less unsatisfactory than appears at first sight.

He concluded:

> On the experience thus gained there can be no doubt that old injuries of the brachial plexus located within an accessible region should be submitted to operation rather than condemned as hopeless—a position which has even led to amputation for the removal of a useless encumbrance. It is only in those cases in which the plexus is torn away from the cord that operation is impossible, and a careful examination on the lines indicated in an earlier part of this lecture will readily distinguish such cases.

Three years later, in 1903, Kennedy[14] of Glasgow reported the results of three cases in which he had performed resection and suture of the upper trunk. The first case was an infant operated on at two months and followed for nine months. The functional result was stated to be excellent, with shoulder abduction to 90 degrees and normal elbow flexion. The other two patients, one of whom was a 14-year-old with an upper-type birth palsy, were not followed long enough for assessment (5 months and 12½ weeks, respectively). On final examination they had not had improvement in voluntary control, but had electrical signs of recovery. In this same paper, Kennedy also alluded to a neurolysis done in 1900 for total neonatal arm palsy. This patient was said to have had complete recovery 14 months postoperatively.

The next 15 years saw increased interest in the surgery of the birth plexus injury and, in 1905, the publication of the first of a series of important papers by Clark, Taylor, and Prout.[7] The results of these, which appeared in 1905, 1907, 1913, and 1920, will be discussed together, since they describe a continuous series of patients that eventually grew to 70 operated cases.[37–39] The most common pathology was described as infraganglionic at the upper trunk. At operation the neuromatous area was sharply excised, and fine silk was used to suture the sheath only, approximating the head and shoulder to eliminate tension. Cargile membrane was wrapped around the suture site to prevent connective tissue ingrowth. Of the first seven infant patients there were two deaths in the immediate postoperative period, one from recurrent diarrhea, and one attributed to status lymphaticus. Three had insufficient or no follow-up, and two were subsequently re-reported by Taylor[37] in 1907. One, an 8-year-old boy, was reexplored because of persistence of medial rotation of the humerus with posterior dislocation of the shoulder. In addition to suture of the suprascapular nerve, the shoulder was reduced, and at ultimate examination two years and seven months following the first operation and six and a half months after the second he noted beginning action of the external rotators (suprascapular nerve) and deltoid and "improved nutrition and growth of the extremity."

The second patient also reported in the first series, a 10-year-old, followed more than three years, had undergone a suture of the suprascapular nerve and a neurolysis of the upper trunk. He was reported to have made significant functional gains and demonstrable improvement in growth of the limb as well as external rotation and supination of the forearm.

A one-year-old patient, not previously reported, was operated upon in 1905. After complete excision of the conglomerate neuroma distal to the foramen there was such a large gap that it could not be closed. Chromic catgut and cargile membrane were used as a scaffolding for the nerves to grow upon. One year later, there was reported to be some power in the deltoids, slight wrist flexion, and "almost normal sensation."

Taylor noted an increasing area of paralysis in most patients postoperatively, but stated that in all cases the lost power was regained with time. On the basis of this series he advocated only operation for the birth palsies, indicating that 6 to 12 months was suitable, and maybe even earlier. By 1919 the series[39] had grown to 70 cases, and he had a control series of 130 patients in whom no operation was performed because of (referring) physician or parental refusal of surgery. The rate of spontaneous recovery in these patients was 1%. Of the operative cases Taylor stated:

> Concerning the functional results, there has been no perfect anatomic or physiologic recovery. With a few exceptions in which the damage has been found to be irremediable, these children have made marked improvement and many of them have attained almost perfect function in the extremity.
>
> In a number of cases . . . physical therapeutics were relied upon by the parents and physician for a period of two to four years and when improvement had ceased for a long interval operation was done and the result was a marked improvement. This improvement therefore "is solely attributable to the operation."

Unfortunately, the documentation of the details of this important series of patients is unavailable, other than the fact of the death of the third patient from intraoperative hemorrhage.

Taylor[39] also reported a series of 14 brachial palsies of the Erb's type in adults in whom, presumably, sutures were done. In seven cases there were one or more root avulsions documented. The results was given as: three lost to follow-up, one "perfect," one "almost perfect," one "good," and one "unsatisfactory" because of having pulled the postoperative dressing apart. No further details are available.

During this same period, others had also been at work. In 1916 Sharpe[35] had reported 56 cases of birth palsy that he had operated upon. He advised operations at one month of age because there was less scarring, the infants were thought to withstand surgery better, and there was no retraction of the torn nerve ends. There were no deaths, but two slight infections. Again, however, the results were reported in vague terms that defied verification. He stated that children operated upon at three months of age had made excellent recoveries (no complete tears of the plexus, whereas those at one month were more severe):

> Half of the children operated on at one month have shown a marked improvement, and in four it may be possible to obtain a normal arm."

In 1920 Sir Harry Platt[28] urged conservative treatment of infantile brachial plexus injury unless complete paralysis accompanied by definite muscular wasting had persisted for at least 12 months. Where the clinical symptoms indicated a lesion in the region of the intervertebral foramen, he considered the case inoperable. As part of the same symposium before the British Orthopaedic Association, H. A. T. Fairbank[9] advised exploration at three months if electrical reactions done under general anesthesia indicated denervation and there was no clinical recovery. He emphasized the importance of suprascapular nerve repair, and advocated a nerve-crossing operation in which the torn C5 was spliced into an intact C7. Of the five cases he operated upon, one had secondary suture of C5 and 6 at 12 months, and at follow-up 13 years later, the paralyzed muscles were acting, although there were contractures. One was probably a case of arthrogryposis and was thought not to be a birth injury. Two others had either no significant functional recovery, and one no follow-up.

The next 15 years saw general pessimism regarding the surgery of traction injuries. In 1915 Sever[34] of Boston said:

> We have had no very brilliant results from the plexus repair. Many of the plexuses that have been operated on have shown absolutely nothing in the way of functional recovery, and nothing could be expected from the type of injury found at the time of operation. A few cases suggest that a plexus operation, always in connection with the muscle operation, may offer a better arm in the end. However, we are not over enthusiastic on this point.

In 1930 Jepson[13] reported:

> There has been no case yet, reported to my knowledge, which has shown an anatomic and physiologic cure from the plexus operation. Even marked improvement is usually lacking. This may in part be due to the fact that the deformities were not first recognized and corrected and the plexus operation done later. Many times the nerve is so badly damaged that it is beyond repair.

In 1934 J. H. Stevens,[36] writing in Codman's book on the shoulder, stated:

> The presumption should be against operating in cases of tension or traction injuries. The chance of suture of a ruptured nerve trunk is a forelorn hope. The main indication for operation is the release of pressure from exudate.

He did, however, advocate immediate operation in all cases of penetrating wounds with paralysis involving the branches of the plexus, and in all cases with arterial complications.

In 1947 Davis and colleagues[8] reported on a mixed group of open and closed injuries of the adult brachial plexus. There were 30 open wounds and 17 due to "blunt trauma." Six of these patients also had associated injury of the spinal cord. A much-quoted statement was made in which they asserted that with time, encroaching scar may impair previously uninvolved parts of the plexus. Operation on the plexus was discussed in a favorable light, and nerve grafts using fresh homogeneous nerves were advocated. Although the authors' series did not in any way provide documentation, they stated:

> The outlook for recovery of function is much improved with prompt surgical repair.

Forrster's series in the German literature in 1929 was quoted in evidence by Davis and colleagues.[8] Twenty-nine sutures and 17 neurolyses had been done on 39 patients with satisfactory results in the majority of them, and, in many cases, complete recovery.

Again, unfortunately, in the six cases reported by Davis and colleagues[8] as having been assessed after adequate followup, there was no detail as to the type of injury or surgery. In three there was complete functional recovery, one was reported as greatly improved, and two had little improvement.

In 1947 Seddon,[31] in his presentation of the results of autogenous grafts in the repair of large gaps in peripheral nerves, detailed four cases of traction injury of the brachial plexus treated by grafts. Three were cable grafts, and he noted that the extent of the damage was such that in no case was an entirely adequate resection performed. One was a failure because of severe muscle atrophy and long delay (21 months) before operation. Another, done at $6\frac{1}{2}$ months, achieved a MRC Gr 2/5 biceps and a little sensory recovery at three years follow-up and was deemed a failure. The third, done at two months, achieved deltoid and biceps of Gr 2 plus/5 with return of sensibility and was called "partial recovery." All three grafts used three strands of superficial radial nerve. A fourth traction lesion, grafted at nine months and using 9.5 cm of radial nerve main trunk, was a failure.

Barnes'[4] study of 63 traction injuries of the brachial plexus in adults was published in 1949. The prognosis of each type of lesion was discussed and conservative treatment was advocated. Evidence was cited against early or late operations. Since the spontaneous rate of recovery of the upper three roots was good in this series, he felt that the necessity of surgery here was unlikely. He suggested, however, that if the upper trunk was damaged, it could be resected and bridged by autogenous grafts. He concluded that the number of cases in which grafting was feasible was few, and that it still had to be proved that functional recovery after grafting was as satisfactory as the results of late reconstructive surgery.

The American experience of surgical treatment of 117 patients who had brachial plexus injury sustained in World War II was documented by Nulsen and Slade[27] in 1956. They concluded that patients with stretch injuries could not be improved.

This pessimistic outlook was also expressed by Tracy and Brannon,[41] who in 1958 described their experiences with 16 adult traction injuries. They explored two patients, and in both found extraspinal lesions not amenable to repair. They concluded that neurological repair of such injuries is usually unrewarding, and they concentrated on reconstruction. They did advocate exploration for prognostic purposes in those patients who showed no improvement within a six-month period and who had negative myelograms.

Thus, the surgical enthusiasm of the beginning of the century had given way to conservatism on the basis of six decades of generally unrewarding experiences. This view was solidified by the painstaking work of Bonney,[5] who in 1959 reported his experience with 20 patients with complete traction lesions, of whom 15 were explored for prognosis. The purpose of the operation was never more than to get better information about the site of the lesion and the severity of the damage than could be obtained by clinical examination. He commented on the difficulty of relating findings at operation, especially in the lesion in continuity, to ultimate prognosis, and, most important, he stated:

> In no case was it possible to contemplate repair of the neural lesion, the extent and complexity of the damage always preventing resection and repair.

There was the solid feeling that evidence for two supraganglionic (preganglionic) lesions signified a bad prognosis for the whole plexus. Bonney concluded:

> Exploration is applied just to those cases in which the lesion is largely postganglionic—hence, a useful proportion of definite results will be obtained. When a postganglionic lesion of one nerve is associated with a preganglionic lesion of two or more other nerves, the likelihood is that there has been severe damage to the former.

Patients with these findings were advised that no recovery could be expected, and that, if elected, amputation could be done at a later date.

In 1963 Sir Herbert Seddon,[32] in the Watson Jones Address to the Royal College of Surgeons of England stated:

> Repair of the brachial plexus has proved so disappointing that it should not be done except for the upper trunk.

It would appear that by all logic the story should have come to an end here. Direct surgical attack on traction lesions of the brachial plexus was unrewarding at best, or even potentially harmful. However, it was precisely at this time that renewed interest in grafting of peripheral nerves arose as a result of significant advances in optics and microtechniques. In a remarkably clear assessment of the status of nerve grafting in 1954, Brooks[6] reported the results of 93 peripheral nerve grafts done over a 12-year period by Seddon and his coworkers. The essentials of technique and theory were described. It remained for the development of the operating microscope and improved suture materials to energize the process anew. In a few centers in the world, new techniques were being developed and used on carefully documented large series of cases. From 1964 to 1972 Millesi of Vienna operated upon 56 patients with brachial plexus injuries, employing autografting and neurolysis. The results[20] were reported in 1973, and it was apparent that gratifying results had been obtained. Comparable results were reported by Samii[29,30] and Narakas.[23,24] Narakas' extensive experience extended to 107 patients operated upon between 1966 and 1977. Lusskin, Campbell, and

Thompson[18] in New York had explored 20 patients for posttraumatic neural deficits of the brachial plexus between 1963 and 1970. Thirteen underwent neurolysis and two with lacerations had grafts that gave useful results. In France, Allieu, reported on his 34 surgically treated cases of traction injury and also detailed the experience of Alnot, Mansat, and Sedel, a total of 99 cases.

So it seems, then, that we have come full circle in almost eight decades of controversy. Modern technology has changed the state of the art, but we must carefully evaluate the available well-documented contemporary series of plexus operations in order to achieve perspective. From such analysis we can develop general principles by which to manage our patients.

Millesi's work,[21] first published in German in 1973, was updated and published in detail in English in 1977. It had been presented in Paris in 1975 at a meeting of the Société Francaise de Chirurgie Orthopédique et Traumatologigue and subsequently published in 1977.[22] The 56 patients were followed at least five years postoperatively. The results are presented here in detail.

There were 20 patients with lesions at root level. The distribution was as follows:

1. 5 roots avulsed	2 patients
2. 4 roots avulsed 1 root ruptured	4 patients
3. 3 roots avulsed 2 roots ruptured	5 patients
4. 2 roots avulsed 3 roots ruptured	1 patient
5. 1 root avulsed 4 roots ruptured	2 patients
6. 1 root avulsed 2 roots ruptured 2 damaged but continuity present	5 patients
7. 1 root ruptured 4 roots damaged but continuity present	1 patient

Two patients with *all five roots avulsed* were operated upon to attempt to restore elbow flexion by means of neurotization with intercostal nerve grafts. In one, scarring prevented the completion of the operation, while the result of the other was excluded from the series. The results in the remaining 18 patients were as follows:

Ten of 18 patients recovered useful function at one or more levels, as follows:

shoulder	5/8 "M3"
elbow flexion	9/18
triceps, biceps	1/18
wrist and finger	2/18

Protective sensibility was reported to have returned in 15 of 19 patients in whom the general nutritional status of the extremity was also improved. In six patients who did not achieve active shoulder control, the tone of the musculature improved to the point where subluxation was prevented.

Eleven patients had *partial palsy due to lesions at root level,* and nine developed useful function as follows for those areas where there was a deficit:

shoulder	3/10
elbow	7/9
wrist	3/7
fingers	3/7

Sensibility was reported as improved in these nine patients.

Complete palsy due to a peripheral lesion was present in 13 patients. Eight developed useful function for those areas with deficits.

shoulder	6/13
elbow	7/13
wrist	5/13
fingers	5/12

In this group of patients there was only one with a complete interruption necessitating nerve grafting. The remaining 12 were treated by neurolysis.

Partial palsy due to a peripheral lesion was present in 12 patients, and ten developed useful function:

shoulder	7/10
elbow	8/9
wrist	3/6
fingers	3/8

In summary, then a useful recovery was obtained following surgery in at least one functional area in 38 of 54 cases (70%).

The experience of Narakas[23,24] of 107 surgical explorations for posttraumatic lesions of the brachial plexus was reported in 1977 at the same symposium. Of these, 60 were followed for more than two years postoperatively. The results are presented in Table 10.1. These results can be further amplified by the diagrams shown in Figure 10.1 of 32 operative cases where suture or graft was used for repair. The results of return of sensibility in these same 32 patients is seen in Table 10.2 from Narakas.

Lusskin, Campbell, and Thompson's report[18] in 1973 described the results of 20 operative interventions for posttraumatic neural deficits of the brachial plexus performed over the years 1963–1970. Nineteen had paralysis, and 17 underwent neurolysis, while two had autografts for lacerations. Of the 11 patients who had neurolysis for treatment of a traction lesion and had long enough follow-up with documented muscle testing, the results were as follows:

Shoulder: Five out of 10 had functional recovery
Elbow flexion: Nine out of 10 had functional recovery

In 1981 Alnot, Jolly, and Frot[3] reported a series of 100 brachial plexus injuries between April 1974 and January 1979. Neurolysis without plexus repair was performed in 25, nerve grafts for one, two, or five roots in 64, and in nine cases, intercostal nerve or spinal accessory nerve transplantation was carried out. Forty-eight cases followed for more than two years were studied to specifically develop therapeutic indications depending on the number of usable nerve roots. They stated that if only one usable root was present, they gave preference to the suprascapular nerve and lateral cord. If two roots were available for grafting, they also added the radial nerve and the posterior cord. They concluded that the results justified this type of surgery and that the best results came from repair of C5 and C6 with reinnervation of the shoulder and elbow.

These authors made the point that shoulder function should not be evaluated before 12 to 15 months and alluded to a function that is difficult to

Table 10.1 Outcome at More than Two Years After Repair of Brachial Plexus Injuries: Narakas Series

		Good*	Fair*	Poor*
Neurolysis	18	5	8	5
Proximal autographs	28	3	16	9
+ Distal sutures	12	7	4	1
Neurotization	2	—	—	2
Total	60	15	28	17

* Good = Normal or almost normal use of the extremity. Bimanual use possible.
Fair = An assistive member of about 50% use. Pain not distressing.
Poor = Limb not practically useful; severe pain; greater than 50% disability.
From Narakas A: Indications et resultats du traitement chirurgical direct dans les lésions par élongation du plexus brachial. Rev Chir Orthop 63:88, 1977.

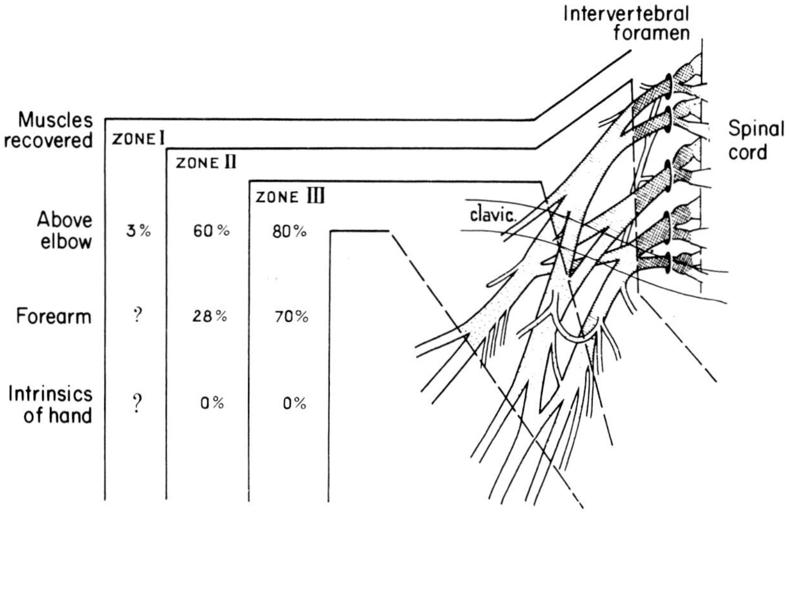

Fig. 10.1. This diagram shows the results of 32 operative cases where suture or graft was used for repair. Compare with Table 10.1. (Reproduced from Narakas A: Indications et résultats du traitement chirurgical direct dans les lésions par élongation du plexus brachial. Rev Chir Orthop 63:88, 1977, with permission.)

Table 10.2 Sensory Results Obtained in 32 Patients with Total Destruction of Nerve Pathways: Narakas Series

		Territory of Musculocutaneous Nerve	Radial Nerve	Median Nerve	Ulnar Nerve
Total		32	25	13	13
Very good	S4 }	29	13	7	1
Good	S3 }				
Satisfactory	S2	—	7	4	4
Poor	S1 }	3	5	2	8
Nil	S0 }				

Best Weber test in median distribution: Children 8 mm, Adults 25 mm
From Narakas A: Indications et resultats du traitement chirurgical direct dans les lésions par élongation du plexus brachial. Rev Chir Orthop 63:88, 1977.

quantitate, the disappearance of inferior subluxation in the previously paralyzed shoulder that did not regain active movement but was regarded as useful. They also urged notice of fatigability of muscles that had been reinnervated. In paralysis involving C5, C6, C7, C8, and T1 with total avulsion of the roots, they had four cases followed more than two years with neurotization using intercostal nerves and had two cases with useful function and two failures. There were three neurotizations of the musculocutaneous nerve with two failures, of which one required secondary amputation and one recovered elbow flexion against gravity. In the case of neurotization of the ulnar nerve, the patient recovered sensibility to the level of the hand. In paralyses of C5, C6, C7, C8, and T1 with irreversible lesions of the inferior roots, the object was to graft C5–6 and sometimes C7 to attempt to reinnervate proximal muscles in the shoulder and elbow, as well as the extrinsic muscles of the hand in certain cases. Their detailed results of 65 grafts for total paralysis in 26 cases followed for 2½ years are given in Table 10.3.

In paralysis involving the upper roots, they reported better results. It was their opinion that these results were better than any possible muscle or tendon transfer. Subsequently, in 1981, the results were also referred to by Narakas,[26] wherein he presented his clinical experience based on 800 cases seen over a period of 15 years of which he operated upon 307. He said that the first three degrees of Sunderland's classification of plexus injury should not be treated surgically and that even fourth-degree injury, interruption of the fascicles with the stumps in contact and well aligned, should not be operated upon. He reserved surgery for the fourth-degree cases of fascicular disruption and fifth-degree, which implies total interruption of the nerve trunk. He also included as potential surgical cases some root avulsions, a few cases of conduction block and internal or external nerve compression syndromes. He stated that if the roots C8 and T1 or their terminal branches were affected, no hand function would be achieved and with the exception of babies, one could not expect intrinsic function. In the upper trunk (C5–C6), good shoulder function (elevation above the horizontal) could not be obtained. He stressed that patients should be realistically informed of the expected results prior to surgery.

Narakas'[26] series of 243 patients was summarized as shown in Table 10.4.

Since in complex severe lesions all functions cannot be restored by neurological reconstruction, Narakas' priorities in repair were elbow control; wrist and finger flexion, then median nerve sensibil-

Table 10.3 Results in 26 Cases of Nerve Graft for Total Paralysis with Follow-up of More than 2½ Years: Series of Alnot et al.

Number of Roots	Number of Cases	Results
1 grafted	13	3 complete failures 2 partial failures 8 useful recovery
2 grafted	9	3 failures 1 not reviewed 5 useful recovery
Upper trunk	2	2 useful recovery
3 grafted	1	1 useful recovery
5 grafted	1	1 useful recovery

Data from Alnot JY, Jolly A, Frot B: Traitement de lésions nerveuses dans les paralysies traumatiques du plexus brachial chez l'adulte. Int Orthop 63:82, 1981, with permission.

Table 10.4 Types of Operations in 243 Patients[a]

Exploration only	4
Emergency exploration	4
External neurolysis only	20
Fasicular neurolysis	14
Autologous grafting	142
Neurotization only	28
Autologous grafting and neurotizations	33
Total	247

[a] Two patients had an emergency exploration with an arterial graft and secondary plexus repair. Two other patients had a two-stage grafting procedure.
From Narakas A: Brachial plexus surgery. Orthop Clin North Am 12:303, 1981, with permission.

ity; shoulder control; and wrist and finger extension. Narakas presented his results along with those of Alnot because both physicians used the same operative techniques and the same criteria of evaluation. Their results are given in Table 10.5. For the incomplete brachial palsies, the combined results of Narakas and Alnot in 34 cases is given in Table 10.6. In Narakas' series of 100 grafted cases, useful results were obtained in 64% of cases for proximal lesions and in 73% for distal lesions. Normal function, excellent results, have never been obtained. Narakas' results of neurotization in 50 patients followed up for more than 3 years are given in Table 10.7.

By comparing a series of patients with lesions of Sunderland's fourth- or fifth-degree and root avulsions, one group treated conservatively and the other group operated upon, Narakas concluded that there are statistical advantages to surgical treatment. In this series, 19 patients with severe injury, who could not be treated surgically, were given conservative treatment. None of them reached a good result, whereas 23% of the patients who were operated upon did so.

In 1982 Sedel[33] reported on 62 patients with posttraumatic brachial plexus palsy operated upon by the same surgeon and followed for a minimum of three years for complete lesions and two years for initially partial lesions. All operations were performed between the second and twenty-fourth month after injury. Postoperative results were based upon clinical examination, the usefulness of the arm, and the patients' occupation. Detailed results are given in the following discussion.

Sedel assessed the usefulness of the arm in five grades:

Grade 1: Manual work can be performed with normal strength.
Grade 2: The limb can perform or assist everyday activities such as cutting meat or tying shoelaces, but is not strong enough for manual work.
Grade 3: Usefulness of the limb is very limited, the forearm can be held against the chest, the flexed wrist can be used as a hook or the whole arm can be used as a paperweight.
Grade 4: The limb is virtually useless, although there is some movement of the elbow and fingers, and this is referred to as an anesthetic, animated arm.
Grade 5: No recovery has occurred, the limb is anesthetic but not animated, but occasionally, because of trophic changes, it is not even anesthetic.

Occupation was graded as follows:

Grade 1: Manual workers were able to resume their previous occupation.
Grade 2: Nonmanual workers returned to their preinjury jobs.

Table 10.5 Complete Brachial Plexus Palsy: Results of Repair of Supraclavicular Lesions in 68 Cases Followed Up For More Than Three Years: Narakas and Alnot (combined results)

			Results	
Number of Grafted Roots	Total Number of Cases	Total Failure	Partial Results	Useful Results
1	21	8	2	11
2	36	3	11	21
3	10	0	2	8
5	1	0	0	1

From Narakas A: Brachial plexus surgery. Orthop Clin North Am 12:303,1981.

Table 10.6 Incomplete Brachial Plexus Palsy: Results of Repair of Supraclavicular Lesions in 34 Cases Followed Up For More Than Three Years: Narakas and Alnot (combined results)

			Results	
Number of Grafted Roots	Total Number of Cases	Total Failure	Partial Results	Useful Results
1	12 6 (C7–C8–T1 undamaged) 6 (C8–T1 undamaged)	1	3	8
2	17 10 (C7–C8–T1 undamaged) 7 (C8–T1 undamaged)	0	4 (1 lost to follow-up)	12
3	5 (C8–T1 undamaged)	0	0	5

From Narakas A: Brachial plexus surgery. Orthop Clin North Am 12:303,1981.

Grade 3: Patients had to change their jobs and could only do nonmanual work.
Grade 4: Patients were unable to work.

In summary, the results were as follows:
For seven patients with complete avulsions

1. One patient was explored and not repaired.
2. Six patients had nerve transfers: three or four intercostal nerves were used in three cases, and a mixed transfer from the intercostal nerves and the accessory nerve was used in three cases.
3. Five patients recovered elbow flexion: one had some recovery in triceps and deltoid, and one in flexor digitorum profundus.
4. Four patients recovered gross sensation in the forearm, and one in the hand. However, the usefulness of the upper limb was poor, and in all cases it was graded 4.

For eight patients with type II lesions with only one root ruptured distally and the remainder avulsed, in which a graft was done from C5:

1. Six patients had an added nerve transfer.
2. Three patients recovered usefulness to Grade 3, three to Grade 4, and two had no recovery, Grade 5.
3. The nerve transfer was occasionally followed by sensitivity, in that the patient felt his chest if one touched his hand.

For seven patients with type II lesions with two roots ruptured distally:

1. In all cases, C5 and C6 were ruptured distally and the remaining roots were avulsed.
2. Following grafting, the limb was Grade 3 in five of these patients, one of whom had a functional hand.
3. One patient had a Grade 4 result, and one a Grade 5.

Sedel had 31 patients with partial palsies, so classified in that at the time of operation they had one or more active muscles beyond the shoulder:

1. Six cases were of the C5–C6 type: two patients had grafts of the upper trunk; one achieved a good result, while the other was fair.
2. Three patients had neurolysis of the upper trunk, with two good results, although they both needed derotation osteotomies of the humerus; one had a fair result.

Table 10.7 Results of Neurotization in 50 Patients Followed Up for More than Three Years

Nerve	Fair	Poor or Nil
Bell's nerve on lateral cord or suprascapular nerve	3	2
Spinal accessory nerve on lateral cord	1	1
Intercostals on C5 and C6	1	2
Intercostals only	6	9
Intercostals on lateral cord or musculocutaneous	8	3
Intercostals on posterior cord, axillary nerve, or suprascapular nerve	4	2
Intercostals on medial cord or median or ulnar nerves	8	
Motor results (FCU, FCR, FDP, FDS)	2	6
Sensory results	4	4
Total	26	24

From Narakas A: Brachial plexus surgery. Orthop Clin North Am 12:303, 1981, with permission.

3. In three patients, the usefulness of the upper limb was Grade 1, in the other three, it was Grade 2.

Nine patients with C5, C6, and C7 palsies had grafts, one with a nerve transfer:

1. In eight patients, recovery was good; two had their shoulders fused, and one had a tendon transfer for radial palsy.
2. The usefulness was Grade 1 in four patients, Grade 2 in four patients, and Grade 3 in one patient.

The three remaining patients with supraclavicular lesions and the 13 cases of partial palsies with infraclavicular lesions were a mixed group with generally better results than in those patients with complete lesions.

Sedel's discussion of the effect of surgical repair indicated that it was favorable in most cases. Of the 32 cases of complete palsies, 26 had repair procedures, and in 22 of these, there was improvement, although four were failures. Of the 23 cases of partial palsies who had major repairs, 20 were improved in at least one area, and three were complete failures. As to the usefulness of the recovery, Sedel stated that major benefit was seen with initially partial palsies. When good elbow movement and some shoulder movement was regained, then simple procedures such as rotational osteotomy or shoulder fusion could be added with benefit. The repair procedures in the complete palsies were less useful; 11 were Grade 3, 12 were Grade 4, and three were Grade 5. Sedel concluded that surgical repair of traumatic brachial palsies does improve the prognosis, and it is more effective for patients who sustain infraclavicular lesions or for supraclavicular lesions when at least two roots can be used for grafting. The results of nerve transfer are functionally disappointing.

INDICATIONS

The lengthy foregoing historical review has, I believe, been necessary to establish not only the reasons for divergence of opinion, but the difficulties involved in comparing the results reported by the various authors and workers in the field. The choice of central neurological repair or peripheral reconstruction must not be viewed as an "either/or" situation, since they must be considered as complementary in the treatment of individual patients. It should further be remembered that all surgical treatment of patients with major injuries to the brachial plexus is palliative, since in no case can a completely normal limb be restored. It is crucial, however, that the surgeon who assumes responsibility for the patient's care be cognizant of all the alternatives of treatment and either be able to accomplish them himself or with the aid of knowledgeable colleagues within the same center. Only in this manner can continuity of care be preserved and treatment accomplished in optimal fashion. This implies, therefore, that specific centers that are capable of providing such care be responsible for it and that an efficient referral system be established. Since the time element is an important determinant in the success or failure of treatment, a concerted educational program must be diffused through the outlying community so that patients can reach the center as soon as their general condition permits.

Obviously it is impossible to detail completely and categorically an infallible algorithm for the care of closed injuries of the brachial plexus that will satisfy every case one encounters. Similarly, these knowledgeable and diligent groups of surgeons, who, over the years, have recorded their truths and subsequent recommendations, will continue to disagree. However, certain generalizations can, I believe, be made.

Because I remain convinced of the distinctive character of the closed infraclavicular injury of the plexus, its identification in all potentially pertinent circumstances must be pursued. The criteria for recognition of this considerably smaller subgroup and the mechanism of injury have been described in detail in Chapter 3. Suffice it to say that, although closed supraclavicular traction injuries may extend to the infraclavicular parts of the plexus, the pathogenesis of the classical infraclavicular injury usually spares the supraclavicular region. With the exception of those infraclavicular injuries accompanied by vascular injury, or those in which there is adequate indication of neurotomesis due to fracture fragments, the treatment of the neural elements in this group is conservative. Peripheral reconstructive surgery is only occasionally required.

The patient with a closed supraclavicular brachial plexus injury resulting in a flail-anesthetic arm remains the greatest problem, but for whom the results of neurological reconstruction make the greatest possible difference (Fig. 10.2). Until twenty

(Text continues on p. 174.)

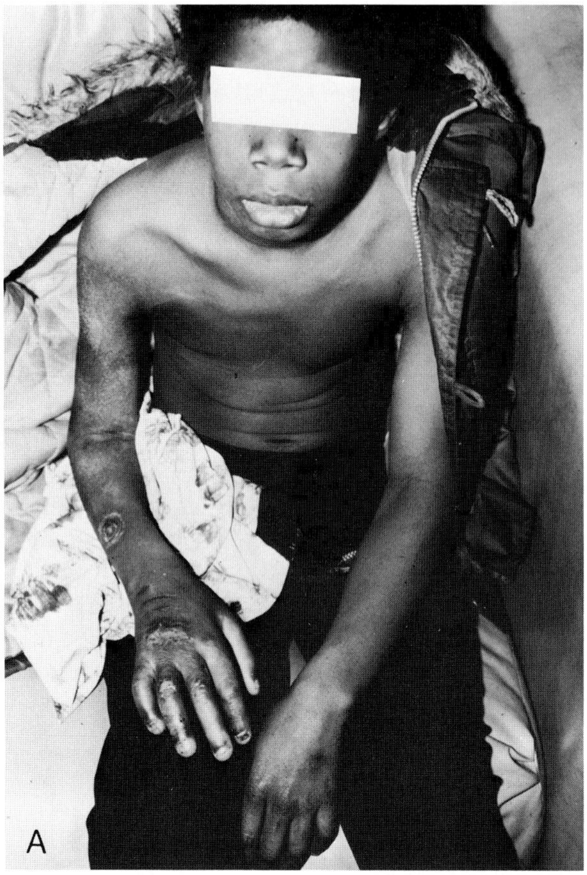

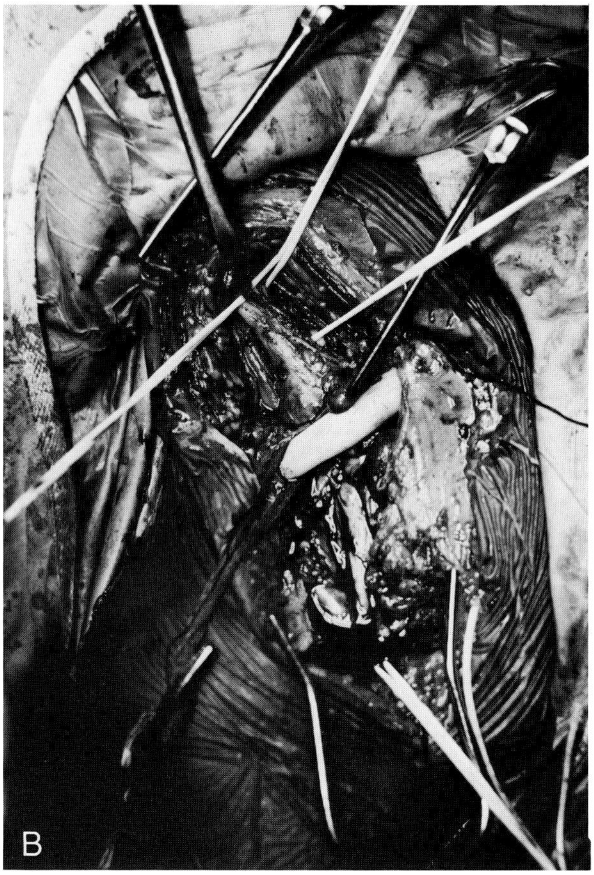

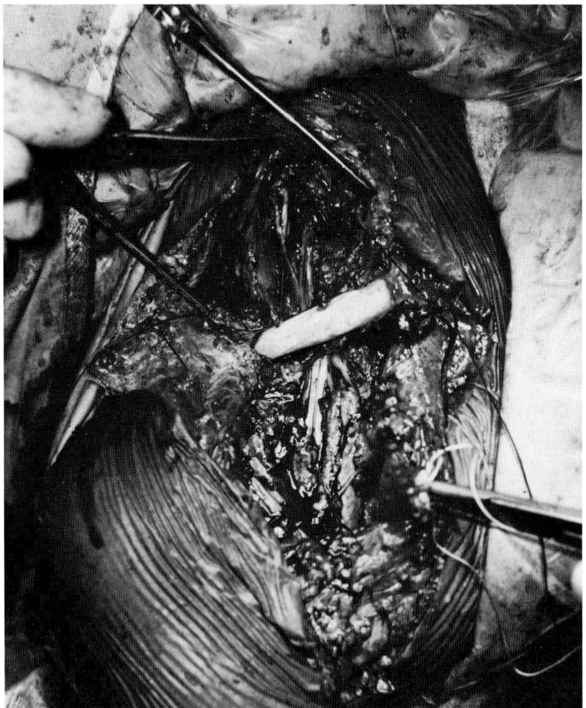

Fig. 10.2. **A**: A 10-year-old boy who sustained a severe traction injury to his right brachial plexus when he fell from the back of a moving bus on which he had hitched a ride. Seen here four months post injury with a flail-anesthetic arm and Horner's syndrome. He already has ulcerations on his arm and hand. Myelogram showed pseudomeningocele at T1. **B**: At exploration, there was a large conglomerate neuroma involving upper and intermediate trunks. **C**: Sural nerve grafts from C5 and C7 to suprascapular nerve, lateral and posterior cords. C6 neuroma extended into the foramen. Clavicle intact.

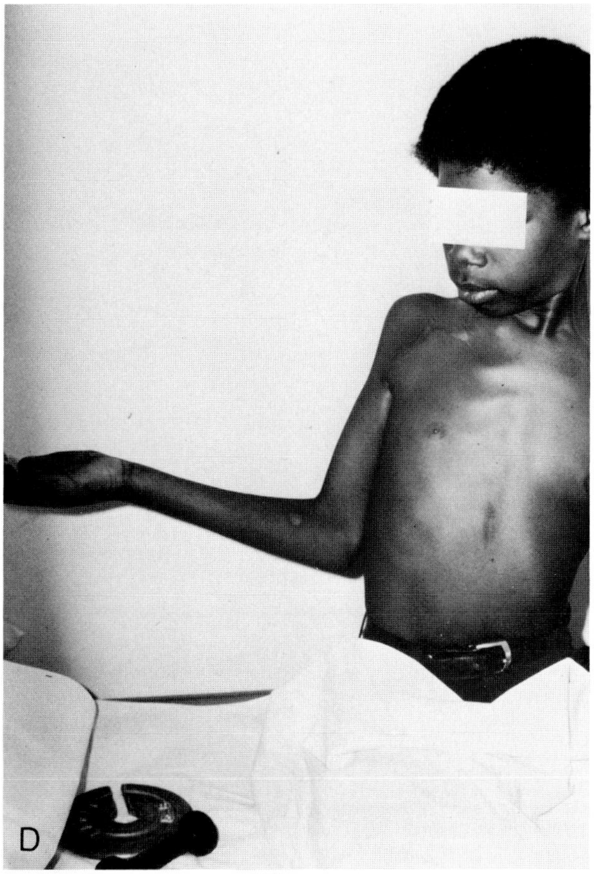

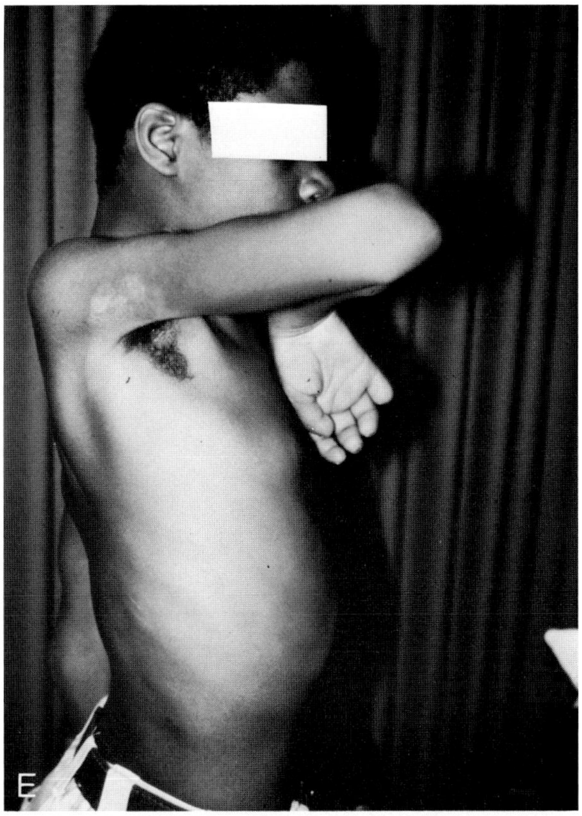

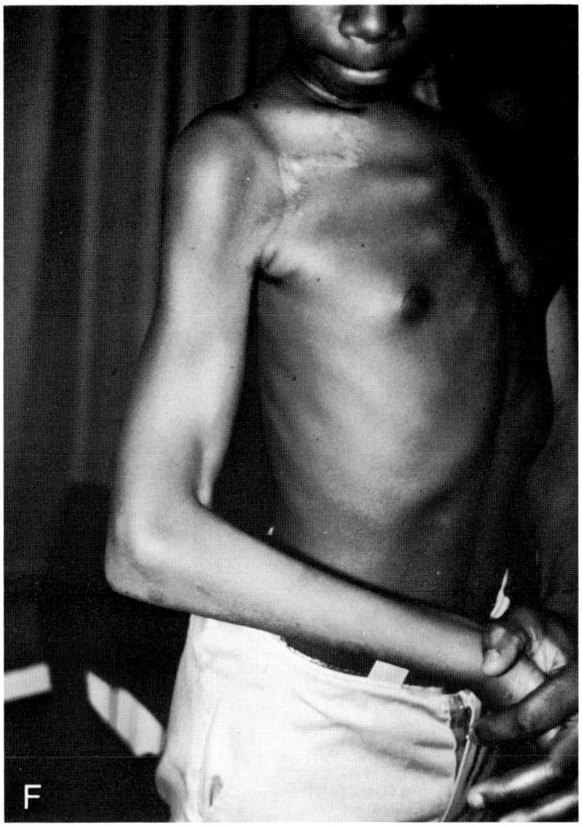

Fig. 10.2 *(continued)* **D**: One year later showing elbow flexion and active lateral rotation. **E** and **F**: Two years postoperatively—deltoid, pectorals, and latissimus have recovered in addition to biceps and lateral rotators. Sensibility much improved in arm, but absent in forearm and hand.

years ago there were essentially just three alternatives for these patients, and there was significant agreement concerning them. The first possibility, and one which many patients and physicians elect even today, is to do nothing aggressive, teach the patient to live one-handed, and protect the limb from injury or from simply "getting in the way" with the aid of a sling. Some may opt for a functional brace. Depending on the patient's socioeconomic circumstances and degree of prudence, this has been, and for some may continue to be, a viable alternative for living with a "dead" arm. To elect this course, however, is to deny any possibility of return of function, and, although it has been pursued for many years, it should not be recommended unless circumstances make the chance of even limited success very unlikely indeed. Some patients may, because of recurrent injury to the limb, trophic changes, or simply a desire to be rid of it, elect to undergo ablation at some time remote from their injury. It should be emphasized, however, if a patient elects to live with the flail, anesthetic arm, that "guardian maintenance" rather than "masterly neglect" is required.

The second alternative, that of surgical reconstruction of the flail, anesthetic arm, has had few champions since Hendry's[12] article describing it in 1949. The amount of surgery that is required to produce a limb of trivial functional capacity, but considerably greater vulnerability than the prosthesis it cannot even duplicate in usefulness, is simply too great a price to pay.

The third approach, amputation, may be combined with arthrodesis at the shoulder, and especially if an elbow with proprioceptive feedback can be preserved, the usefulness of the limb will be greatly enhanced, even if cutaneous sensibility over the stump is minimal or absent. We have yet to experience stump breakdown in approximately 18 patients so treated over the past 20 years. Furthermore, for those patients who have had active elbow control reestablished by means of nerve grafts wherein no hand function is present or expected, a below-elbow prosthetic fitting can be quite useful (Fig. 10.3). This subject will be discussed in detail in Chapter 11.

For those patients who find none of the three classical approaches applicable to their situation, there is little question that surgical treatment of the plexus itself offers benefits that no other method can provide. I believe that this approach should be pursued whenever there is a potential for truly functional improvement. Although in partial paralyses there is usually some retained sensibility, and at least some potential for redistribution of available motors, the patient with a complete lesion of the plexus has nothing with which to work. Very often, there may be a severe pain problem as well. If we assume that myelography and other indirect methods of analysis indicate total root avulsion, the functional outlook for neurotization by means of providing axons from intercostals or a portion of the spinal accessory nerve is guarded. Although the sacrifice of three or even four intercostal nerves is relatively safe, the chance of loss of a significant portion of the innervation of the trapezius is, in my opinion, a very large price to pay, despite assurances by some authors that it can be avoided in most cases.[2]

For those patients with complete plexus injuries due to a combination of supra- and infraganglionic lesions, the potential for gain from any procedure will depend largely on the available axon population with which to reconnect the distal elements of the plexus and their end organs. Even though a root may not appear to be avulsed from the cord, it may be damaged in the region of the intervertebral foramen proximal to the scalene muscles, in which case the number of viable and available axions will be negligible. Hence grafts done in this area have a poor prognosis. Assuming the availability of root stock upon which to graft, the object would be to connect these axons with those elements innervating the motors with the best chance of recovery of function. Generally, these are the elbow and, to a lesser degree, the shoulder. The forearm and hand have a considerably poorer outlook for motor recovery. The statistics of several surgical centers have already been detailed, and it is generally conceded that not only is the prognosis for spontaneous recovery of elbow flexion better than that of the shoulder following traction lesions, but the results of grafting follow suit. That this is a result of the larger number of motor units normally present in the biceps as compared with the deltoid has been suggested by Allieu.[1]

In addition, it must be remembered that recovery of the deltoid alone is not sufficient to produce a functional shoulder. I do not accept as a "good" or "satisfactory" or "useful" result a shoulder that is merely capable of voluntarily reducing an inferior subluxation or one that has better tonus following

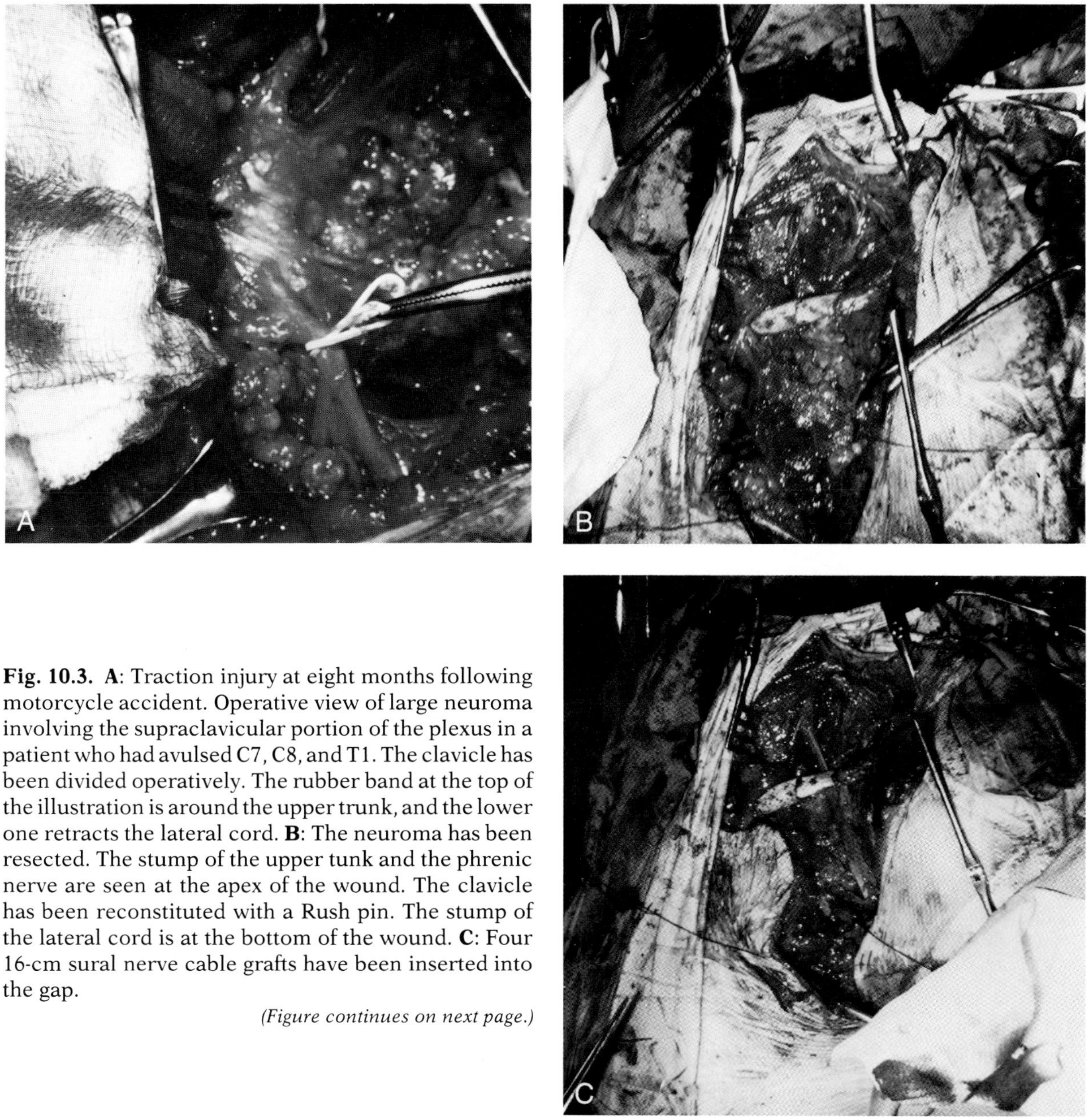

Fig. 10.3. **A**: Traction injury at eight months following motorcycle accident. Operative view of large neuroma involving the supraclavicular portion of the plexus in a patient who had avulsed C7, C8, and T1. The clavicle has been divided operatively. The rubber band at the top of the illustration is around the upper trunk, and the lower one retracts the lateral cord. **B**: The neuroma has been resected. The stump of the upper tunk and the phrenic nerve are seen at the apex of the wound. The clavicle has been reconstituted with a Rush pin. The stump of the lateral cord is at the bottom of the wound. **C**: Four 16-cm sural nerve cable grafts have been inserted into the gap.

(Figure continues on next page.)

nerve grafting. In order for a shoulder to be rated as "useful," it should be able to support the limb at the horizontal against moderate resistance and to allow the hand or terminal device to reach the opposite axilla and both ipsilateral trouser pockets. Since patients with shoulder fusions can achieve these ends, there exists a readily applicable benchmark, and it should be applied. Unless there is control of lateral rotation because of reinnervation of supra- and infraspinatus through the suprascapular nerve, the shoulder will be unstable, and function, even with a good deltoid, will be restricted to shrugging or overcoming inferior subluxation. It is for this reason that the results of neurological reconstruction for the shoulder are not only worse than those for the elbow flexion (a considerably simpler function), but the

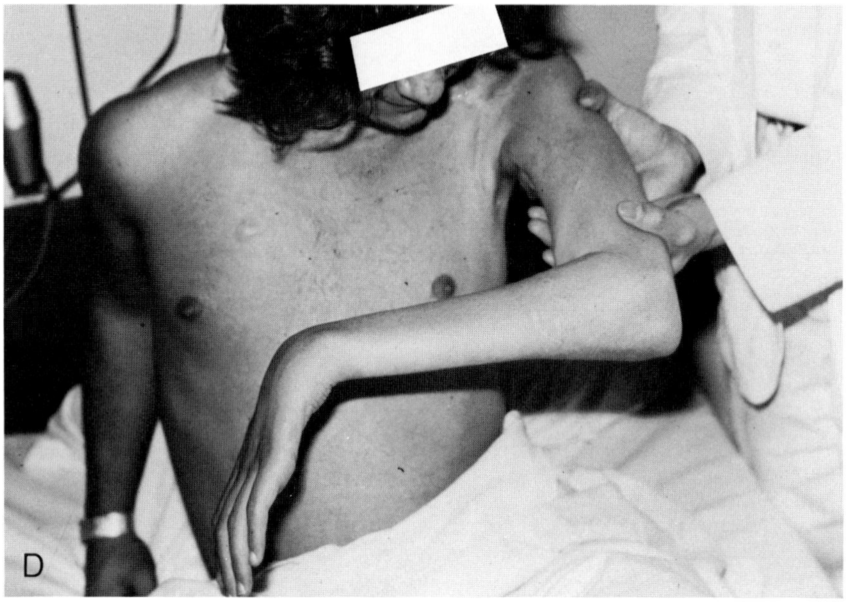

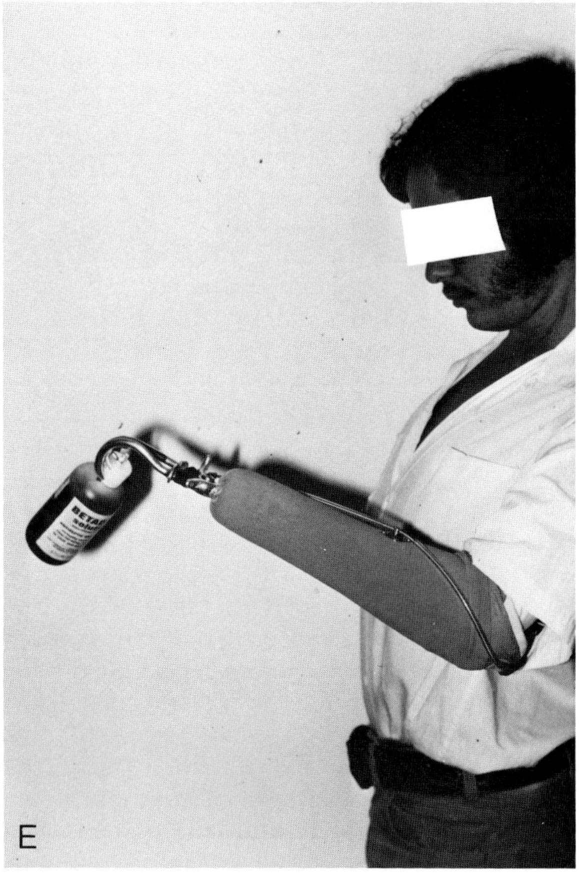

Fig. 10.3 *(continued)* **D**: Eighteen months postoperatively, the patient has regained elbow flexion. No other function returned. **E**: Patient underwent amputation through the forearm and shoulder fusion. He uses the prosthesis daily.

manner in which those results are reported must be more carefully scrutinized.

The optimal situation in a neural reconstructive procedure would be to reconstitute, if possible, everything available. Practically, it comes down to using the C5, 6, 7 outflow the bridge to the lateral and posterior cords. The lower trunk, C8 and T1, is of questionable value as a source of axons, even if it is technically possible, since the chances of functional motor recovery from this maneuver are remote in adults. Occasionally the flexor carpi ulnaris, and sometimes a profundus, may be reinnervated. Even though the results of the neural procedures done for the flail-anesthetic upper extremity in terms of motor function may be minimal, anything that is obtained is more than would have been gotten by any other method, since we are dealing with total loss of the plexus. They should be evaluated not only from the point of view of postoperative neurological testing, but from the more complex yet more important perspective of whether the patient can actually use the limb better than before the surgery.

Of greatest importance is the possibility of return of sensibility and alleviation of trophic changes. Since even in partial lesions there is no way of restoring these functions by peripheral reconstruction, nerve grafting or repair constitutes a clearly superior approach in this area.

The timing of such surgery is of great importance for a number of reasons. Obviously, one would not want to commit the patient to a long and probably fruitless period of "waiting for something to happen." Specifically, the longer the elapsed time since injury, the greater the scarring to be dealt with at surgery, and, more importantly, the operative results reported by most authors have indicated that the first three to six months give the best chance of success. After 18 months the chance of functional recovery is slim. Therefore, if the patient is seen immediately with a complete traction lesion, all diagnostic maneuvers, including myelography and electrodiagnostic studies, should be completed by two months. If there are no signs of recovery by three months, one should proceed with surgical exploration, prepared to graft or provide axons for neurotization if necessary.

For the patient with a partial lesion, the choice of alternatives of management becomes less categorically defined, and more related to which part of the plexus has been damaged. Here again, reference to the reported series reveals that the outlook for recovery of the lower trunk lesion is poor. Since no responsible author has claimed recovery of intrinsics in adults, and most admit that finger flexion is unlikely to result from direct repair at this level, I consider the peripheral reconstructions to be most appealing, since the results are generally predictably good. Function is restored within weeks of surgery, and although sensibility cannot be regained, its deficit on the ulnar aspect of the hand and forearm are of relatively lesser importance. For the patient with a complete C8, T1 lesion, then, surgical reconstruction of the hand could commence immediately after the lesion had been thoroughly documented.

For the patient with an incomplete lesion that paralyzes the outflow of C5, C6, or C5, C6, and C7, the outlook for spontaneous recovery of function is considerably better than the whole plexus lesion. Probably this relates to the lower incidence of root avulsions at these levels. However, this group is also the most difficult in terms of alternatives of treatment, despite the fact that the injury per se is much less catastrophic to the patient himself. From the point of view of critical loss of sensibility, although there is a deficit in the important radial side of the hand, it is rarely complete enough to make that hand "blind." If wrist and finger extension are lost, with additional motor deficits above the elbow, the problem is no worse than that of an isolated peripheral radial nerve lesion, and the solution is, in my opinion, in conventional tendon transfers, which have an extremely high rate of success. Whatever loss of active elbow extension occurs is lessened in its consequences by the ability to use gravity for extension, although, admittedly, there are circumstances where this maneuver does not suffice. The means of restoring active elbow flexion by peripheral reconstruction have already been described. Although none of them can result in motor power that is normal or nearly so, again, they can be used with a predictably high rate of producing a functioning elbow, and the time between operation and the end result is considerably less than the time taken for reinnervation of the muscles supplied by the musculocutaneous nerve. On the other side of the argument, the results of neurological reconstruction are most favorable at this level and can even approach normal function, which tendon transfers cannot do (Fig. 10.4).

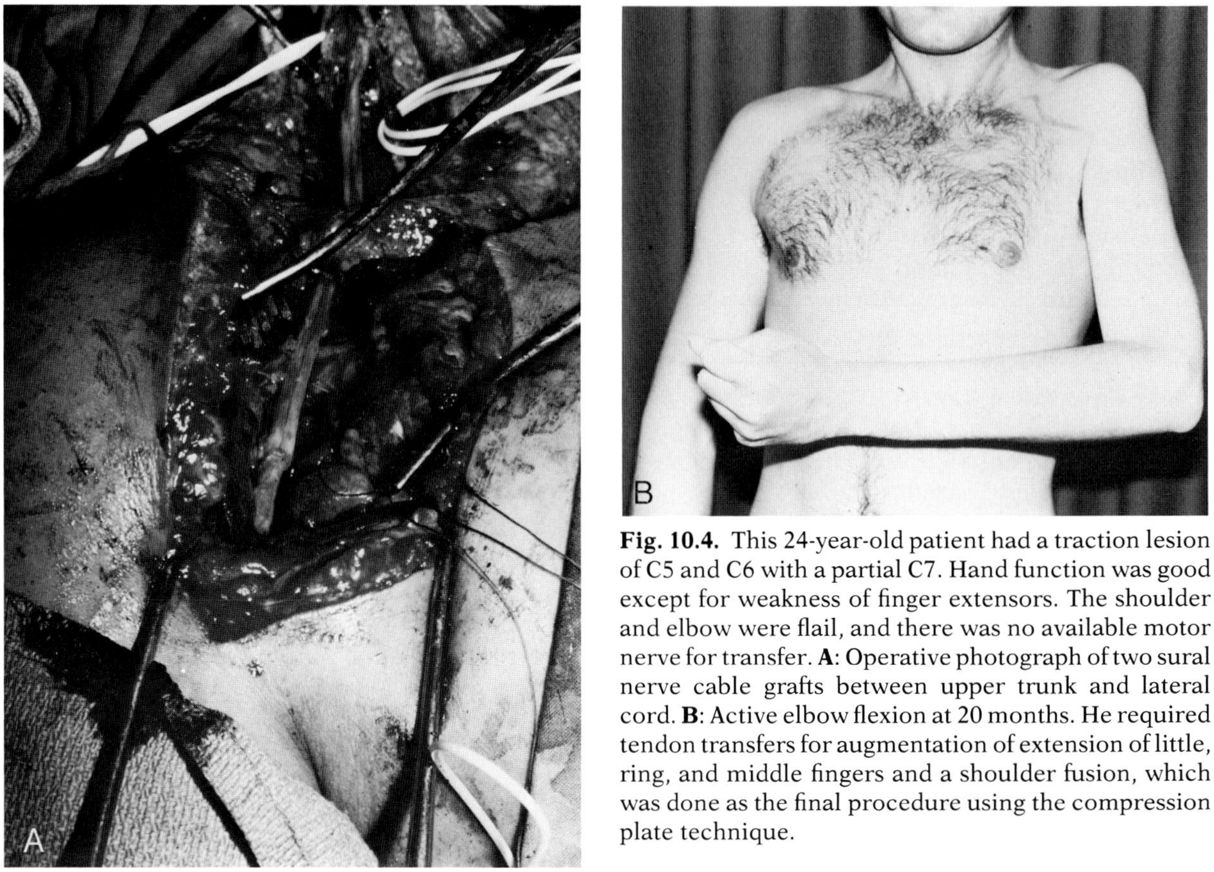

Fig. 10.4. This 24-year-old patient had a traction lesion of C5 and C6 with a partial C7. Hand function was good except for weakness of finger extensors. The shoulder and elbow were flail, and there was no available motor nerve for transfer. **A**: Operative photograph of two sural nerve cable grafts between upper trunk and lateral cord. **B**: Active elbow flexion at 20 months. He required tendon transfers for augmentation of extension of little, ring, and middle fingers and a shoulder fusion, which was done as the final procedure using the compression plate technique.

Shoulder function is the most complicated, and therefore the most potentially controversial, problem in this group of patients, and has already been discussed. According to Allieu,[1] even in those patients in whom the useful grade of recovery is not obtained, the recovery of deltoid tonus may make the procedure worthwhile in some cases where fusion is rejected. He therefore tends to offer the patient neurological reconstruction rather than fusion for the shoulder. However, Allieu and colleagues[2] caution that in a patient with a lesion of the upper trunk in whom elbow flexion has recovered, endoneurolysis of that trunk is contraindicated for fear of losing the function of the biceps and brachialis as against the poor chance of lessening the shoulder paralysis by direct surgical attack.

Arthrodesis of the shoulder can be done at a later date if neurological reconstruction fails. In most of my patients it has been used as a primary procedure with very gratifying results.

The timing of operative intervention requires reemphasis, since most authors are agreed that delay of more than six months post injury will diminish the chance of functional recovery. Those patients with nondegenerative lesions, or neurapraxias, will have begun to recover by six weeks, and in most the degree of recovery will be substantially ahead of what might be otherwise expected. For the patient with a lesion in continuity, in the period between two and three months, regeneration has begun and conservative therapy is indicated. If, in three to six months, regeneration continues, conservative treatment is employed, but for those without signs of regeneration or advancement, if surgery is to be done on the plexus, it should be done then. In formulating these guidelines, Millesi[21] admits that those cases in which regeneration has had a late start, some will undergo surgery when they might have gone on to recover spontaneously. He therefore states that with meticulous microsurgical technique he does not hesitate to explore the plexuses. The late phase of direct repair, which Millesi designates at six to 12 months, has a considerably poorer prognosis for recovery following direct repair, although, if the patient is young, there is still a sufficient chance to make the intevention worthwhile. For those patients who have been documented as having stopped their recovery in this period when it had been proceeding satisfactorily before, neurolysis is indicated. However, these patients are not common.

Although most authors have done grafts and neurolyses in patients seen after one and one-half years, the percentage of failures in this group has been so high as to make the procedure considerably less worthwhile.

OPERATIVE TECHNIQUE

The normally complex anatomy of the brachial plexus may be so distorted by traction injury and scarring that it may be practically unrecognizable. Reconstructive surgery may, therefore, be extremely difficult. It should not be attempted by occasional operators, or those not prepared to deal with all the problems that may arise. The critical prerequisites are sound knowledge of anatomy and familiarity and training in technique rather than certification in any particular surgical specialty. In addition, the primary surgeon should have available a technically able assistant or alternate who can take over when he is fatigued. This is particularly true after the dissection required for the exposure of the lesions has been done, which may take as long as four to five hours. Having then to do the nerve graft sutures under high magnification can be very difficult indeed. Being able to rest briefly while the other surgeon continues is a big advantage. Also, because of the possibility of intraoperative vascular injury, contingency arrangements to meet these situations must be firmly made prior to the procedure. Pneumothorax may occasionally occur intraoperatively, particularly when dissecting in the region of the first rib. It is easily managed by tube thoracostomy.

The anesthetic management of these long and difficult cases is best done by those well accustomed to similar problems. Hypotensive anesthetic techniques are really of no advantage, since one would be well advised to be aware of even seemingly trivial bleeders. In cases where electrical stimulation is to be employed intraoperatively by the surgeon, it is imperative that the anesthetist refrain from using neuromuscular blocking agents that would prevent normal responses. Also he or she should be made aware if somatosensory evoked potentials or other neurophysiologic measurements are to be made.

Position on the operating table should provide maximal exposure, not only over the plexus itself, but for potential harvesting of grafts, or whatever other techniques may be required. The surgical exposure will be described in detail in the next section. The semisitting supine position has the advantage of avoiding pooling of blood in the depths of the wound where it would obscure the field. For those surgeons who have had the aggravating and tedious experience of having to procure two sural nerves from a patient lying in the supine position, the simple expedient of beginning the operative procedure with the patient prone to harvest the grafts before they are needed is helpful (Fig. 10.5). Obviously, subsequent developments may prove them unnecessary, but this will not occur often.

The supine position on the operating table with a pillow beneath the ipsilateral scapula to bring the shoulder forward, and the head turned to the opposite side will allow for just about every conceivable maneuver that will be required. Elevation of the back of the table to low Fowler's position will be of advantage. The ipsilateral hemithorax and axilla as well as the upper extremity are sterilely prepped and draped into the field as are both lower extremities. Only in this way will an adequate supply of donor sites for nerve grafting be assumed. The arm may be abducted on a narrow arm board for access to it and the axilla. It is advisable to insert an indwelling catheter into the urinary bladder for the duration of the procedure.

OPERATIVE APPROACH

The skin incision must provide access to both supra- and infraclavicular parts of the plexus. It begins at the midpoint of the posterior border of the sternomastoid muscle and drops vertically to the midpoint of the clavicle although medial inclination of this part of the incision will help to reduce hypertrophic scarring. Preliminary infiltration of the skin in the line of the incision with a dilute solution of

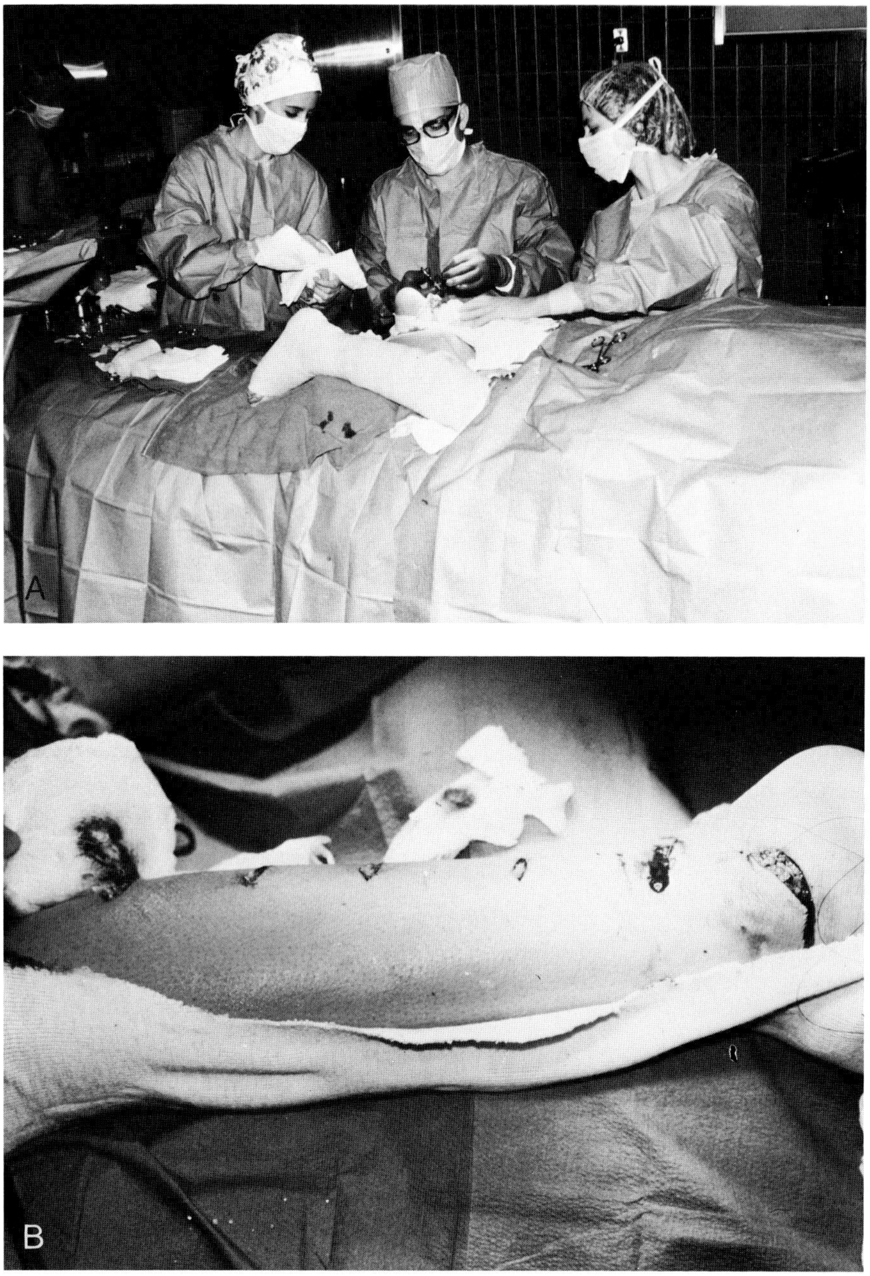

Fig. 10.5. A: The prone position to harvest the sural nerves. **B**: Multiple short transverse incisions are used in the leg. They heal with minimal scarring.

vasopressor can be of help in diminishing the bleeding in this area. Care must be taken to identify and protect the cutaneous branches of the cervical plexus as well as the highest structure in the incision, the spinal accessory nerve. The external jugular vein will usually have to be ligated and divided for exposure as will the suprascapular and transverse cervical vessels that cross the plexus perpendicularly. The omohyoid muscle must also be divided, but the two ends should be tagged for reapproximation over the plexus or grafts at the end of the operation. In a dissecting room specimen this part of the procedure will be relatively straightforward. In a patient who has had a significant traction injury to the brachial plexus, the normal interval between the anterior and middle scalene muscles may be virtually impossible to define because of the scarring, and one may be hard-pressed to identify the neural elements. Painstaking dissection and the use of the nerve stimulator will usually provide the solution, since the phrenic nerve may almost always be stimulated to produce contraction of the ipsilateral hemidiaphragm. The nerve can then be followed proximally on the surface of the anterior scalene to define the fourth cervical and subsequently fifth cervical roots. Dissection is carried to the intervertebral foramina, and when possible, the root collateral branches are identified. By continuing the dissection distally, the remaining neural elements may be either identified or verified as being absent. If further dissection becomes impossible in one area because of impenetrable scar, then dissection should shift to another area. Because the entire plexus must be seen in order to verify that the infraclavicular portion is indeed intact, the nerves must be followed down behind the clavicle. The incision is prolonged distally across the clavicle, then laterally a thumb's breadth distal to it to reach the deltopectoral groove over the coracoid process. The interval is readily identified by the presence of the cephalic vein, which should be ligated and removed to prevent annoying bleeding during the course of the procedure. The neurovascular sheath may be traced proximally from the brachium and axilla by appropriate extension of the incision, usually made technically easier by often normal conditions of the structures at that level.

The problem of the management of the clavicle in this situation has been met in a variety of ways. The most obvious, but not necessarily the best, way is to simply divide it obliquely with a Gigli saw while protecting the great vessels and nerves that lie beneath it. The cut ends may then be turned forward to provide exposure. At the end of the procedure the osteotomy may be aligned and reapproximated by means of a compression plate. There is a significant risk of nonunion or even osteomyelitis of the clavicle as reported by Lusskin, Campbell, and Thompson.[18] Predrilling the clavicle before osteotomy may facilitate the osteosynthesis with a compression plate. Most experienced surgeons today will exert considerable effort to avoid dividing it. With a mobile shoulder girdle, it is usually possible to lift the clavicle forward and work effectively beneath it. The access to C8 to T1 are more difficult with an intact clavicle, however. The pectoralis major and minor will be temporarily partially detached to gain further exposure. It is imperative that neither the nerve supply nor the substance of the pectoralis major be damaged during its mobilization, and that it be carefully replaced at the end of the procedure to prevent loss of this important muscle. The omohyoid, although functionally insignificant, can serve as a soft-tissue buffer between the clavicle (and fracture callus if it has been osteotomized) and the nerve grafts crossing just beneath it.

The intricacy of the surgical manipulations required in attempting repair of the traumatized brachial plexus dictate that microsurgical instruments, suture materials, and techniques be employed. Magnification will vary considerably, depending on whether the gross identification of the neural elements or their meticulous separation from scar is being done. Thus, provision for a wide range of optical capabilities is necessary. Some surgeons find that the operating microscope with zoom capabilities answers all of their needs. Others find that the size and varied topography and depth of the surgical field make the use of the microscope cumbersome and prefer the eyeglass mounted operating telescopes for part of the dissection. These are readily available in 2.5 – 6 × magnification. Although 8 × glasses can be ordered, they are considerably harder to adapt to than the 6 ×. As with all such highly magnified situations, a prefocused headlamp must be used concomitantly.

Suture material and needles continue to be improved, but 9 : 0 and 10 : 0 nylon are quite satisfactory for most situations one is likely to encounter.

Because of the nature of the traction injury, direct suture will almost never be feasible even with attempted mobilization and posturing of the neck and shoulder. This maneuver should not be done, since when normal mobility is resumed, either a rupture of the suture line or an additional traction lesion will result. Under the existing limitations of technology, suture of roots avulsed from the spinal cord is not possible. The nerve root ruptured in the foramen is a problem because, although it may appear to present a viable source of axons for distal connection, the retrograde damage inflicted on the cell bodies may simply be so great that regeneration is impossible. An atrophic proximal stump, without any evidence of neuroma formation, is a poor prognostic sign, since in all likelihood there will be few viable axons present. The finding of available axons even within the confines of a traumatic pseudomeningocele has been reported by Millesi.[21] The use of somatosensory evoked potentials intraoperatively[17] and improved diagnostic imaging preoperatively makes the performance of laminectomy for verification of the integrity of the nerve roots at the spinal cord level unnecessary. The results of nerve grafting of the plexus at varying distances from the intervertebral foramen has already been discussed: those grafts done at the level of the scalene muscles have a poorer outlook than those done more distally. It follows that, in addition to viable axons with good regenerative potential proximally, the distal connections must be chosen on the basis of which of them have the best theoretical and statistically demonstrated chance of restoring useful function. According to this principle, the preferred ultimate distal connection will usually be the outflow of the lateral and posterior cords. Obviously, any situation in which a more proximal structure can serve as the distal site of suture will be desirable but much less frequently encountered in a major traction injury. Special effort ought to be made to reconstruct the suprascapular nerve, since without this component of the rotator cuff, the shoulder mechanism is usually ineffective, even in the presence of a functioning deltoid. The outflow of the C8 and T1 has had such a statistically poor record of repair that one can only hope for recovery of the flexor carpi ulnaris under the most favorable circumstances, and this may prove useful. Nevertheless, I can find little enthusiasm for attempting lower trunk reconstruction.

Nerve grafts, in addition to viable axons proximally, will ultimately require connection with reference to the intraneural topography of those axons. Some work in this area has already been done by Narakas[26] and others,[19] but more is required. It should be realized that only generalizations can be drawn from the maps of intraneural topography, for each plexus is quite individual in terms of fine detail.

There is no longer any question that fresh autogenous nerve grafts are superior to anything else that has been tried. The problem becomes a practical one of how much and what the patient can spare. The theoretical consideration of the superiority of multiple cables of cutaneous nerves over main trunk nerves for their ease of revascularization may be offset by the larger size of the available Schwann tubes in the main trunk as well as the technical advantage in having a single structure to inset rather than a number of smaller ones. Certainly if a main trunk is available by reason of a forearm that is to be amputated anyway, then the selection is narrowed. One might excise a segment of denervated ulnar nerve in an otherwise intact forearm in which the prognosis for recovery of its motor and sensory function is hopeless. However, the nerve should be reduced in diameter by epineurotomy and stripping of some fascicular groups to avoid central necrosis of the grafts. One could also excise the medial cutaneous nerve of the forearm on the ipsilateral side in the arm. The donor nerve of choice in my experience has been the sural nerve which in the average-sized adult can provide in excess of 30 cm of useful graft. Although the superficial radial and lateral cutaneous nerve of the forearm are available, I have hesitated to harvest them for fear of aggravating an already impoverished sensory nerve supply to the upper limb.

Once it has been established by inspection and palpation that the potential point of attachment of the nerve graft proximally and distally is free of scar, then the length of the graft must be estimated so that it can be cut to size and sutured in place. Tension on the grafts must be avoided. Since the head has usually been turned to the other side for exposure and the shoulder is generally resting in neutral position or even depressed because of the semisitting position of the operating table, the gap is probably at its maximal. To allow for shrinkage, an additional 15% is added to the required length of the graft. Since group funicular suture is usually not possible in this situation, the available axonal cross-sectional area proximally and the distal nerves are connected by intercalated cables with epineural suture, respecting the axial alignment as much as possible with general reference to intraneural topography. As little suture material as possible is used consistant with attaining accurate placement of the grafts. Often a single suture will suffice, and the cables will then adhere due to tissue fluid. There is no evidence that any type of wrapping of the suture line will enhance the degree of recovery by protecting against scarring. Although I did use plasma clot in a few cases, I have not continued to use the method.

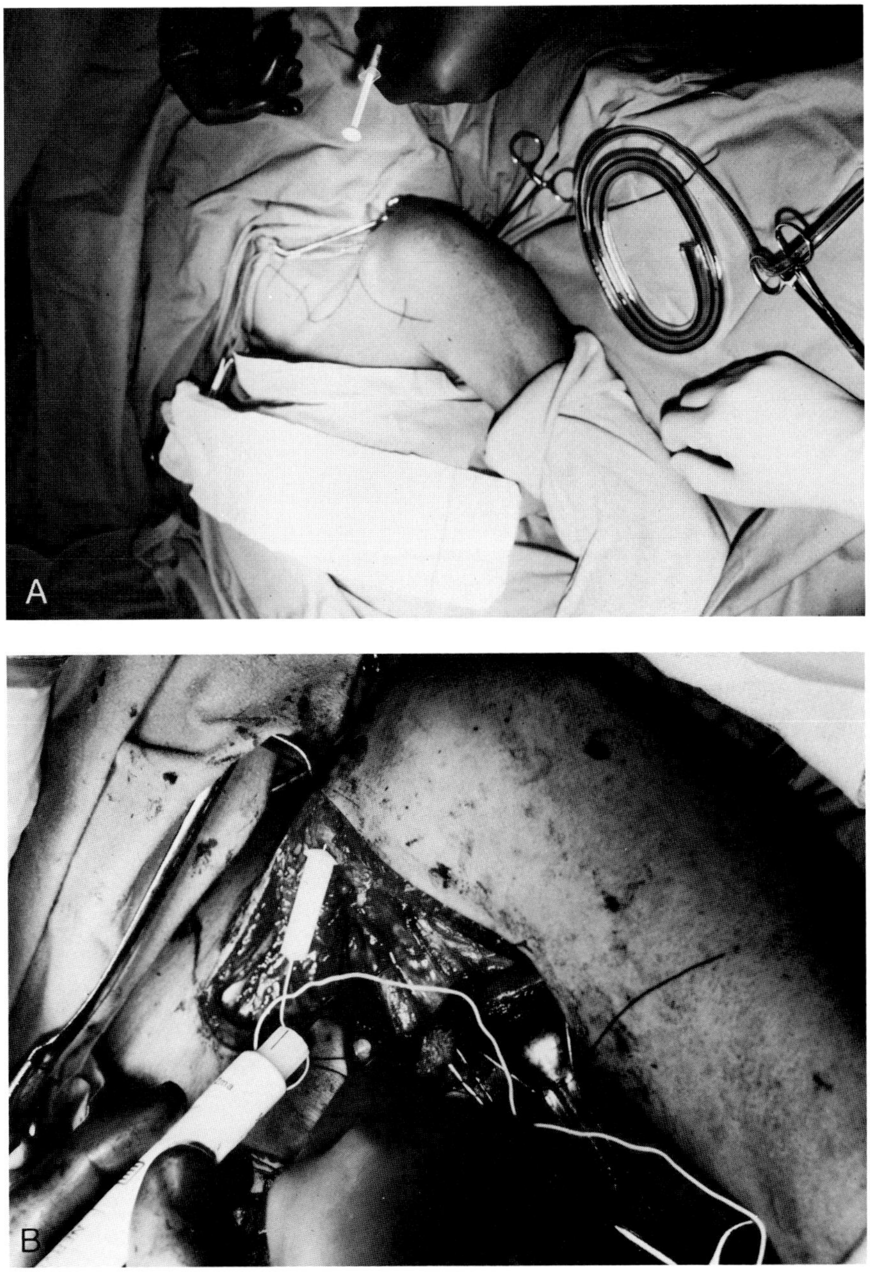

Fig. 10.6. Operative photograph of a patient with a severe traction lesion of the left brachial plexus at eight months with no clinical evidence of recovery and a normal myelogram. There was a strong Tinel's sign in the posterior triangle of the neck. **A**: The incision. **B**: Use of the nerve stimulator during neurolysis.

(Figure continues on next page.)

Neurolysis

The general indications for neurolysis have already been discussed. A patient whose progression of recovery has been positively documented to have stopped or reversed is a candidate for neurolysis. The management of the neuroma-in-continuity, as in peripheral nerve surgery in other areas, is the most difficult problem of all, if for no other reason than that the stakes are higher. There is a very definite risk of making the deficit greater, especially with endoneurolysis, no matter how delicately it is done. One would not, as emphasized by Allieu and coworkers,[2] attempt neurolysis of the upper trunk in a patient who had regained elbow flexion without shoulder

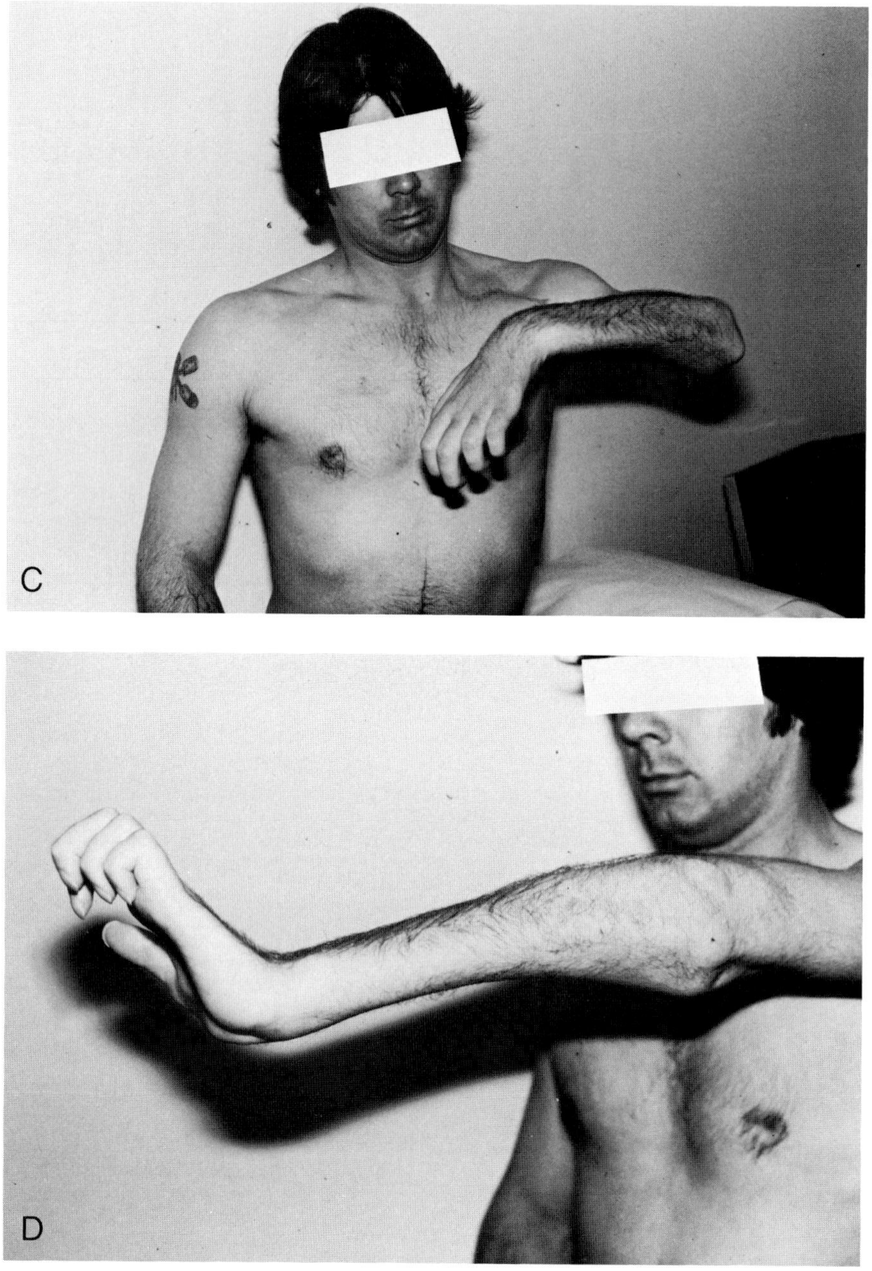

Fig. 10.6 *(continued).* **C** and **D**: Result at two years.

abduction for fear of losing that which had already recovered. In their series of 14 neurolyses, there were only two cases in which recovery absolutely attributable to the neurolysis could be documented. If neurolysis is done, it should be external, with great precision, delicacy, and magnification as well as the nerve stimulator (Figs. 10.6, 10.7). Whether it is reasonable as treatment for the intractable pain of brachial plexus injury remains controversial, and, in my view, unsubstantiated. The use of intraoperative physiological measurements of nerve conduction such as somatosensory evoked potentials and nerve action potential measurement are useful and important adjuncts to what can be clinically determined by

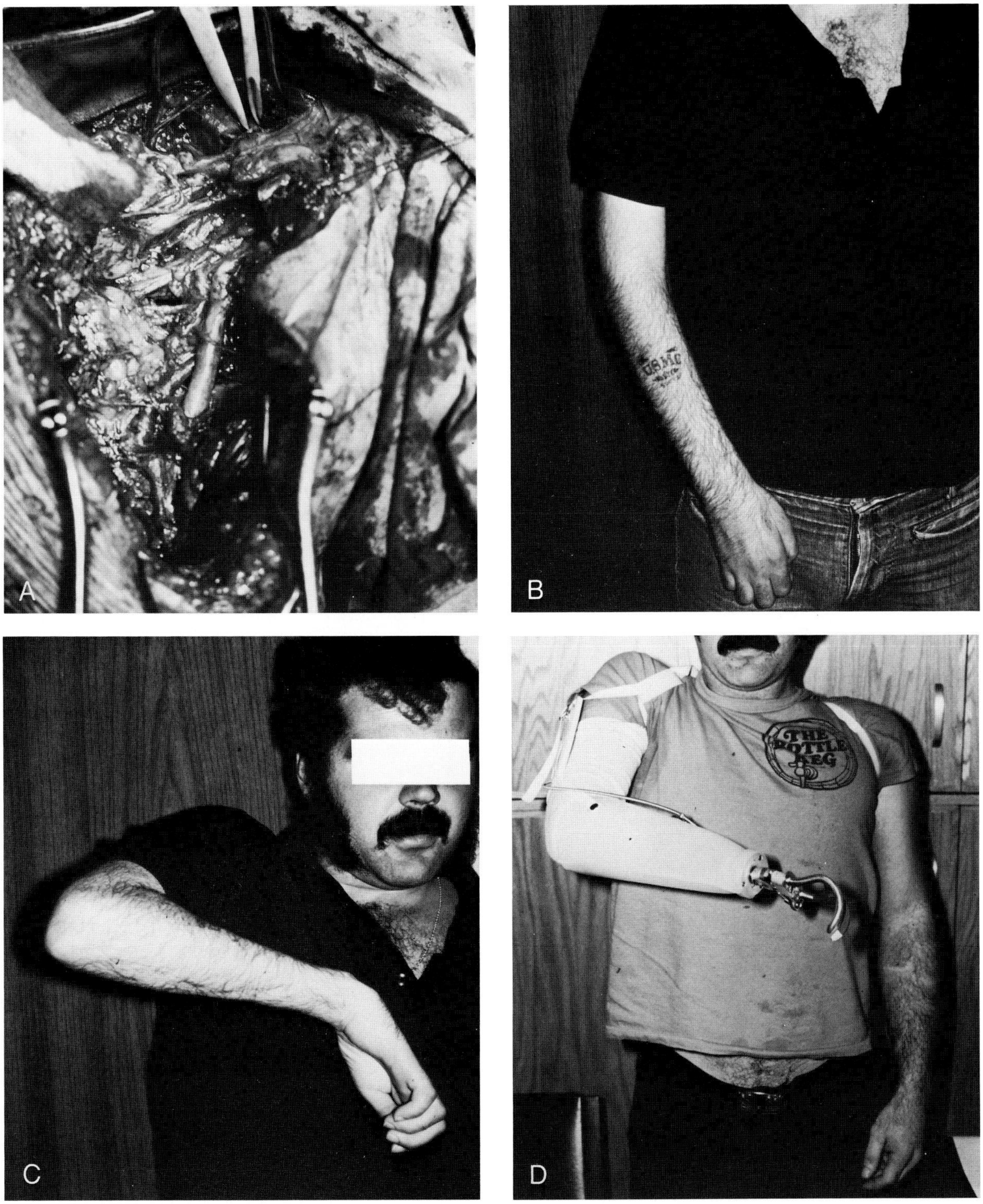

Fig. 10.7. This patient had a flail-anesthetic arm due to a traction injury. Myelography showed pseudomeningoceles at C8 and T1. Exploration performed at six months. **A**: Operative photograph. The clavicle has been divided and retracted for exposure. The scarring is tremendously difficult to define from the neural elements. The thrombosed subclavian artery has been displaced medially by scar. During neurolysis electrical stimulation demonstrated peripheral muscular contraction, so only neurolysis was performed. **B** and **C**: Result at two years. **D**: At four years, no hand function had returned. The patient requested forearm amputation and prosthetic fitting. Result was very functional and patient used it habitually.

inspection, palpation, and even trial section with histological analysis.[15]

Neuroticization

For the patient with a totally flail and anesthetic limb as a result of complete avulsion of the brachial plexus, the only possibility of regaining any function, albeit limited, is to provide a remote source of axons. Historically, although nerve-crossing operations have been reported as long ago as 1903 (Harris and Low[11]), they have not been popular. Seddon and Yeoman[43] in 1961 successfully grafted intercostals III and IV to the musculocutaneous nerve using the ulnar nerve as a free graft from a forearm amputation specimen. Hence there is adequate precedence for neurotization. The experience of the Japanese (Tsuyama and Hara,[42] Kotani et al.[16]) as well as Millesi,[21] Narakas[23–26] and others has reaffirmed that the procedure can be done successfully.

The use of the spinal accessory nerve as a donor has a significant disadvantage in that if the function is lost to the trapezius, it cannot be replaced by any other means and it is vital to the action of the shoulder complex. Even use of part of the nerve has the potential for weakening the muscles. This disadvantage is not a feature of intercostal nerve graft, however, and the loss of three intercostal nerves is well tolerated. Whereas Yeoman and Seddon took the intercostals as close to the intervertebral foramen as possible, using a costotransversectomy approach, subsequent surgeons have not found this necessary. Obviously, if the entire intercostal nerve is dissected out to the midline, an intercalated graft will not be necessary, but then much of the motor supply will have been dissipated. A reasonable compromise appears to be to transect the intercostal nerve at the anterior axillary line and then cable graft to the musculocutaneous nerve. Fewer than three intercostals provide an inadequate axonal population to achieve functional elbow flexion. Although initially the elbow flexion is tied to respiration and may occur involuntarily with coughing or sneezing, it is possible to achieve independent action for voluntary elbow flexion. Whether such restoration of elbow flexion actually enhances the habitual functional use of the limb is questionable. If such grafts are done to restore sensibility in an anesthetic hand, the localization of stimuli applied to the reinnervated skin is to the chest wall. It does not convert with time.

Postoperative Care Following Surgery of the Brachial Plexus

As has been stressed, the grafts should be long enough to allow full motion of all joints in the neck, shoulder joint complex, and arm without causing rupture or additional traction lesions of the plexus. Therefore, immobilization is required, usually in no more than a sling, for only three weeks postoperatively. This gives the reattached muscles ample opportunity to heal.

Complications of Brachial Plexus Surgery

The complications of surgery of the brachial plexus have been alluded to in other chapters devoted to various aspects of the problem. They will be summarized here for the convenience of the reader.

Certainly the length of the operative procedure should predispose to infection, yet this has rarely been reported as a complication, and then, usually having to do with the osteotomized clavicle. Nevertheless, prophylactic antibiotics would seem indicated for these long operations. The problem of nonunion of the clavicle has been described.

It is indeed fortunate that modern anesthesia has advanced to the point where a 10- or 12-hour procedure can be safely done, but it also imposes upon the surgeon the obligation to assume that he has adequate anesthetic coverage and that the patient's general condition will allow prolonged anesthesia. A massively traumatized or multiply injured patient is a poor candidate for the additional trauma involved in a reconstruction of the brachial plexus. It can always be done as a secondary procedure, particularly if the primary indication for surgery was the presence of a vascular lesion. Just as certainly, the potential for vascular injury exists in all traction injuries with extensive scarring. The development of well-vascularized collateral circulation can make exploration hazardous. Similarly, the proximity of the pleura to the lower trunk of the plexus must be remembered when dissecting in that area.

The problem of aggravation of the existing neurological deficit by subsequent surgical intervention, especially neurolysis, remains one of the most unfortunate complications. Hence the potential gain must be carefully weighed against the risks in every surgical candidate. A deficit that is improving cannot be "hurried along" by even the most well-intentioned and carefully executed neurolysis—it can only be made worse!

The scarring from the operative incision can be distressing, particularly in the vertical limb in the neck, and is somewhat unpredictable. A more oblique incision here will tend to minimize hypertrophic scarring. Closure of the platysma with care and the use of subcuticular suture can also be of benefit.

Finally, the morbidity attributable to the donor sites of the nerve grafts is usually not significant, unless the deficit created either increases the functional deficit (not a problem with sural nerve grafts), or results in a tender and adherent neuroma. For this reason, for example, the proximal stump of the donor nerve should be taken high enough to allow it to be covered with adequate soft tissue, and at least to be located far enough away from adjacent joints so as not to be disturbed by their motion. This is particularly important for the sural nerve at the ankle. Although it would be rare to have need for a short graft in brachial plexus reconstruction, if such were the case, a length great enough to insure clearance of the mobile skin adjacent to the ankle would be advisable.

REFERENCES

1. Allieu Y: Exploration et traitement direct des lesions nerveuses dans les paralysies traumatiques par élongation du plexus brachial chez l'adulte. Rev Chir Orthop 63:107, 1975
2. Allieu Y, Privat JM, Bonnel F: Les neurotizations par le nerf spinal (nerf accessorius) dans les avulsions radiculaires du plexus brachial. Neurochirurgie 28:115, 1982
3. Alnot JY, Jolly A, Frot B: Traitement direct de lésions nerveuses dans les paralysies traumatiques du plexus brachial chez l'adulte. Int Orthop 63:82, 1981
4. Barnes R: Traction injuries of the brachial plexus in adults. J Bone Joint Surg 31B:10, 1949
5. Bonney G: Prognosis in traction lesions of the brachial plexus. J Bone Joint Surg 41B:4, 1959
6. Brooks D: The place of nerve grafting in orthopedic surgery. J Bone Joint Surg 37A:2, 1955
7. Clark LP, Taylor AS, Prout P: Study on brachial birth palsy. Am J Med Sci 130:670, 1905
8. Davis L, Martin J, Perret G: The treatment of injuries of the brachial plexus. Ann Surg 125:647, 1947
9. Fairbank HAT: Birth palsy: Subluxation of shoulder joint in infants and young children. Lancet 1:1217, 1913
10. Flaubert M: Mémoire sur plusiers cas de luxation. Rep Gen Anat Physiol Pathol 3:55, 1827
11. Harris W, Low VW: The importance of accurate muscle analysis in lesions of the brachial plexus. Br Med J 2:1035, 1903
12. Hendry AM: The treatment of residual paralysis after brachial plexus injury. J Bone Joint Surg 31B:42, 1949
13. Jepson PN: Obstetrical paralysis. Ann Surg 91:724, 1930
14. Kennedy R: Suture of the brachial plexus and birth paralysis of the upper extremity. Br Med J 1:298, 1903
15. Kline DG, Nulsen FE: The neuroma in continuity: its pre-operative and operative management. Surg Clin North Am 52:1189, 1972
16. Kotani T, Toshima Y, Matsuda H, Suzuki, et al: Postoperative results of nerve transposition in brachial plexus injury. Orthop Surg (Tokyo) 22:963, 1971
17. Landi A, Copland SA, Wynn-Parry CB, Jones SJ: The role of the somatosensory evoked potentials and nerve conduction studies in the surgical management of brachial plexus injuries. J Bone Joint Surg 62:492, 1980
18. Lusskin R, Campbell JB, Thompson WAL: Post-traumatic lesions of the brachial plexus. Treatment by transclavicular exploration and neurolysis or autograft reconstruction. J Bone Joint Surg 55A:1159, 1973
19. Mansat M: Anatomie topographique et chirurgicale du plexus brachial. Rev Chir Orthop 63:20, 1977
20. Millesi H, Meiszl G, Katzer H: Zur Behandlung der Verletzungen des Plexus brachialis. Vorschlag einer integrierten Therapie. Burns Beitr Klin 220:429, 1973
21. Millesi H: Surgical management of brachial plexus injury. J Hand Surg 2:367, 1977
22. Millesi H: Indications et resultats des interventions directs paralysie traumatique du plexus brachial chez l'adulte. Rev Surg Orthop 63:82, 1977
23. Narakas A: Lesions dans les elongations du plexus brachial. Rev Chir Orthop 63:44, 1977
24. Narakas A: Indications et resultats du traitement chirurgical direct dans les lésions par élongation du plexus brachial. Rev Chir Orthop 63:88, 1977
25. Narakas A: Surgical treatment of traction injuries of the brachial plexus. Clin Orthop 133:71, 1978
26. Narakas A: Brachial plexus surgery. Orthop Clin North Am 12:303, 1981
27. Nulsen FE, Slade HW: Peripheral nerve regeneration, VA medical myelograph. In Woodhall B, Beebe GW (eds): A Follow-up Study of 3,656 World War II Injuries. Chap 9. p 389. Recovery following injury to the brachial plexus. 1956
28. Platt H: Opening remarks on birth paralysis. J Orthop Surg 2:272, 1920

29. Samii M, Kahl RI: Clinische Resultate der autologen Nerven Transplantation. Melssunger Med Mitteil 46:197, 1972
30. Samii M: Modern aspects of peripheral and cranial nerve surgery. In Krayenbuhl H (ed): Advances in Technical Standards in Neurosurgery. Vol 2. p 53. Springer-Verlag New York, 1975
31. Seddon HJ: The use of autogenous grafts for the repair of large gaps in peripheral nerves. Br J Surg 35:151, 1947
32. Seddon HJ: Nerve grafting. J Bone Joint Surg 45:447, 1963
33. Sedel L: Results of surgical repair of brachial plexus injuries. J Bone Joint Surg 64B:54, 1982
34. Sever JW: Obstetrical paralysis. Etiology, pathology, clinical aspects and treatment with report of 470 cases. Am J Dis Child 12:541, 1916
35. Sharpe W: The operative treatment of brachial plexus paralysis. JAMA 66:876, 1981
36. Stevens J: Brachial Plexus Paralysis. In Codman EA: The Shoulder. G. Miller, Brooklyn, NY, 1934
37. Taylor AS: Results from the surgical treatment of brachial birth palsy. JAMA 48:96, 1907
38. Taylor AS: Conclusions derived from further experience in the surgical treatment of brachial birth palsy (Erb's type). Am J Med Sci 146:836, 1913
39. Taylor AS: Brachial birth palsy and injuries of similar type in adults. Surg Gynecol Obstet 30:494, 1920
40. Thoburn W: Obstetrical paralysis. J Obstet Gynecol Br Emp 3:454, 1903
41. Tracy JF, Brannon EW: Management of brachial plexus injuries (traction type). J Bone Joint Surg 40A:1031, 1958
42. Tsuyama N, Hara T: Intercostal nerve transfer in the treatment of brachial plexus injury of root-avulsion type. Proceedings of the 12th Congress of the International Society of Orthopaedic Surgery and Traumatology, Tel Aviv. Exerpta Medica, Amsterdam, 351, 1972
43. Yeoman PM, Seddon HJ: Brachial plexus injuries: Treatment of the flail arm. J Bone Joint Surg 43B:493, 1961

11

Peripheral Reconstruction of the Upper Limb Following Brachial Plexus Injury

Although the function of the human upper limb is an extremely complex subject, it can be essentially summarized as follows:

The parts proximal to the wrist serve to position and stabilize the hand in space. Without the prehension of the hand and its sensibility, the remainder of the limb is deprived of much of its raison d'être, and without the means to reach, grasp is of little use.

For the patient with injury to the brachial plexus, either all or part of these interrelated functions may be temporarily or permanently lost. Since it is rare for a patient with an extensive posttraumatic lesion to spontaneously achieve total recovery, it is necessary to review the available armamentarium with which to favorably influence the functional outcome. Such deliberations must be functionally directed and not confined to the simple recapitulation of a list of techniques. Rather we should ask: What does the patient lack, what does he need, and how can we attempt to achieve those ends?

First we must determine when spontaneous recovery is unlikely or highly improbable. This state can be said to exist if by means of all available methods of evaluation we have established that the nerves have been irrevocably destroyed, or sufficient time has elapsed without the appearance or further progression of functional recovery. One cannot, especially within the first 12 months of the injury, make such a determination absolutely unless there has been incontrovertible verification, by means of direct operative intervention, of nerve destruction, even though indirect methods may provide strong presumptive evidence. At one year post injury, a patient with no evidence of continued proximal recovery would be unlikely to experience distal function within the distribution of a particular spinal nerve under consideration. Although some benefit may result from operative reconstruction of the nerves at or after this time, in adults the results are sufficiently poor as to make them usually of considerably less value.

Generally, since the observed functional deficits encompass both motor and sensory loss, in planning reconstruction we must determine what is available to restore that loss. Unfortunately, no peripheral reconstruction can return sensibility lost by brachial plexus injury. This, in turn, may seriously compromise the result of any procedure done for restoration of motor control. If neurological reconstruction can ameliorate the deficit with reasonable predictability, and if there is no great risk to existing function, then the nerves themselves should be repaired.

The experience of reconstructive surgeons in the treatment of motor loss due to poliomyelitis has provided techniques of proven worth to improve motor function, but they must not be adapted without reservation to the plexus-injured patients. An upper limb paralyzed by polio has normal sensibility—therefore its usefulness with even minimal voluntary control can be significant. By contrast, an insensate limb with the same motor pattern may be less than useless, since it is vulnerable to injury that may only become apparent after it has sustained significant damage. Even the possibilities of augmentation of function by means of external orthoses are limited by this "weakness of insensate flesh."

The judicious combination of tendon transfers when possible, and arthrodesis when preservation of motion is not, is the subject of peripheral reconstruction.

The rationale and sequence of reconstruction must be thoroughly understood by the patient as well as the surgeon, since maximal cooperation is necessary for a satisfactory result. If the hand and forearm are intact, then, beginning distally, one would address the problem of the elbow. If a Steindler flexorplasty[58-60] is to be done, it is technically easier if the arm can be abducted freely at operation to allow access to the medial side of the elbow. A fused shoulder would make this very difficult indeed. If, however, a pectoral transfer is planned, it requires either a shoulder under good voluntary control, or one that is solidly fused, and so the shoulder joint would, in this case, be operated upon first. Furthermore, the functional interdependence of these joints is seen in the agumentation of elbow flexion by a shoulder that can be forward flexed or abducted to eliminate the effect of gravity at the elbow. A strong elbow flexor can materially lessen the demands made on the shoulder.

For the patient with a potentially useful hand, but one which needs one or more operative procedures, these should be done, whenever possible, as the initial stage of reconstruction. Aside from practical considerations of positioning the hand at operation, since it is the most important part of the upper extremity (assuming it can be saved), its outcome will often determine whether subsequent operative stages will be initiated. Furthermore, one can often learn much about the ability or willingness of the patient to cooperate in the program—which might radically alter what is done later.

THE SHOULDER

The shoulder joint complex provides the balanced combination of mobility and stability that allows us to position the hand in space. Unfortunately, this most mobile of all joints is frequently impaired by the effects of brachial plexus injury. Not only is the innervation very much at risk, but the complexity of its normal muscular function makes successful surgical reconstruction very difficult. In a normal shoulder the range of motion under voluntary control should permit us to place the hand anywhere on the surface of the body except for a small area between the scapulae, assuming the distal joints are unimpaired. Normally, although backward reach is restricted, that to the side and in front is limited only by the combined length of the fully extended segments of the arm, forearm, and hand.

Observation of many patients with brachial plexus injury has established to my satisfaction (or chagrin) that even the most elegantly reconstructed limb is no longer used habitually as the preferred or dominant limb if it once was. Of course, one might argue that if the treatment rendered had been good enough, this would not be true. Nevertheless, it has been my experience in the vast majority of cases. We shall assume that the other limb is normal, and all that follows is predicated on this condition. If it is not, then various compromises must be accepted: With unilateral impairment, much of the normal global range of the involved shoulder is no longer used for function. It would be unlikely for such patients to reach out to the side or above the head with the impaired limb while the other, normal, one, remained idle. The tasks requiring extremes of strength, dexterity, or position will be accomplished by the normal limb, with the impaired one as an assist. Therefore, the weaker limb must be capable of steadying something, holding it, or transferring it to the other hand. For all activities except those involving working above shoulder level, the "global requirement" of the impaired limb is substantially reduced to one approximating the baseball batter's "strike zone." This extends from the level of the axillae to the top of the knees. The width of the zone is considerably narrowed as well, extending from the lateral side of the normal shoulder, obliquely across the midline of the body at the umbilicus on the paretic side, and posteriorly to where the back trouser pocket would be located. Reconstructive procedures should be considered within this space.

Tendon Transfers for Treatment of the Paralyzed or Weak Shoulder

It should be appreciated why arthrodesis has been the accepted method of management of the paralyzed or weak shoulder. Extensive experience has shown it to achieve a predictable result in most patients, without requiring ultrarefined technique on the part of the operating surgeon. Historically, most of the patients so treated gratefully accepted the limitations of the result in return for control, albeit restricted, of the shoulder. Attempts to retain mobility of the glenohumeral joint by means of tendon transfer have had a long and uneven history. According to Steindler,[60] in 1901 Hoffa thought of using the trapezius to substitute for the paralyzed deltoid, and this was reported by Lange[32] in cases of birth palsy. Mayer[36] later refined the technique with a fascial cuff and silk suture to elongate the tendon. The results have been indifferent. In 1906 Hildebrand[26] used the entire pectoralis major folded on itself and attached to the lateral third of the clavicle and acromion. In 1932 Ober[41] inserted the long head of the triceps and the short head of the biceps into the acromion. The idea of double substitution for the paralyzed deltoid was originated in 1927 with Spitzy[56] and Mau,[35] who employed the pectoralis minor and the trapezius, and to Ansart,[2] who used the pectoralis major, the teres major, and the latissimus dorsi. These early workers realized, as had Mayer, that substitution for an isolated, single muscle deficit (deltoid) produced considerably better functional results than when multiple muscles were paralyzed about the shoulder. In 1950 Harmon[24] described multiple transfers for the paralysis of the deltoid accompanied by paralysis of the external rotators. Prior to that, in 1939, L'Episcopo[34] had reported on the restoration of lateral rotation by posteriolateral transfer of latissimus dorsi and teres major in Erb's palsy.

Harmon's procedure was quite extensive. The latissimus dorsi and teres major were transferred for lateral rotation. Abduction was aided by anterior shift of the origin of the posterior deltoid, if it was preserved, and the clavicular portion of the pectoralis major to the acromion, if this was spared. The long head of the triceps and short head of the biceps were transferred to the acromion as in Ober's operation. The results were reported to be good.

All of these clinical trials and their results simply reaffirmed what was learned by kinesiological studies of the shoulder joint from anatomic and functional research (Inman et al.[29]) as well as observation of cases of paralysis; the shoulder was too complex to be conquered by a simplistic approach using a single transfer.

Much of the previous experience was correlated in 1967 by Saha,[48] who published his extensive monograph entitled "Surgery of the Paralyzed and Flail Shoulder." Drawing on his previous work on the theory of the shoulder mechanism, he reviewed the biomechanics and described the functional classification of muscles elevating the shoulder. He emphasized that, in addition to a prime mover or elevator, the shoulder joint required "gliders," muscles to steer the head during elevation so that different areas of articular surface could be centered on the glenoid, and, finally, "fixators" to stabilize the head during motion. On the basis of these concepts and mathematical calculations, he described a series of tendon transfers specific for each type of weakness about the shoulder. Some of the procedures were adaptations of those previously described, and others were new. The clinical study involved over 100 cases of upper limb paralysis from polio, and he stated that the methods were equally applicable to brachial plexus injuries. Arthrodesis was decried as largely unnecessary. He argued that indications for fusion have been shown by his work to be ideal indications for providing an actively mobile shoulder. Although the report is illustrated by a number of well-detailed and sometimes spectacular clinical cases, there are no statistics or end results for the entire series, which makes it rather difficult to compare these results with the work of others. In my opinion, this is an extremely important monograph. There is no doubt that many of the procedures do work well. For the patient who has partial paralysis, we should certainly analyze the situation with a view toward preserving a mobile shoulder if at all possible. The L'Episcopo procedure,[34] described in Chapter 5, does work well in adults (Fig. 11.1). The transfers described by Harmon,[24] as well as other multiple transfers, can give surprisingly good results in selected patients (Figs. 11.2, 11.3).

Whether the procedure described by Saha for the flail polio shoulder using the upper two digitations of serratus anterior, the levator scapulae, and a modified trapezius transfer is applicable to the brachial plexus palsy remains to be seen. It is undoubtedly a surgical tour de force, requiring far more expertise than shoulder fusion. In the plexus injury even when the C5–6 outflow in the limb is totally paralyzed, it is most often found that the lesions are infraganglionic, so that theoretically the serratus anterior and levator scapulae should be unimpaired and available for transfer. Presumably, if the procedure did not work and the serratus and trapezius were not unduly compromised by the surgery, then a fusion would be available as a salvage procedure. I have never done this operation, nor have I had the oppor-

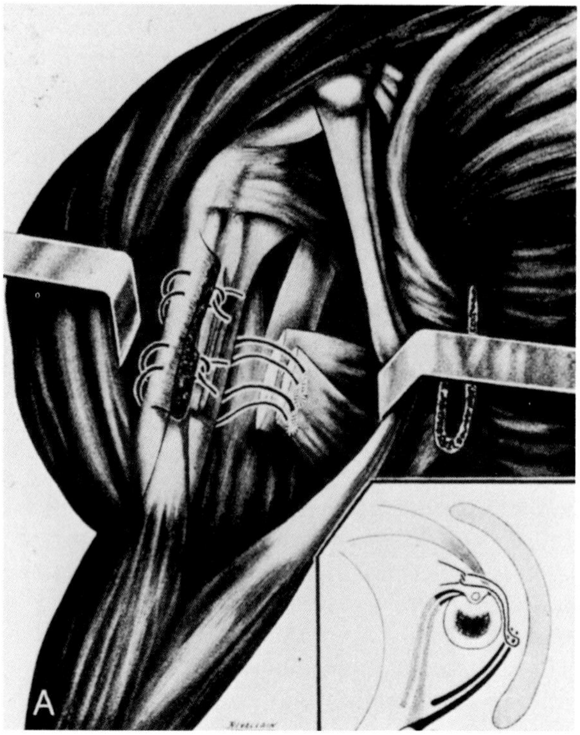

Fig. 11.1. A: The tendons of the teres major and latissimus dorsi detached and rerouted posterolaterally, here sutured to the stump of the pectoralis major, which has been released. (Reproduced from D'Aubigne M, Benassy J, Ramadieu JO (eds): Chirurgie orthopédique des paralysies. Masson, Paris, 1956.) **B**: Child with adduction and medial rotation contracture of right shoulder due to Erb's palsy. **C**: Postoperative immobilization.

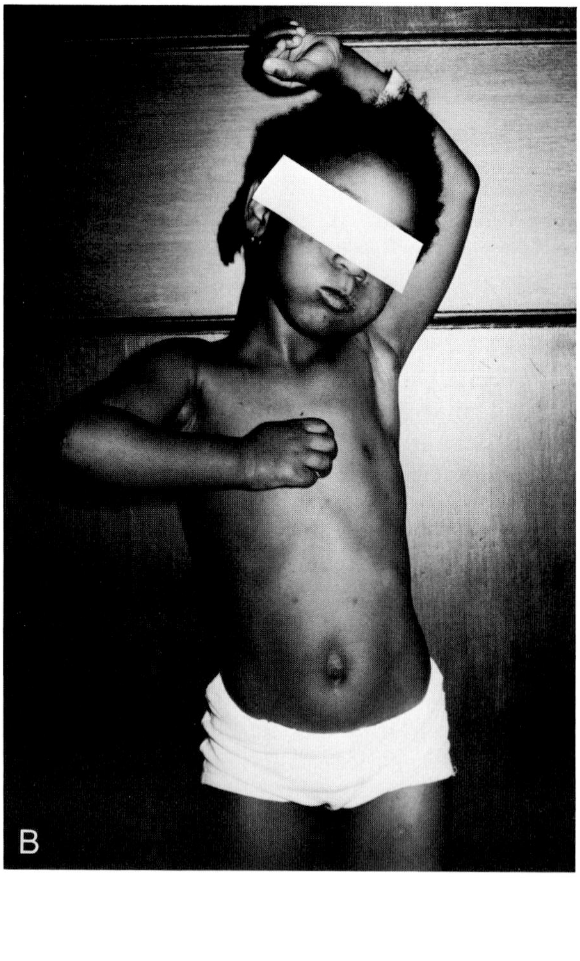

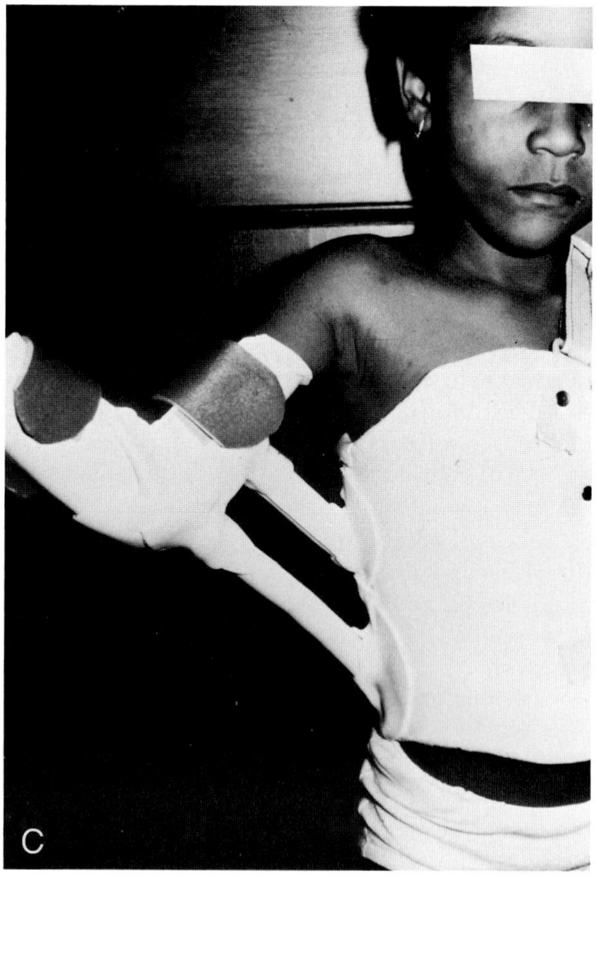

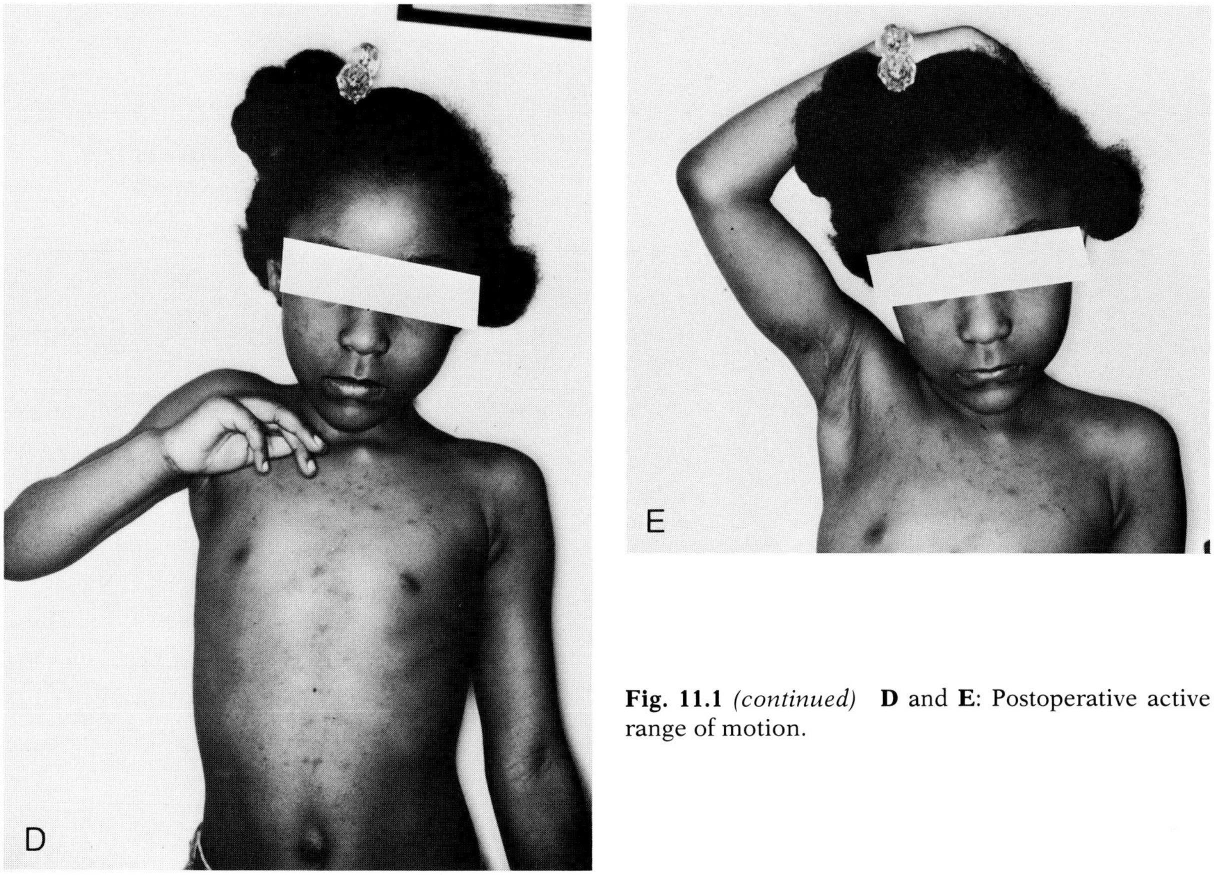

Fig. 11.1 *(continued)* **D** and **E**: Postoperative active range of motion.

tunity to review the results of surgeons who have had experience with it.

Arthrodesis of the Shoulder

The classical approach to the problem of the flail shoulder has been arthrodesis of the glenohumeral joint. Most of the clinical experience has been in the treatment of patients with the residua of poliomyelitis, and as has already been stated, although there are similarities between the two groups, the differences must be emphasized. Since many of the polio patients were stricken and treated in their growing years, the effect of growth on the final position achieved for the fusion was inadvertently incorporated into the recommended position at surgery. The widely quoted and accepted position for fusion advocated in the 1942 report of the Research Committee of the American Orthopaedic Association[4] was as shown in Figure 11.4.

This position, using as reference points the long axis of the humerus and the vertebral border of the scapula, worked well in the growing patient, especially if no internal fixation was used at surgery. With time and skeletal remodeling, the excessive abduction tended to diminish. For the fully grown individual, by contrast, excessive abduction remained, and resulted in chronic stretch of the serratus anterior muscle, and an aching, weak shoulder that could not comfortably carry the arm at the side. Furthermore, the laterally rotated arm tended to position the forearm and hand away from the body in an unnatural and awkward position (Fig. 11.5).

Realizing the difficulties, Rowe[47] in 1974 reevaluated the position of the arm in arthrodesis of the shoulder in the adult. He reviewed the literature, studied eight patients with arthrodesis of the shoulder, and concluded that the amount of abduction usually recommended is excessive for adults in whom internal fixation is used at surgery. He advised

(Text continues on p. 197.)

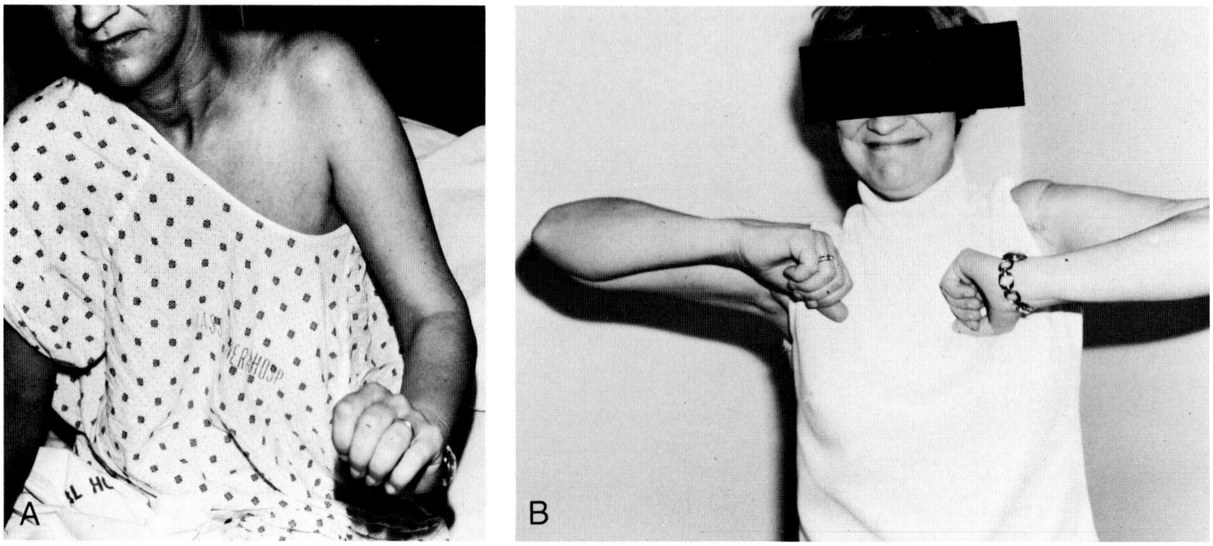

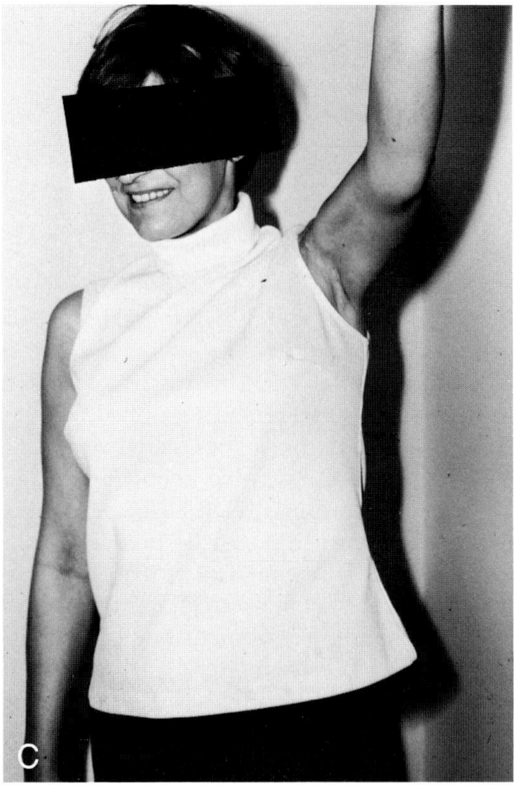

Fig. 11.2. **A**: Shoulder paresis due to knife wound of upper trunk of left brachial plexus, after unsuccessful attempt at nerve repair. Operative procedure consisted of
(1) excision of paralyzed anterior deltoid and rotation of posterior and middle deltoid anteromedially
(2) transfer of long head of biceps to acromion
(3) posterolateral transfer of latissimus and teres major
(4) lateral shift of clavicular pectoralis major
B and **C**: Postoperative range of motion.

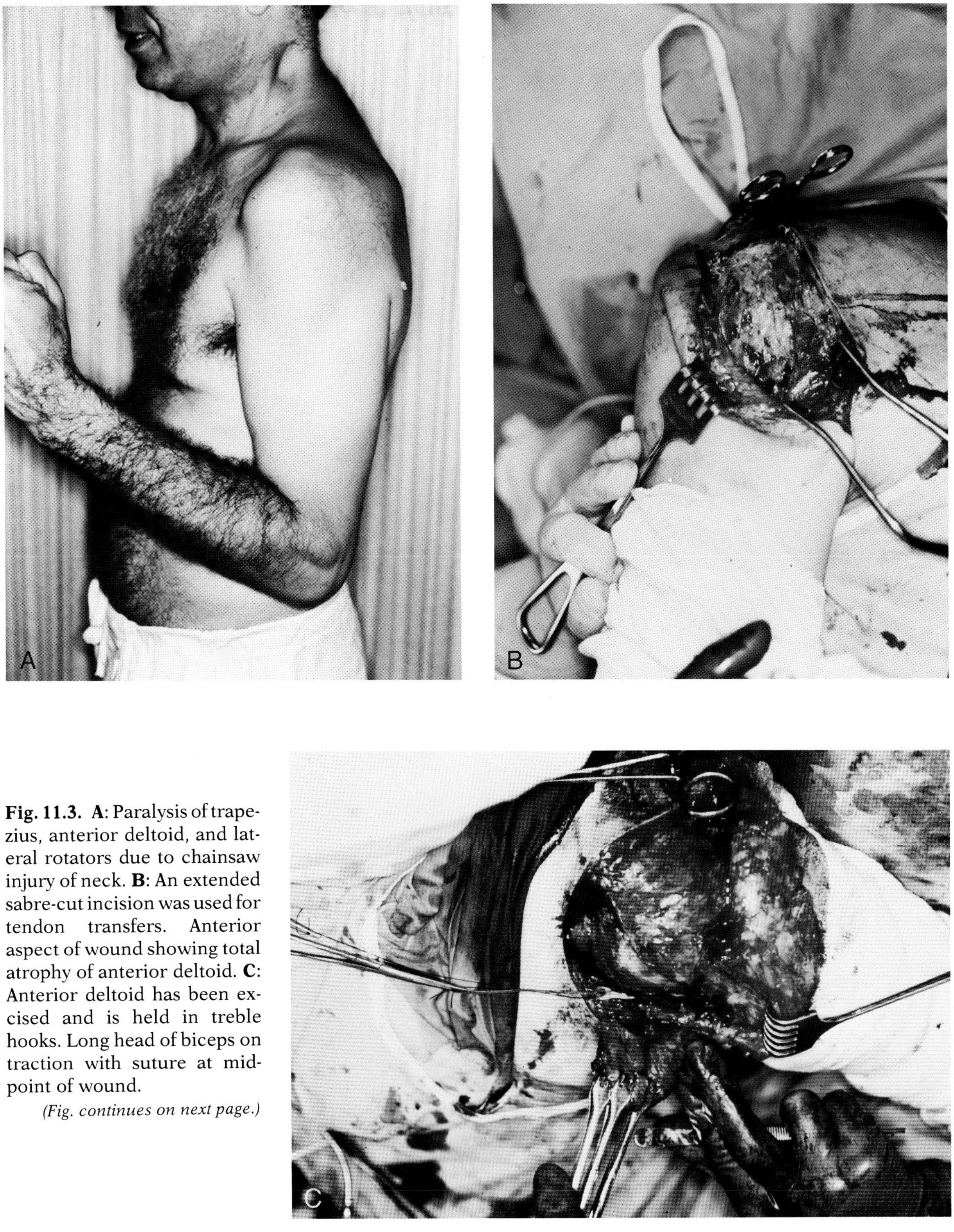

Fig. 11.3. **A**: Paralysis of trapezius, anterior deltoid, and lateral rotators due to chainsaw injury of neck. **B**: An extended sabre-cut incision was used for tendon transfers. Anterior aspect of wound showing total atrophy of anterior deltoid. **C**: Anterior deltoid has been excised and is held in treble hooks. Long head of biceps on traction with suture at midpoint of wound.

(Fig. continues on next page.)

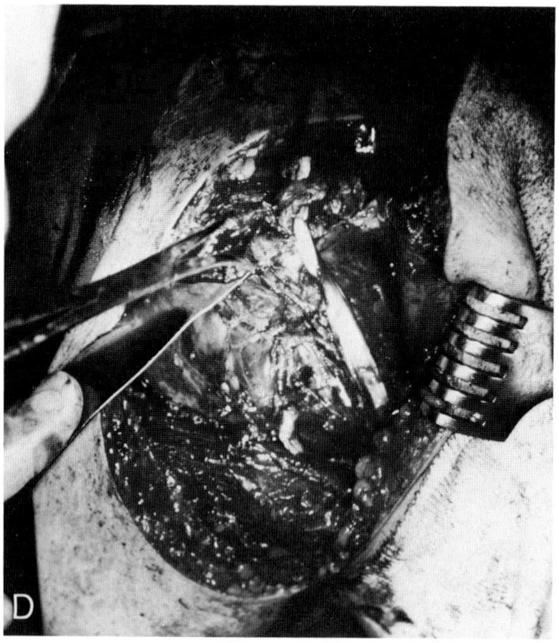

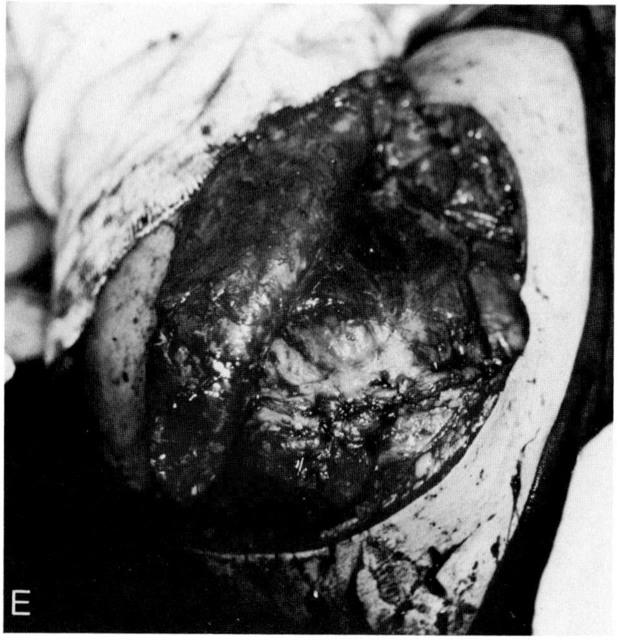

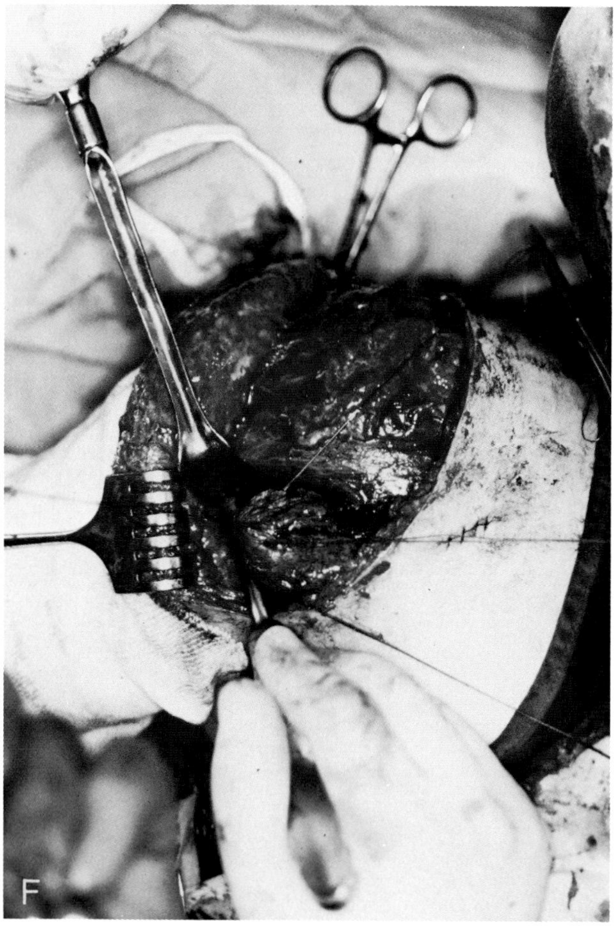

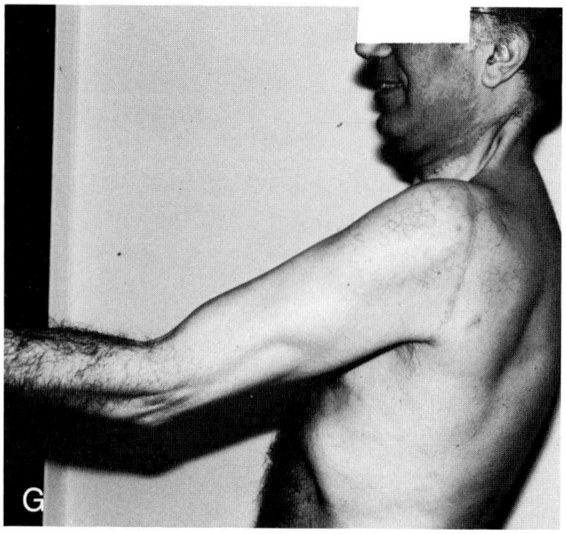

Fig. 11.3 *(continued)* **D**: Long head of biceps has been tenodesed to anterior edge of acromion. **E**: Posterior and middle deltoid have been rotated anteriorly. **F**: The detached latissimus dorsi and teres major on tension with sutures. Richardson retractor under edge of posterior deltoid; rake holding skin flap. **G**: Postoperative glenohumeral control. Total elevation hampered by scapular winging due to trapezius palsy. Scapular stabilization to ribcage was done giving further improvement in function.

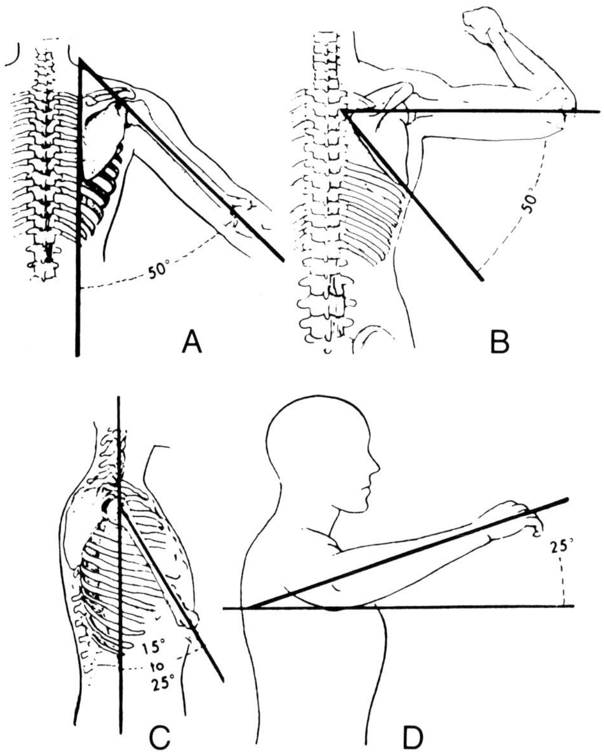

Fig. 11.4. Position for arthrodesis of the shoulder, AOA 1942. (Reproduced from Barr JS, Freiberg JA, Colonna PC and Pemberton PA: A survey of end results on stabilization of the paralytic shoulder (report of the research committee of the American Orthopaedic Association). J Bone Joint Surg 24:699, 1942.)

determining abduction of the arm from the side of the body to clear the axilla (15 – 20 degrees) and forward flexion of 25 – 30 degrees with internal rotation of 40 – 50 degrees (Fig. 11.6). With this position, a patient with a solidly fused shoulder would be able to reach the midline of the body, the face and head, the side and back trousers pockets, anal region, and feet. In addition, the arm would rest comfortably at the side. Excessive strain on the scapulothoracic musculature would be avoided (Fig. 11.7).

I believe that Rowe's observations and recommendations concerning shoulder fusion are correct. In addition to optimal position, one must consider the condition of the scapulothoracic musculature with reference to the ability to control the shoulder – arm complex once the fusion has been done. In a sense, because the lever arms and movements are actually increased following fusion, the demand on the muscles controlling the scapula is supernormal, whereas they are often weakened by injury, denervation, or disuse. The minimal motor picture compatible with good control of a fused shoulder requires a trapezius and serratus anterior in the "good" to "normal" range. In addition, it is desirable, but not essential, to have a functioning levator scapulae and rhomboids to provide smooth antagonistic muscle action. It is fortunate that most patients with severe brachial plexus injuries do not also sustain injury to the spinal accessory nerve so that the trapezius remains intact. Although the serratus anterior derives it innervation from C5, 6, and 7, it is usually preserved because the branches are root collaterals, and, unless the lesion is supraganglionic, they are usually spared. The occasional patient with less than adequate scapular musculature may benefit from shoulder fusion if for no other reason than to alleviate an annoying subluxation at the glenohumeral joint or to eliminate having to wear a sling (Fig. 11.8).

There are numerous techniques that have been described to achieve fusion of the shoulder, but, since this monograph does not purport to be a complete treatise on reconstructive surgery of the paralyzed upper limb, only those facets of the procedure germane to the patient with brachial plexus injury will be stressed, and the two techniques presently used by the author will be described in detail.

Techniques for Shoulder Fusion

The procedure that I have used largely unmodified for the past ten years is as follows.

The patient, under general endotracheal anesthesia, is in the full lateral decubitus position, injured side up. The entire upper limb, shoulder, base of the neck, and hemithorax are sterilely draped to allow for free manipulation of the arm during surgery and identification of the vertebral border of the scapula. This landmark will be the reference point against which the alignment of the humerus will be measured. The affected arm will be supported throughout the operation on a padded, sterile Mayo stand. It can be shifted as necessary to maintain the glenohumeral joint in precisely the correct position for fusion, because once the internal fixation has been placed, it cannot be easily changed. The wire loop technique described by Carroll[15] has interesting possibilities for achieving correction of position if necessary in the

(Text continues on p. 200.)

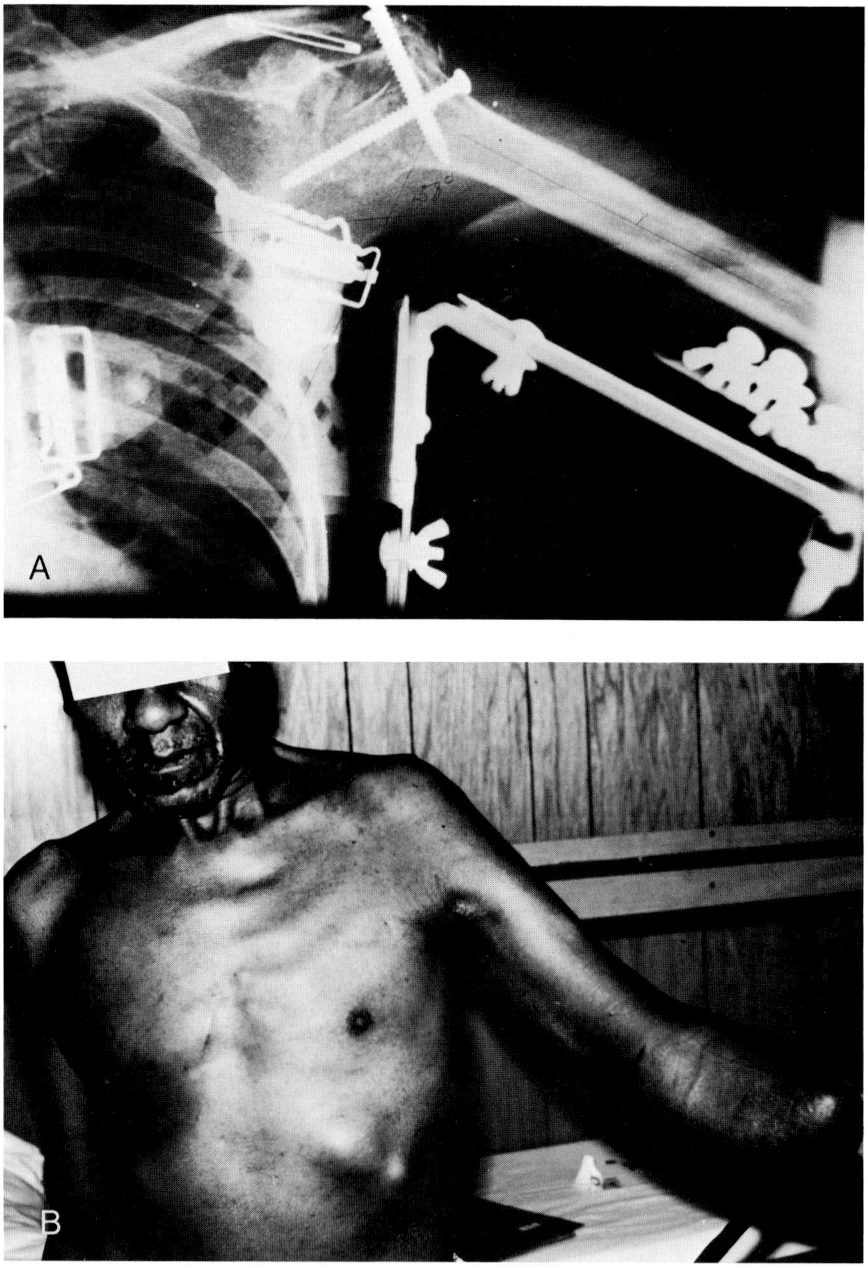

Fig. 11.5. **A**: Radiograph of shoulder fusion done in 58 degrees of abduction and lateral rotation. A forearm amputation was also done. Patient had been treated elsewhere. **B**: Clinical appearance from the front.

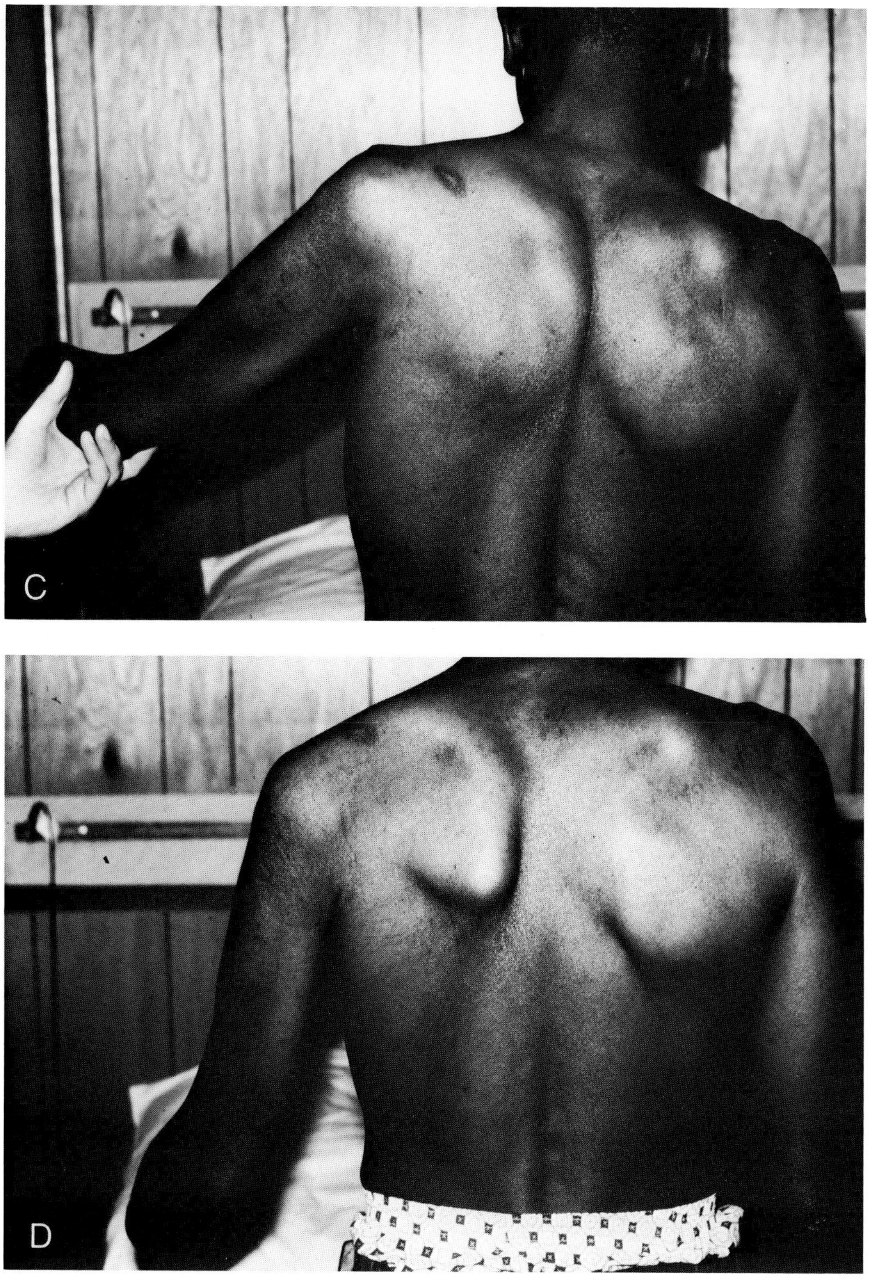

Fig. 11.5 *(continued)* **C**: Positioning the scapula to match the right one in neutral position leaves the arm abducted. **D**: Attempting to bring the arm to the side causes winging of the scapula and pain due to stretch of the muscles. Osteotomy beneath the fusion was required for correction.

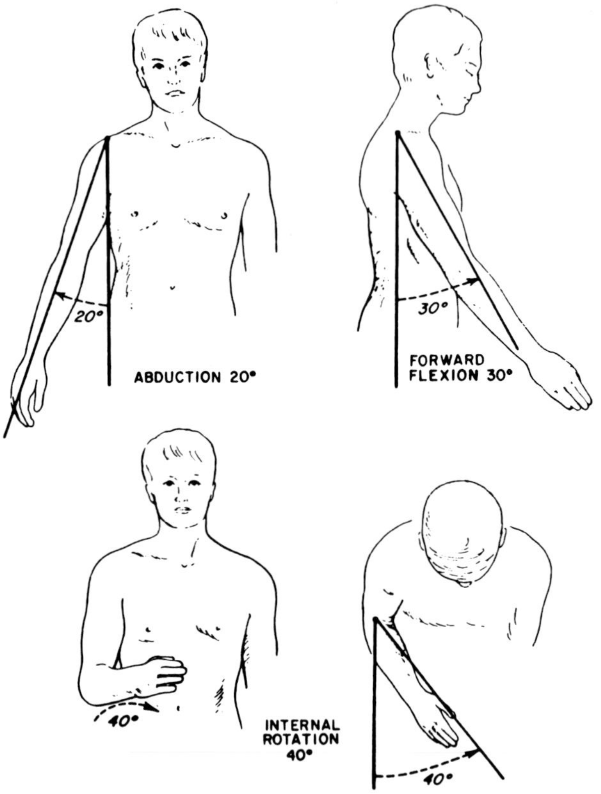

Fig. 11.6. The recommended position for arthrodesis of the shoulder according to C. R. Rowe. (Reproduced from Rowe CR: Reevaluation of the position of the arm in arthrodesis of the shoulder in the adult. J Bone Joint Surg 56A:913, 1974, with permission.)

immediate postoperative period, but I have not used it. Although initially I favored a straight lateral approach to the shoulder joint (to avoid anterior scarring which might interfere if a pectoral transfer were done), I have discarded it in favor of the posterior approach. This technique gives excellent access to the joint as well as to the proximal humerus, spine of the scapula, and glenoidal neck. There are no significant anatomic structures at risk, and the atrophic deltoid and rotator cuff muscles are easily traversed. The skin incision extends the length of the spine of the scapula, a finger breadth below it, and then curves along the posterolateral aspect of the acromion and down over the lateral aspect of the proximal humerus in the midline. The cautery is used to create an inverted U flap of muscle that exposes the joint and the subacromial bursa, which is excised. The capsule and ligaments of the glenohumeral joint are incised transversely, revealing the humeral head and the glenoid. It is wise to decorticate the latter first, since to do the reverse would be to obscure the field due to the raw bone bleeding down onto it. A $1\frac{1}{4}$-inch osteotome is used to reduce the glenoid to a planar surface of cancellous bone after the labrum has been circumferentially resected with the cautery. Then the position of the humerus is established, and an identical second osteotome is used to produce the corresponding parallel surface on the humeral head. It should be possible to achieve contact over the entire glenoidal surface so that no gaps remain when the two bones are fitted together. If the position and the fusion site are deemed satisfactory, then the internal fixation is chosen. If a plaster shoulder spica is to be used postoperatively, and it usually is, then cancellous compression screws are chosen. The bone of the humeral head is usually quite porotic, so that for the average adult I use 6.5-mm diameter, 75- to 80-mm long cancellous screws, half threaded, with washers to prevent their sinking into the bone. Both head and glenoid are predrilled, but not tapped, and the screws are introduced from the region of the greater tuberosity medially into the glenoid. Depending on the size of the bones, three to five such screws may be used, being careful to seat the threaded ends firmly in the relatively denser bone of the glenoidal neck (Fig. 11.9). In some patients it may be possible to translocate the head cephalad and decorticate both the undersurface of the acromial process and the superior surface of the head to afford another, extraarticular, site for fusion. It may be secured either by an additional cancellous screw or heavy wire. No additional bone grafts other than what can be salvaged from the decortication are required, and at this point there should be no visible or palpable gap at the fusion site. The scapula and arm should move solidly as a unit.

Closure is in layers over a suction drain, the arm being supported by the padded Mayo stand. At the end of the procedure the patient is placed in an adjustable abduction brace or sling and pillow splint (Fig. 11.10), since to attempt to apply a neat and comfortable plaster shoulder spica to an anesthetized patient is almost impossible.

In the first few days postoperatively, when the patient has recovered enough to stand comfortably,

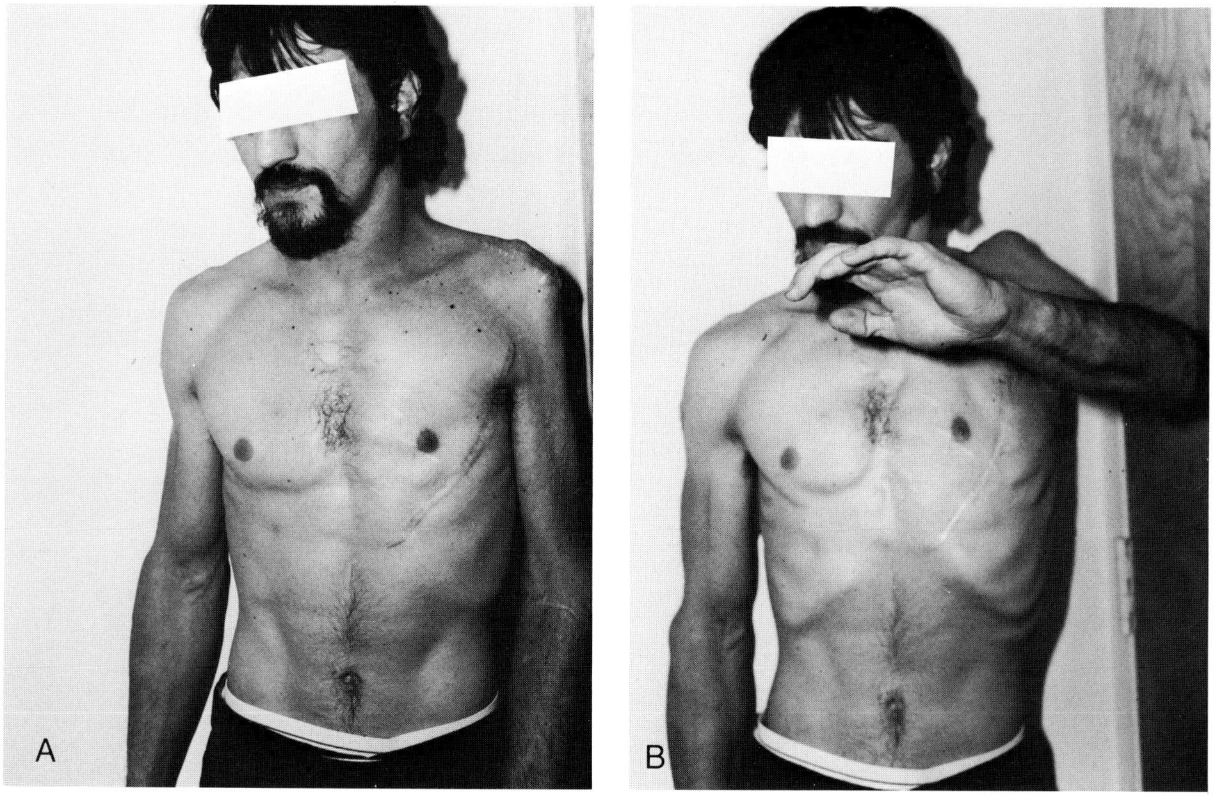

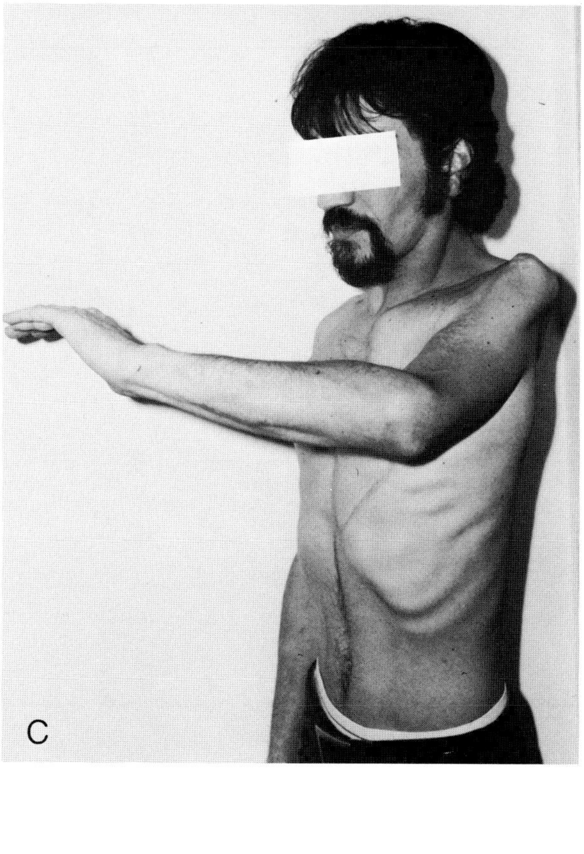

Fig. 11.7. A–F: C5, C6, C7 traction injury of the left brachial plexus with flail shoulder and elbow as well as wrist and finger extensor paralysis. Shoulder fusion and Clark's pectoral transfer have been done, as well as tendon transfers in the hand. Patient was employed as a mechanic.

(Figure continues on next page.)

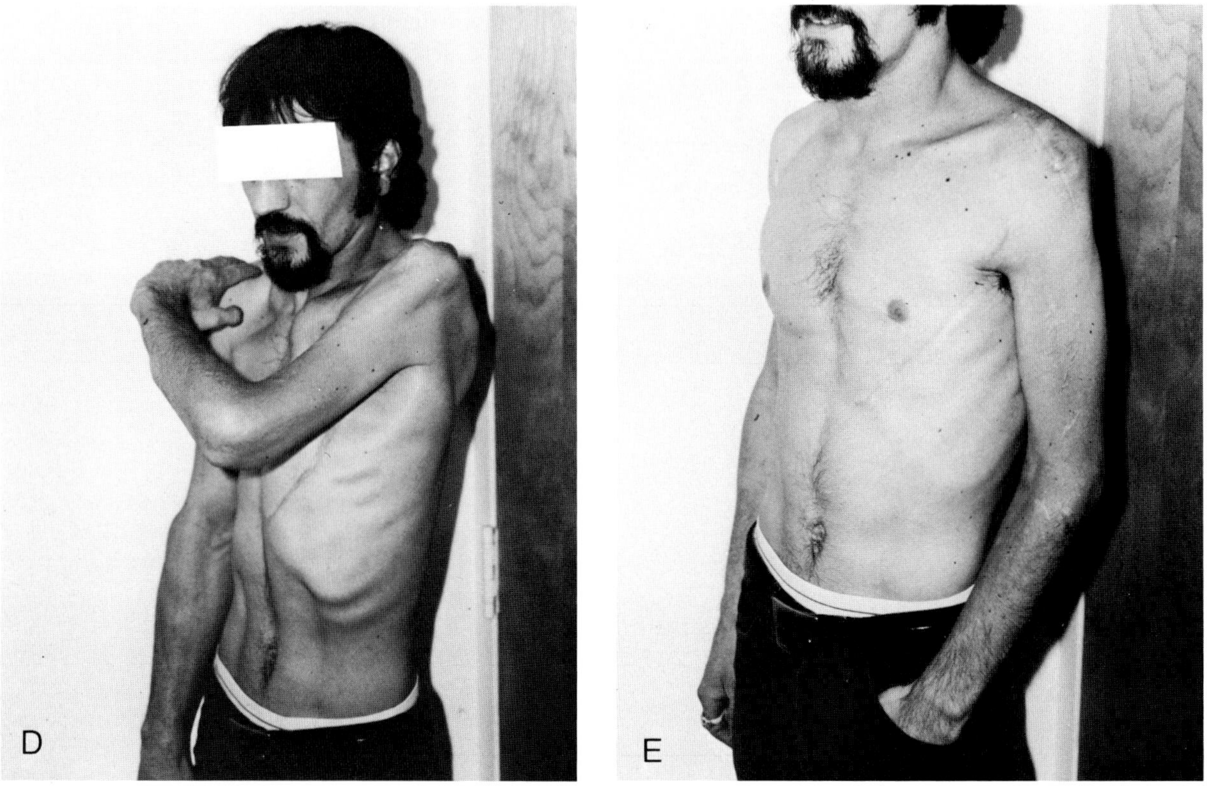

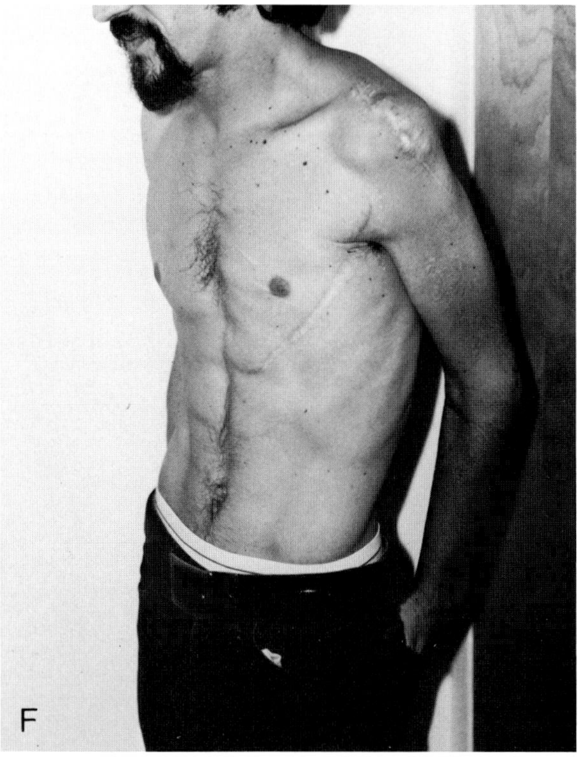

Fig. 11.7 *(continued)*

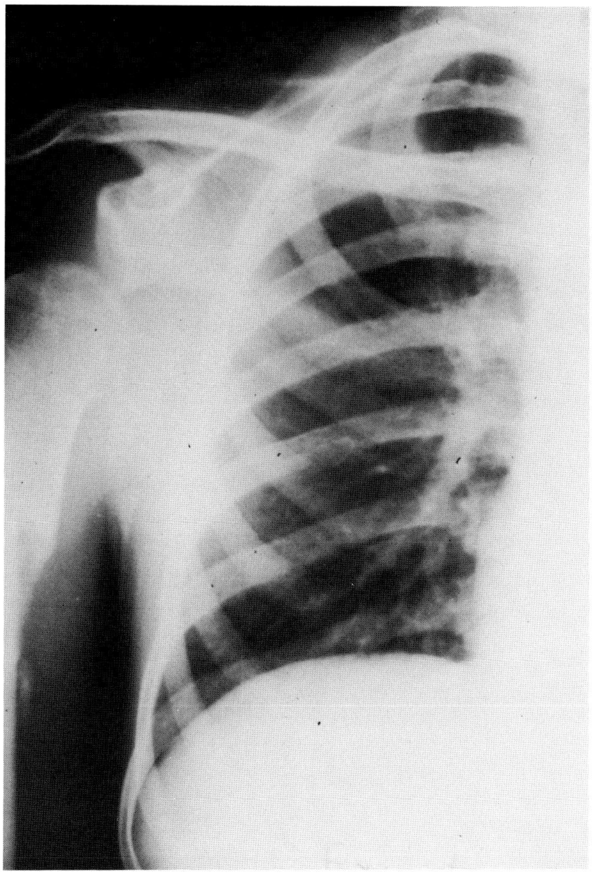

Fig. 11.8. Glenohumeral subluxation due to paralysis.

the spica is applied (Fig. 11.11). It is generally removed at 12 weeks for tomographic examination of the fusion site. Usually the fusion is clinically solid by that time, but assessment by means of plane radiographs is difficult. Therefore, the tomograms are of considerable help in demonstrating bony fusion.

In carefully selected patients who are thoroughly reliable, the spica may be eliminated by the use of a compression plate technique similar to that suggested by the A.O. group.[39] A 10-hole plate is contoured to extend from the spine of the scapula to the lateral aspect of the proximal humerus. An additional buttress plate is applied posteriorly from the head across to the neck of the glenoid. This procedure is considerably more time-consuming and difficult, but worthwhile if the patient is to be spared the aggravation of having to wear the spica (Fig. 11.12). A light plastic brace may be used to immobilize these patients, and it is considerably more comfortable than a plaster, but I do not allow them to go totally unsupported for at least 8 weeks. I cannot overemphasize the importance of patient cooperation if this technique is to be used, since there is a very real danger of loosening the fixation and failure of fusion if the patient allows stress on the fusion site. Of the 10 patients in whom I have done this plating procedure, two have had delayed union. One of these resumed

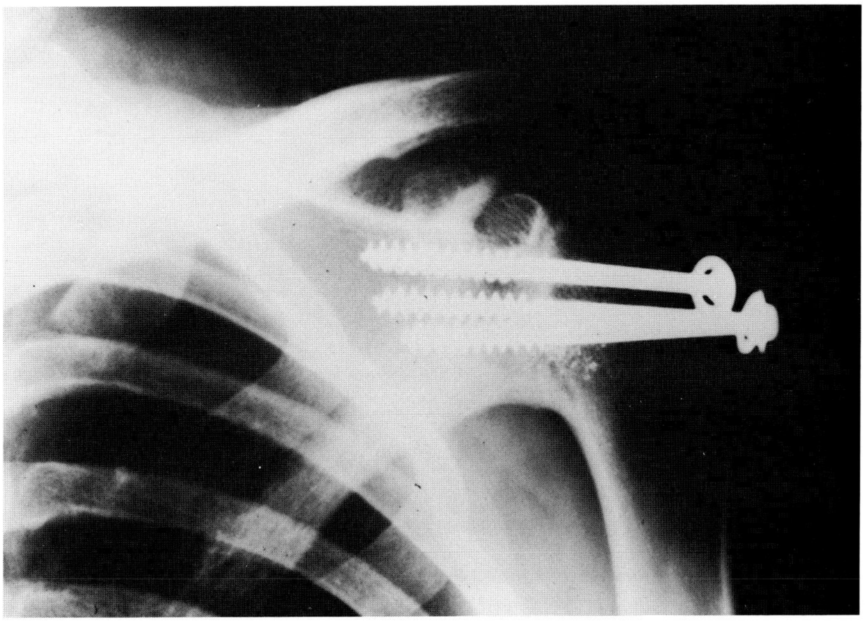

Fig. 11.9. Glenohumeral fusion using cancellous screws with washers. Note that the threads are all past the fusion site so that compression is assured.

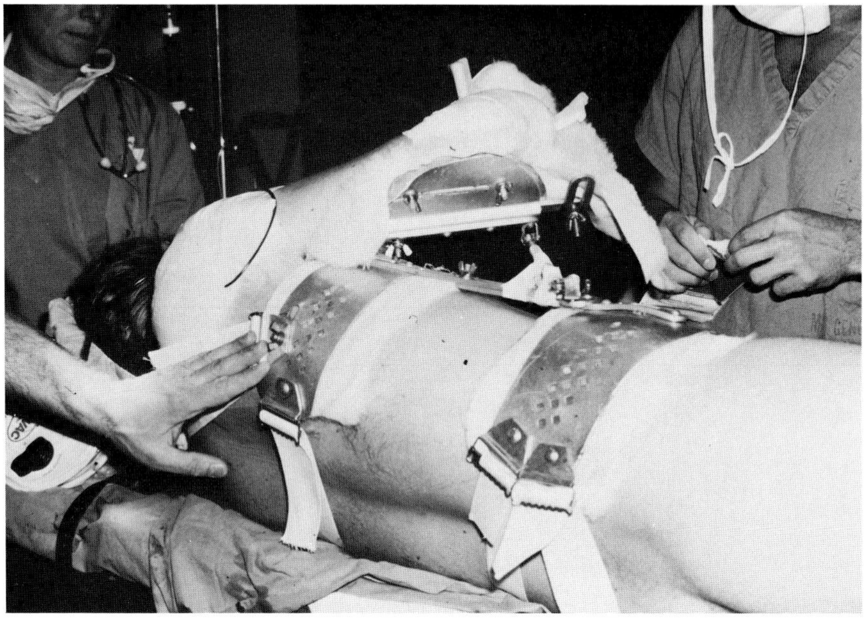

Fig. 11.10. The adjustable abduction brace must be carefully padded to avoid pressure sores. In this case, a forearm amputation was done at the same time.

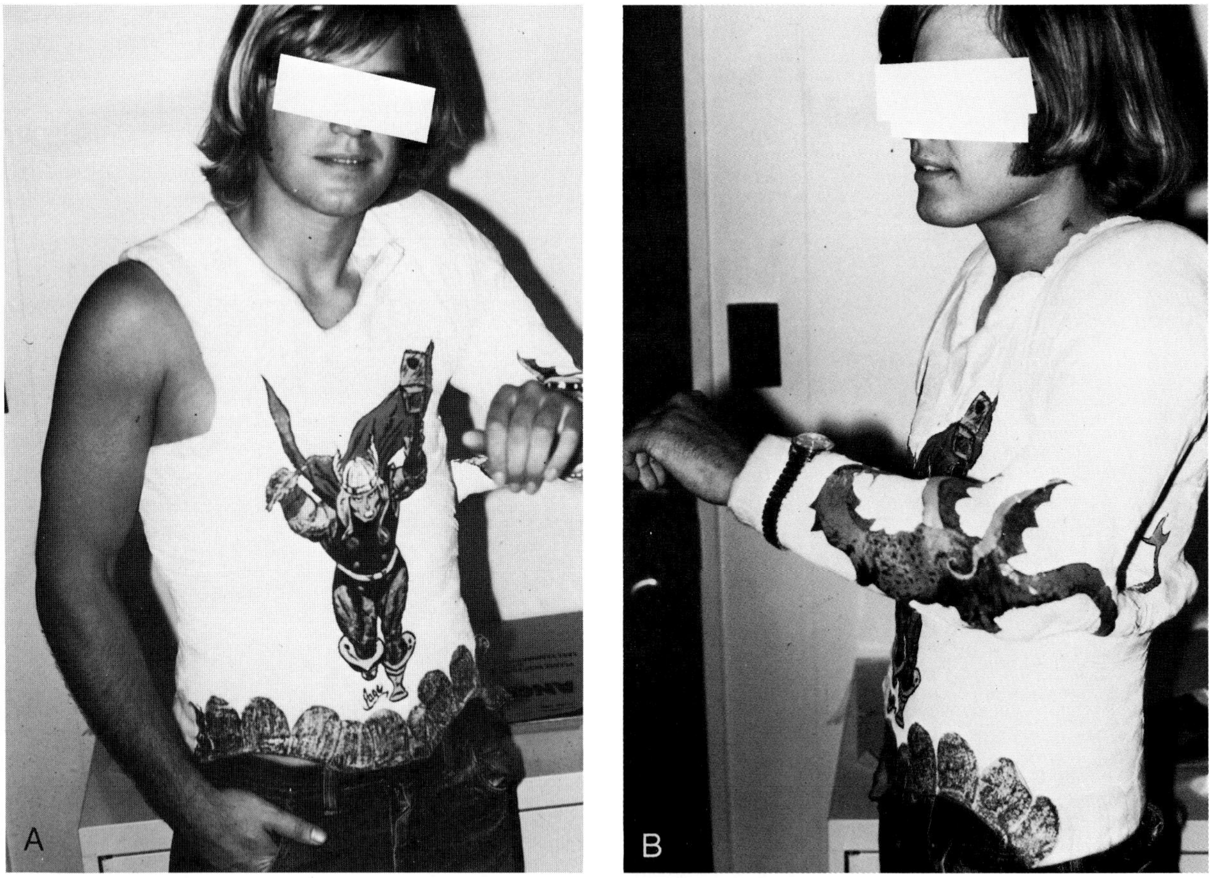

Fig. 11.11. A and **B**: The spica must rest on the iliac crests lest it lever on the arm and distract the fusion site. Artwork is optional.

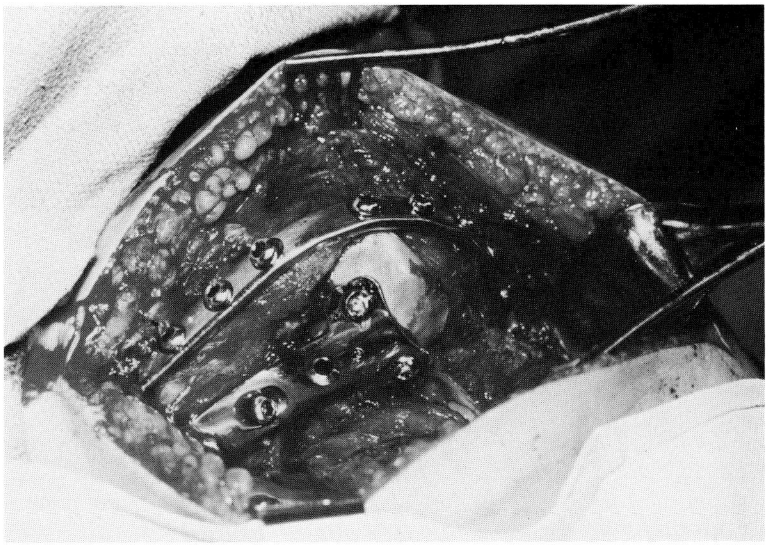

Fig. 11.12. Shoulder fusion using compression plate technique.

his job as a piano mover two weeks postoperatively, and the other rode his motorcycle strenuously in the immediate postoperative period. Both patients eventually achieved solid fusion with further immobilization. In patients who have little subcutaneous tissue and significant atrophy of the muscles overlying the scapula there is a risk of skin breakdown over the plates as shown in this patient (Fig. 11.13), who, incidentally, did not have a brachial plexus injury, and who ultimately consolidated her fusion despite an exposed plate. Postoperatively the shoulder fusion patients may have some difficulty with elbow stiffness but are usually mobilized easily (Fig. 11.14). For the patient with a significant elbow problem that would be adversely affected by immobilization, a jointed elbow in the spica is usually not totally satisfactory, and compression plate technique may prove quite helpful.

(Text continues on p. 210.)

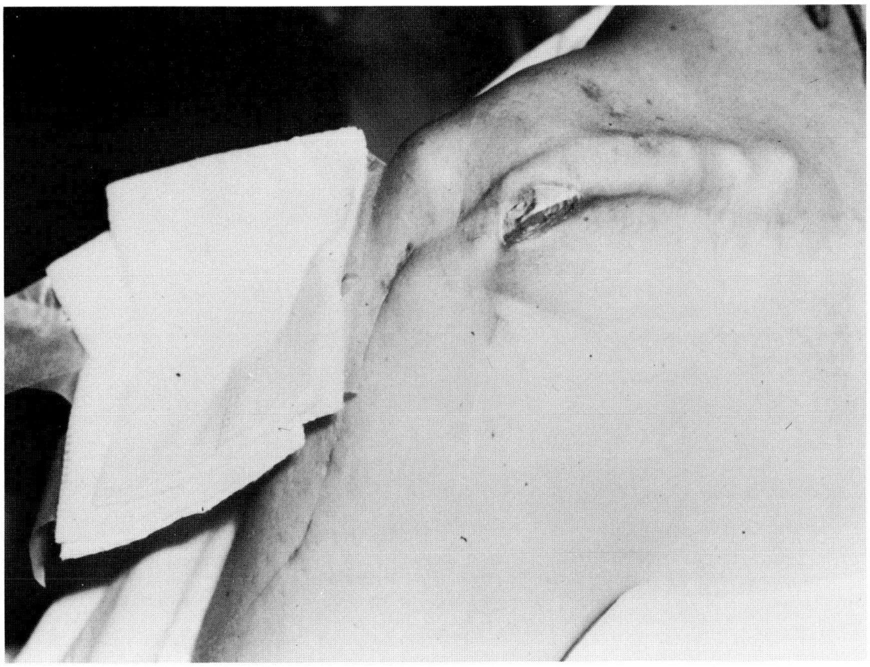

Fig. 11.13. The exposed plate in an elderly patient with poor subcutaneous tissue. The fusion consolidated, despite removal of the plate at six weeks.

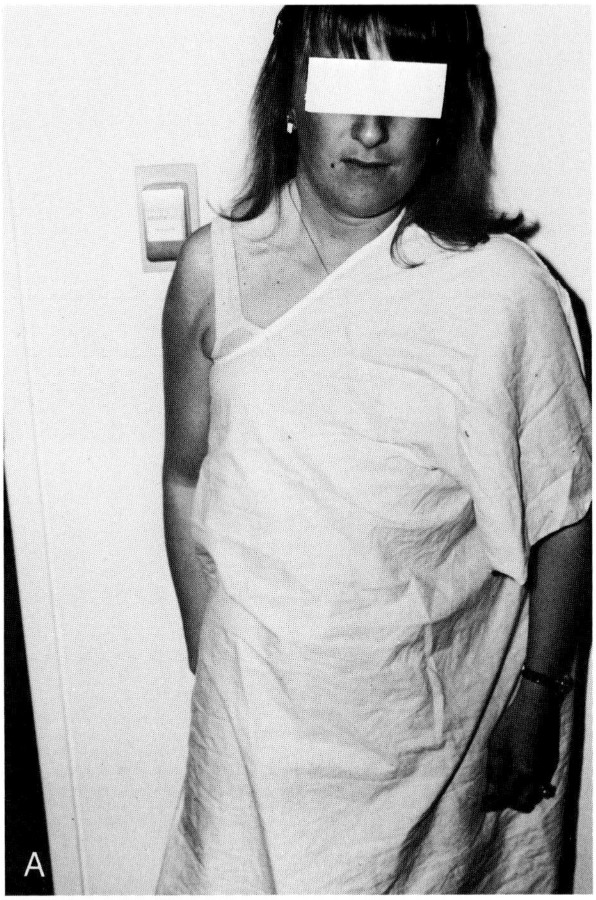

Fig. 11.14. A – D: This patient had a partial C5, C6 traction lesion with a nonunion of a fracture of the midshaft of the clavicle that was painful. The clavicle was plated and grafted, and the shoulder was fused at the same time, using compression screws.

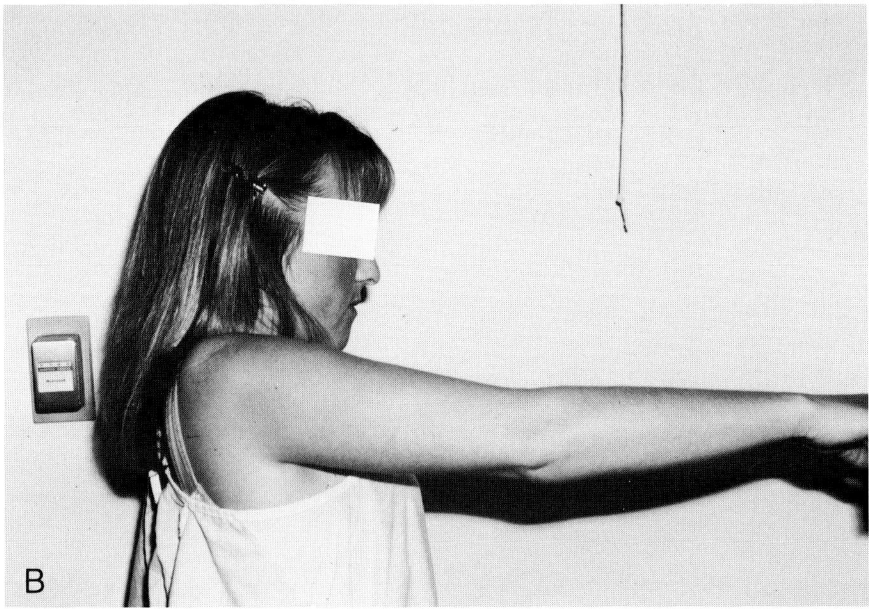

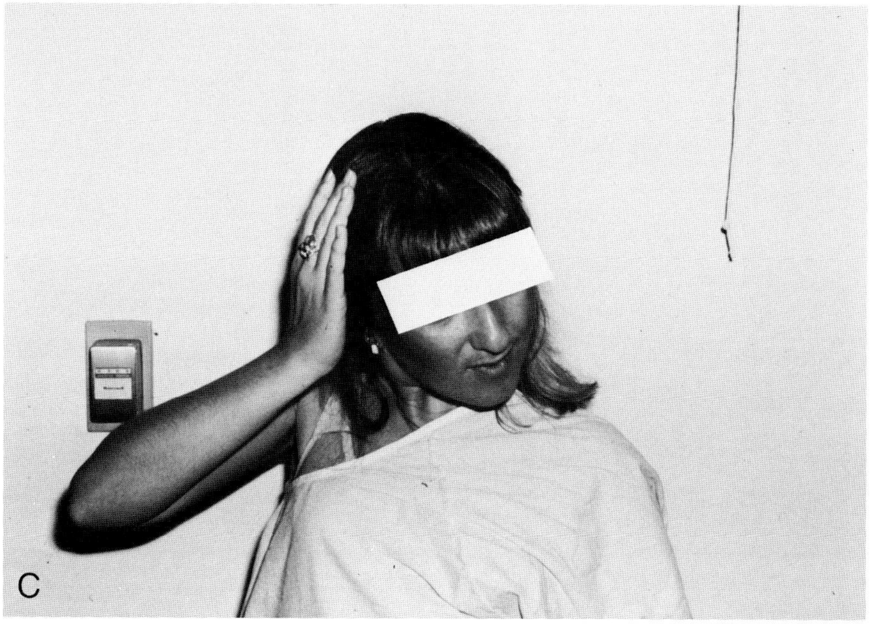

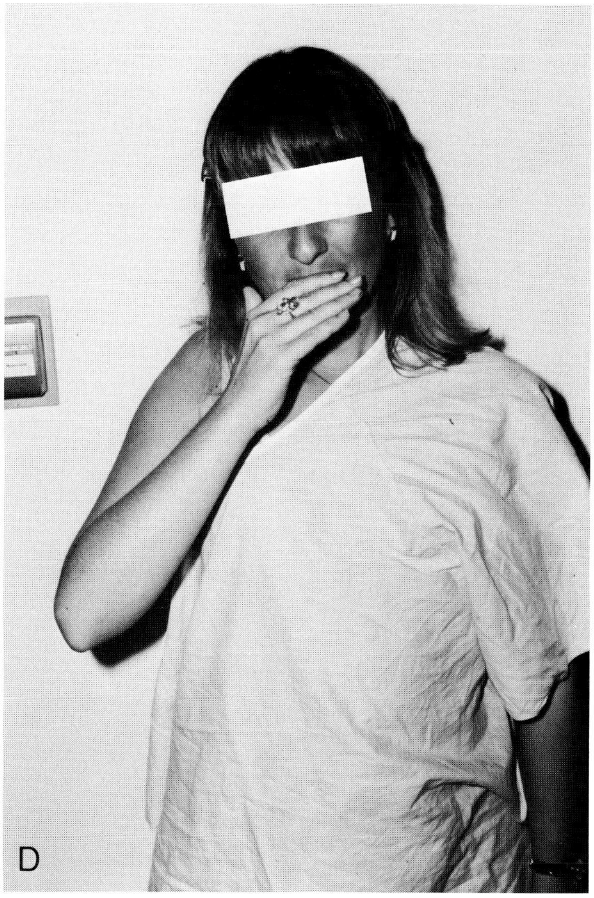

Fig. 11.14 *(continued)* Postoperative range of motion.

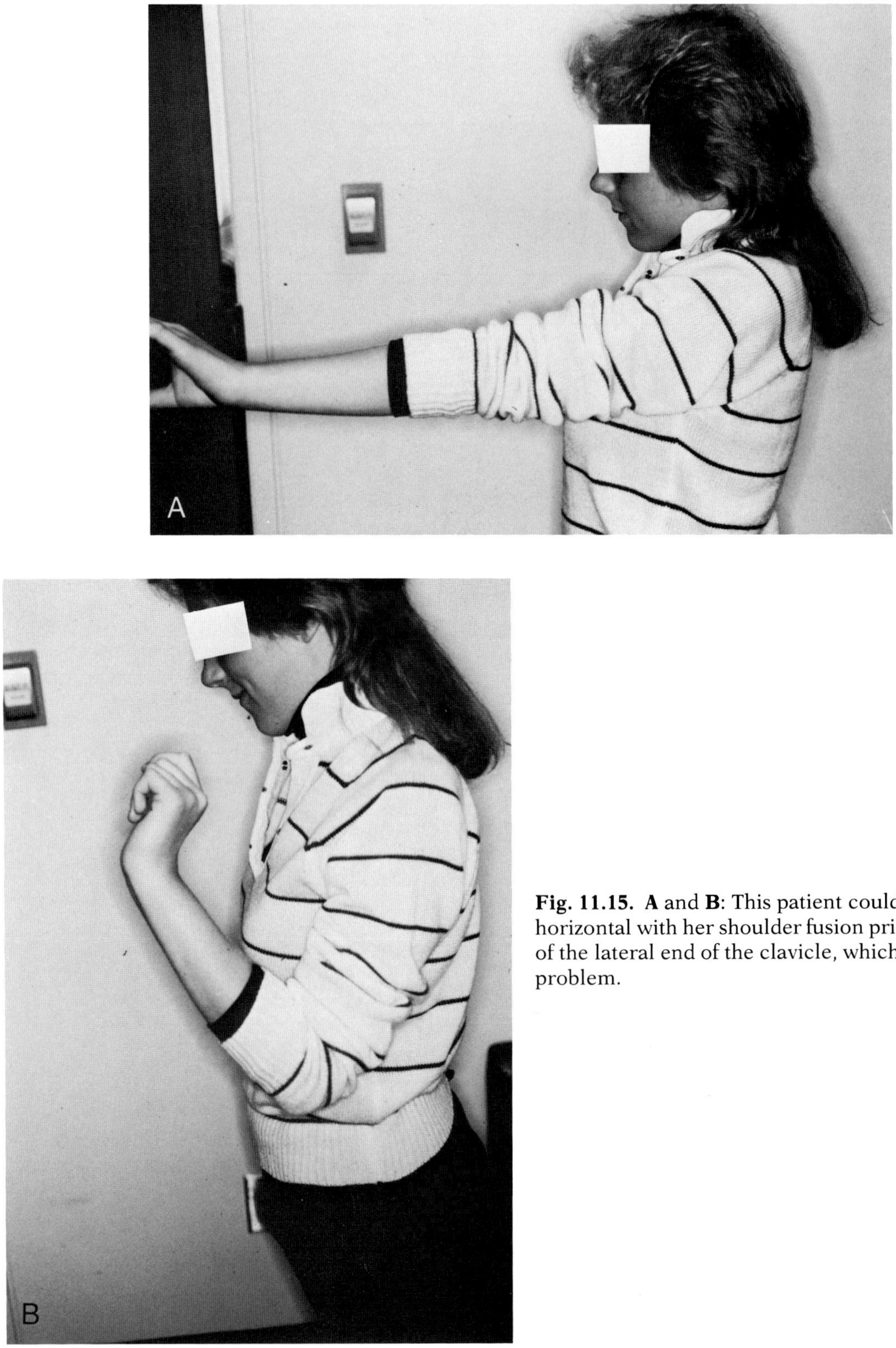

Fig. 11.15. **A** and **B**: This patient could not reach the horizontal with her shoulder fusion prior to resection of the lateral end of the clavicle, which corrected the problem.

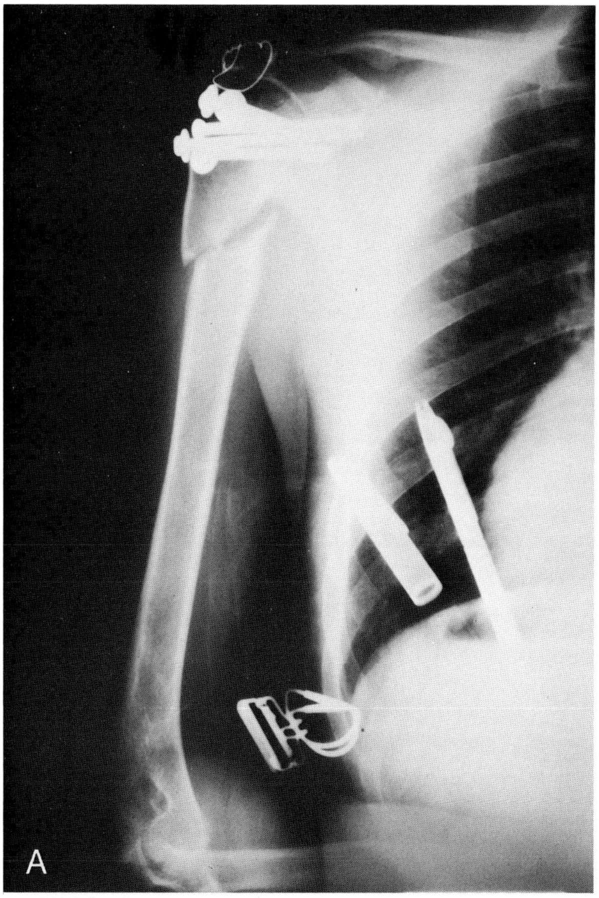

Fig. 11.16. **A**: Fracture of the humerus beneath a shoulder fusion incurred during a fall from the parallel bars in gymnastics. **B**: Solid healing after eight weeks of immobilization in a spica.

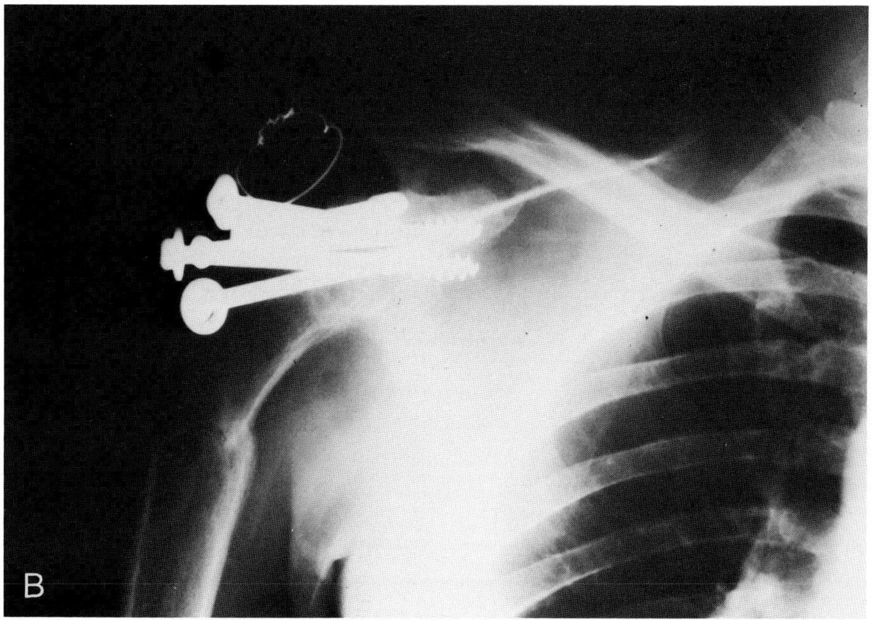

A small but useful increase in range of motion of the scapulohumeral complex may be achieved by resection of the lateral half inch of the clavicular as suggested by Milgram[38] (Fig. 11.15). The integrity of the coracoclavicular ligaments must, however, be preserved, lest a disastrous quadrupedal scapula result.

The benefits of arthrodesis performed according to these principles have proved satisfactory to most of the patients I have so treated. The annoyance of not having a truly mobile arm is significant, but less so if it is under control. The theoretically increased risk of fracture of the arm occasionally becomes reality, but usually if such fractures do occur, they are distal to the site of fusion in the proximal humerus and heal readily with conservative management (Fig. 11.16).

In only one patient has the internal fixation broken after solid healing of the fusion had occurred. This same patient, after successful repair of his fusion, was allegedly assaulted and had his Clark's pectoral transfer ruptured (Fig. 11.17).

THE PARALYTIC ELBOW

If the shoulder complex is thought of as the means of achieving stable position of the limb in space, then it falls to the elbow to lengthen or shorten the limb as necessary for placement of the hand. A poorly controlled shoulder will impose an additional burden on the elbow, whereas one that can easily bring the limb into the "functional space" can compensate for limited range of elbow motion or even motor power by altering the plane of joint motion so as to eliminate the effect of gravity. A horizontally oriented forearm needs little power to achieve flexion.

Just as the shoulder and elbow are linked in the kinesiological chain, their motor control for flexion shares a common origin, the outflow of the upper trunk of the plexus, C5 and C6. Even though the flexor-pronator and extensor-supinator muscles of the forearm span the elbow and act as supplementary elbow flexors, without the major flexors, brachialis and biceps, if the brachioradialis (C5–6) is also paralyzed, then the elbow loses voluntary flexion. Active control of elbow extension is also important, not only to achieve smooth flexor action, but for pushing or steadying objects ahead of the body or working with the arm above the horizontal. For the patient on crutches or one rising from a chair, it is vital. Although elbow flexion is the more important of the two functions, and most surgical procedures have been directed toward its restoration, the effects and limitations imposed by lack of voluntary extension must not be overlooked in planning reconstructive procedures.

Since mobility is the major consideration at the elbow, and since certain compromises or limitations are inherent in the paralytic limb, it is necessary to define where in the approximately 140 degrees of motion in the sagittal plane we ought to concentrate our efforts. Obviously, if full extension can be gained or preserved without prejudice, then so much the better. Small limitations of extension (less than 25 degrees) are of no functional significance and are not obvious in causal observation. Although one may discuss the importance of each few degrees of range, it may be generally said that a controlled range of from 60 to 120 degrees is probably the minimum for good function.

The tendon transfers that have been developed to restore active elbow flexion are varied, not only in terms of the donor muscles, but in the techniques evolved to transmit their power. The use of each of them has had its enthusiastic proponents, a list of whom would constitute a roster of the giants of reconstructive upper limb surgery. However, just as the cynic would quickly remind us that "there is no free lunch," none of these procedures is ideal or without some kinesiological side effect. It therefore behooves the reconstructive surgeon to be aware of these problems.

In general terms, as with all transfers done to restore active motor power, the substitute muscle must have adequate power to perform the function of the paralyzed one. The term "adequate" must be defined not only in terms of cross-sectional area, potential contractile force, and excursion, but also with reference to the patient and his needs. Brachial plexus-injured patients are usually neurologically unimpaired in their other limbs and are otherwise normal individuals. Therefore, they are more likely to expect (whether justifiably or not) strong function from their transfers. For this reason, the muscle chosen must have as close a "match" in terms of potential power as possible.

Fig. 11.17. A: Nonunion allowed to persist by the patient for a year after a fall. Subsequently healed following refusion and graft. **B**: (Same patient as in **A**.) Rupture of Clark's pectoral transfer with retracted muscle. **C**: Knitted Dacron "artificial ligament" used to repair the retracted muscle. A fair clinical result was obtained, which is to be reinforced by a Steindler flexorplasty.

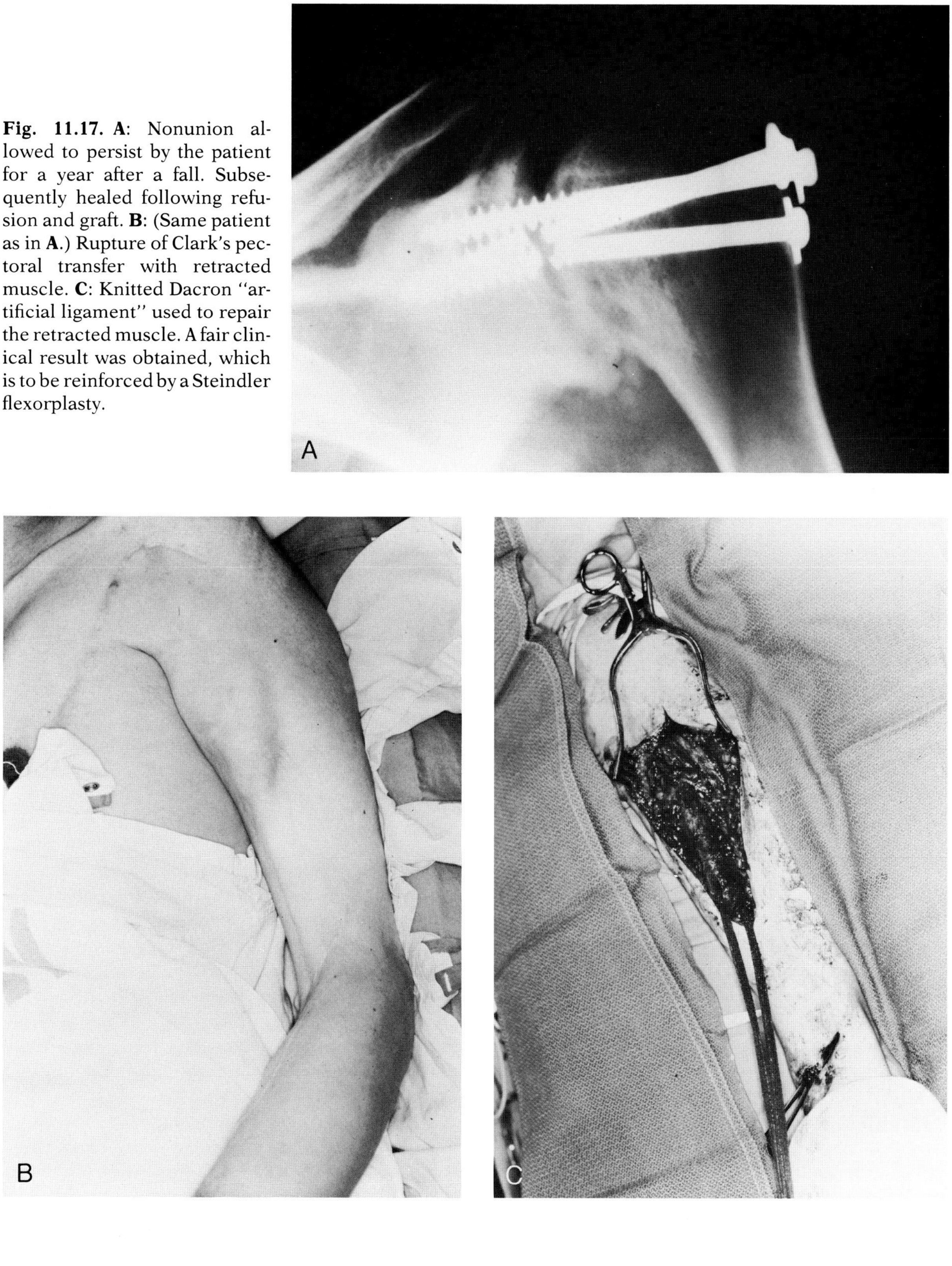

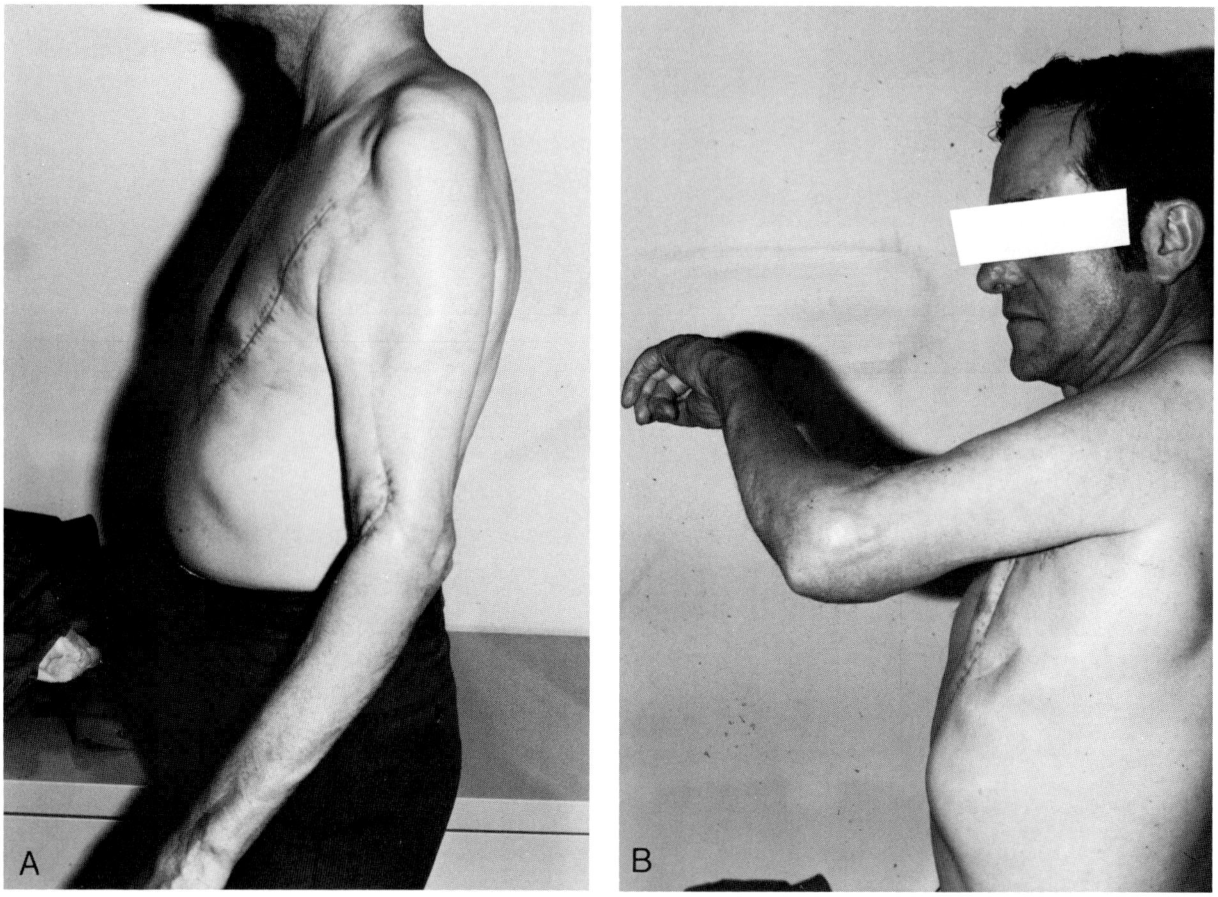

Fig. 11.18. **A** and **B**: This patient had, in addition to a C5, C6, C7 traction injury to the brachial plexus, an open fracture of his left elbow that left him with only 60 degrees of range of motion, despite intensive physiotherapy. Nevertheless, his shoulder fusion and pectoral transfer plus tendon transfers for his hand made it possible for him to return to work in a shipyard. His job included climbing ships' ladders, which he did without difficulty.

The muscles that are usually considered as potential substitutes are as follows:

1. Sternomastoid
2. Pectoralis major
3. Pectoralis minor
4. Forearm flexor-pronator group (Steindler)
5. Triceps
6. Latissimus dorsi

In addition to contractile power, the potential motor for tendon transfer has to be scrutinized from several other points of view. Excursion and alignment of the transfer ultimately are determined by the point of attachment to the lever system, hence they will relate to development of force. For the elbow in particular, the effect on the forearm and hand are of considerable importance. Restoration of active supination is desirable, a habitual pronation attitude or one that appears dynamically with grasp will detract from the functional usefulness, as will an unstable or flexed wrist. An excessive flexion contracture at the elbow as a result of a flexorplasty, while potentially augmenting its power, can be both functionally and cosmetically objectionable. All of these factors must be considered for each patient about to undergo reconstruction. It is axiomatic that, for any of these transfers, the passive range of motion of the elbow must be in the functional range preoperatively in order to have a satisfactory result. Sometimes, because of local trauma to the elbow, something less must be accepted (Fig. 11.18).

Sternomastoid Transfer

The method of restoration of active elbow flexion using the sternomastoid prolonged by a fascial graft and routed subcutaneously to the bicipital tubercle of the radius was originated by Bunnell.[11] Not only does it function as a flexor, but supination is restored as well. The strength and excursion of the muscle are adequate and the mechanical alignment of the transfer is good. The disadvantages, I believe, are significant, in that the bulk of the transfer produces an ugly web in the neck when it contracts, and some patients must stabilize the head or even rotate it to the other side for maximal power of elbow flexion. Obviously, if this occurs, it may interfere with eye-hand coordination and introduce an ungainly motion. Nevertheless, I have had the opportunity to examine several of the patients with polio who had had the procedure done by Dr. Robert Carroll[14] in New York, and I was very favorably impressed by their power of elbow flexion. Ordinarily I do not consider it in cases of paralysis of elbow flexion due to brachial plexus injury.

The Steindler Flexorplasty

In 1918 Steindler[59] first reported the now classic procedure of flexorplasty, which, over the years, has been used more than any other for restoration of voluntary elbow flexion. The flexor-pronator muscles arising from the medial epicondyle of the humerus, that is, pronator teres, flexor carpi radialis, palmaris longus, flexor carpi ulnaris, and flexor superficialis, exert a flexor effect at the elbow joint, which they cross, although the perpendicular distance from them to the axis of joint motion is short and the rotational moment correspondingly small. In addition, the combined work capacity of these muscles (contraction length $\times$ cross-sectional area $\times$ 3.6 kg/cm^2 of cross section) is 0.72 kg as opposed to 3.6 kg, the combined working capacity of the brachialis, biceps, and brachials.[21] Steindler reasoned that, by transposing the origin of the epicondylar muscles to a more proximal point, the moment for elbow flexion could be increased sufficiently to permit voluntary control, as countless clinical cases have proved[59] (Fig. 11.19). However, in addition to the expected lack of power on theoretical grounds, most patients find their transfers adequate for achieving elbow flexion against gravity, but incapable of lifting much weight. Kettlecamp and Larson's[30] detailed analysis of the results of a series of 15 Steindler flexorplasties revealed that nine patients could lift one pound through 110 degrees, and the maximum weight that could be lifted by the best result in the series was 6 lb. Nevertheless, the result can be useful if there is no alternative that would be likely to produce stronger elbow flexion. If the muscles used for transfer are not "normal" or "good" power, then the patient will tend to clench the fist to recruit the flexors superficialis to increase the power, and this will tend to diminish the functional use of the hand as the elbow is flexed. Preoperative assessment of the patient's ability to achieve elbow flexion using this finger-flexion maneuver, the Steindler effect, with the arm held horizontally, will generally predict how well the transfer will function in the antigravity position (Fig. 11.20). If no flexion can be achieved with gravity eliminated preoperatively, then it is unlikely that the transfer will be functionally strong postoperatively. The tendency of the forearm to pronate as the elbow is flexed is a functional disadvantage of this transfer (Fig. 11.19 E, F), and several modifications have been designed to offset the problem. Steindler[59] suggested transfer of the flexor carpi ulnaris to the radius for its supinatory effect and endorsed Mayer's[37] modification incorporating bone from the medial epicondyle with the muscle that is ultimately inset into a hole in the anterior surface of the humerus rather than into the medial intermuscular septum as originally described. Bunnell[11] prolonged the transfer with a fascial graft more laterally. The concomitant transfer of the extensor-supinator muscle origin up from the lateral epicondyle was practiced by Seddon and Brooks.[53] A disadvantage of this modification is that it is likely to cause a permanent flexion contracture at the elbow of 60 degrees or more. A flexion contracture of the elbow increases flexor strength by increasing mechanical advantage, but there is disagreement over just how much of a contracture is acceptable. Mayer and Green[37] felt that with a successful flexorplasty there should be no more than 15 degrees and used extensive bracing to achieve it. Carroll and Gartland[14] accepted 40 degrees, while Steindler deemed 60 degrees as acceptable. Kettlecamp and Larson felt that flexorplasties were more satisfactory with a flexion contracture between 30

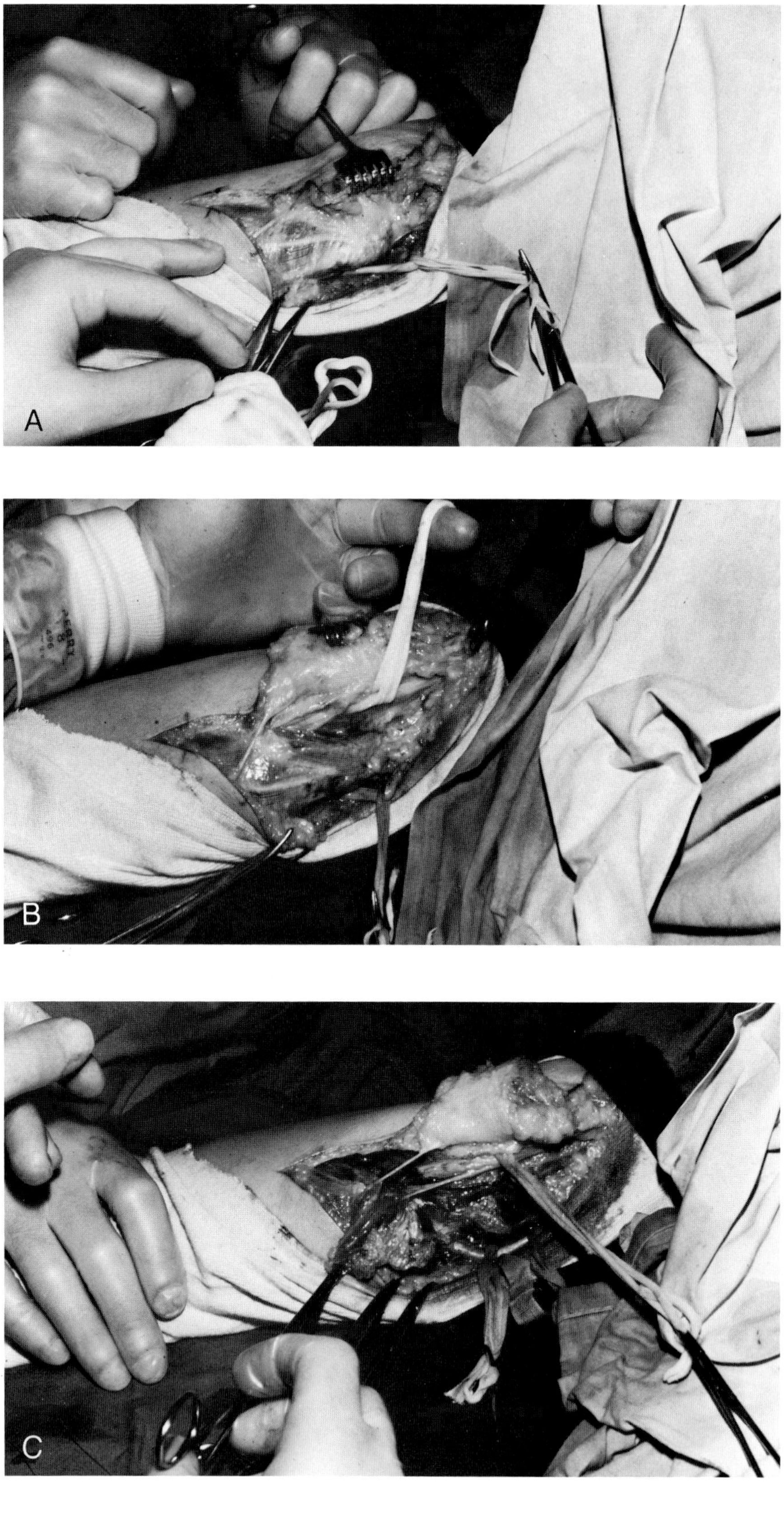

Fig. 11.19. The Steindler flexorplasty. **A**: The ulnar nerve isolated and gently retracted. **B**: The median nerve. **C**: The flexor-pronator muscles have been mobilized. Note the branch of the median nerve to the pronator coming off at the level of the tape retractor and the medial cutaneous nerve of the forearm crossing the field parallel and above it distally. Both of these branches must be sought and preserved.

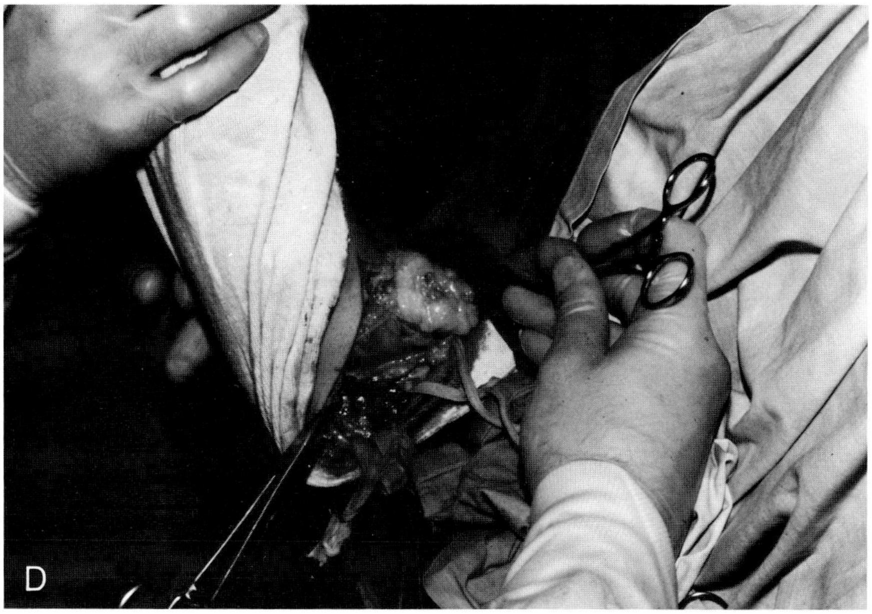

Fig. 11.19 *(continued)* **D**: The flexor-pronator mass has been advanced 6 cm proximally with a 1-cm portion of the osteotomized medial epicondyle. It will be fixed to the midanterior aspect of the humeral shaft with heavy nonabsorbable sutures through two drill holes. The proximal edge of the transfer will be further sutured to the brachialis muscle and periosteum. The nerves will be protected to avoid kinking or injury during closure. **E** and **F**: The result. This patient also underwent shoulder fusion and tendon transfers for his hand. Note pronation attitude of forearm.

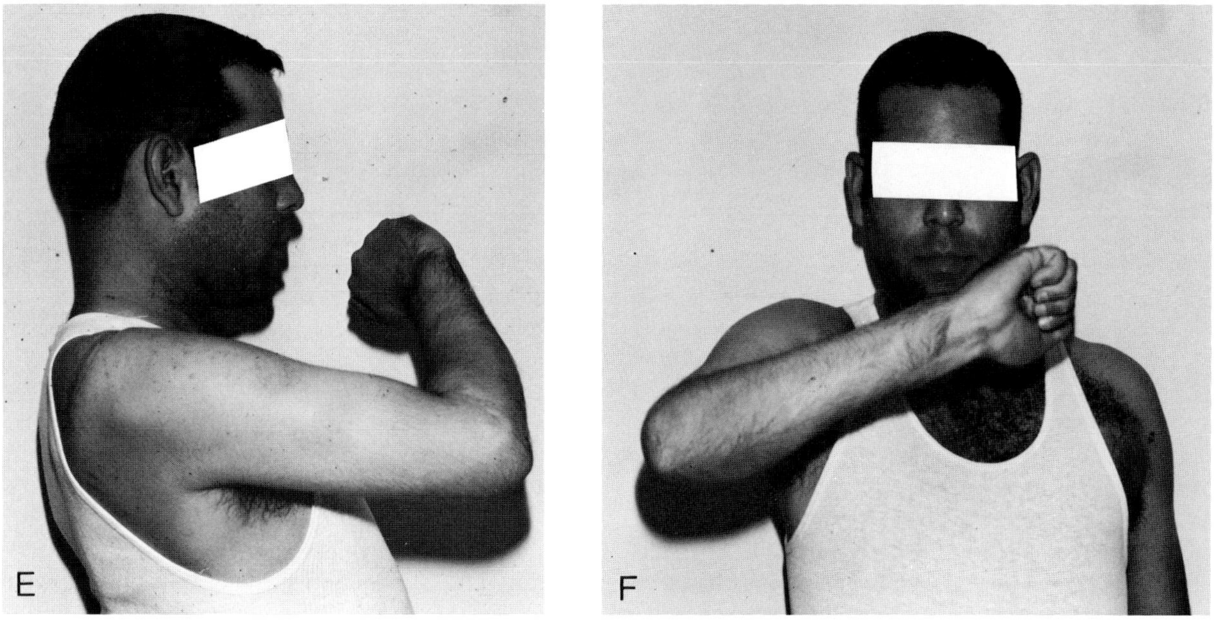

and 60 degrees, and made no attempt to reduce the contracture by bracing in the postoperative period.

The Pectoral Transfers

In 1917 Schulze-Berge[50] transplanted the tendon of insertion of the pectoralis major directly into the belly of the biceps. The procedure was modified in 1918 by Hohmann,[27] in 1928 by Rivarola,[45] in 1930 by F. Lange,[32] and in 1951 by M. Lange.[33] The alignment and method of attachment of the transfers were not satisfactory, however, even though the mass of muscle and excursion are more than adequate to replace the anterior brachial musculature.

In 1945 J. M. P. Clark,[19] a British army surgeon,

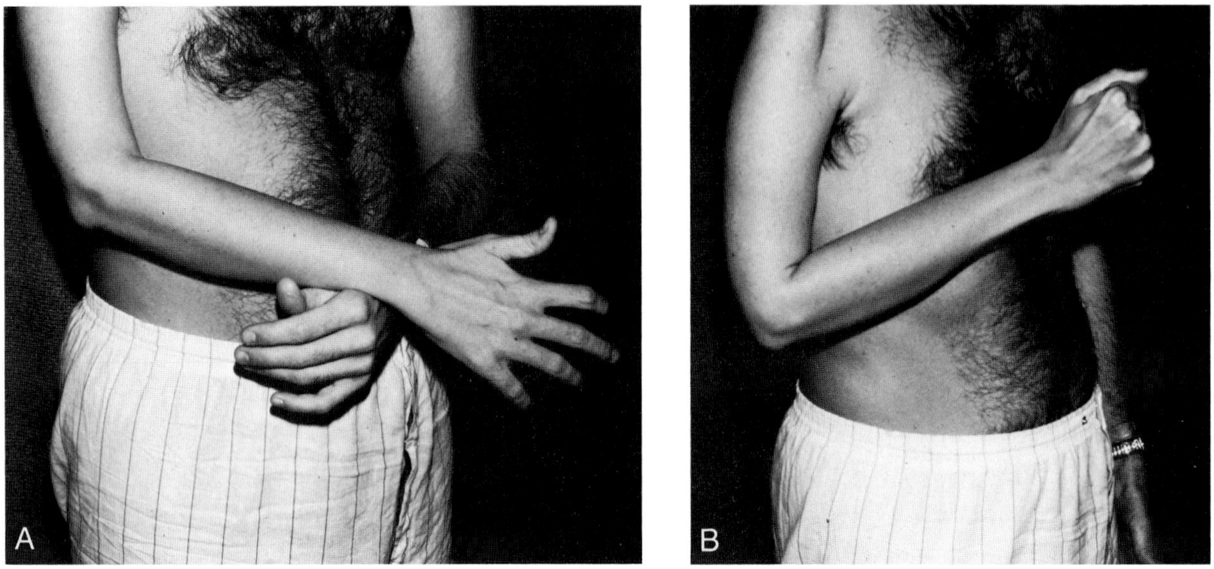

Fig. 11.20. **A**: Adult patient with elbow flexor paralysis due to birth palsy. He habitually shook hands by deftly bringing his left hand up beneath his right forearm to present his right hand. **B**: Elbow flexion achieved by tight finger flexion.

undertook to replace a biceps and brachialis lost due to a war wound complicated by gas gangrene. The patient, a German prisoner of war, had a normal shoulder and full passive elbow motion. Clark detached a portion of the sternocostal head of the pectoralis major and rotated its origin subcutaneously down the arm to be attached to the biceps tendon in the antecubital fossa. The lateral anterior thoracic nerve and its accompanying vessels were preserved intact with the pedicle of muscle, which then functioned quite well as an elbow flexor (Figs. 11.21, 11.22). In 1955 Schottstaedt, Larsen, and Bost[54] modified the technique in order to improve alignment and length-tension relationships, and completely detached the sternal head of the muscle and its insertion so that the latter could be advanced to the coracoid on its pedicle. d'Aubigne[20] used a similar attachment. In 1979 Carroll and Kleinman[18] presented a further modification, wherein the acromion was used as the new origin of the transplant, and reported good results. A variation using the clavicular head of the pectoralis major in those patients who had this part preserved and the sternal paralyzed was previously described by Brooks and Seddon.[9] The paralyzed biceps brachii was surgically stripped of its blood supply so that it was converted into a tendon-like structure to transmit the pull to the forearm. Unfortunately, this procedure has limited application in the brachial plexus population and does not usually produce strong elbow flexion.

The Clark pectoral transfer has met with rather indifferent acceptance despite what would appear to be basically sound advantages. Aside from technical failure caused by damage to the neurovascular pedicle or compromise of the muscle itself, the problems stemmed from incorrect length (tension) or the absence of shoulder control. Clark's original patient had a normal shoulder—the usual patient lacking active elbow flexion due to brachial plexus injury also has no control of the glenohumeral joint. Therefore, when the transfer is activated, it tends to produce unwanted adduction and medial rotation of the humerus rather than the desired elbow flexion. Reestablishment of shoulder control by tendon transfers or stability by means of arthrodesis eliminates this annoying problem, and it should be accomplished before the transfer for elbow flexion is done.

A further benefit of pectoral transfer, in addition to good power of flexion, is the restoration of supination of the forearm and the avoidance of a severe flexion contracture at the elbow. The cosmetic appearance of the atrophic arm is also enhanced.

(Text continues on p. 220.)

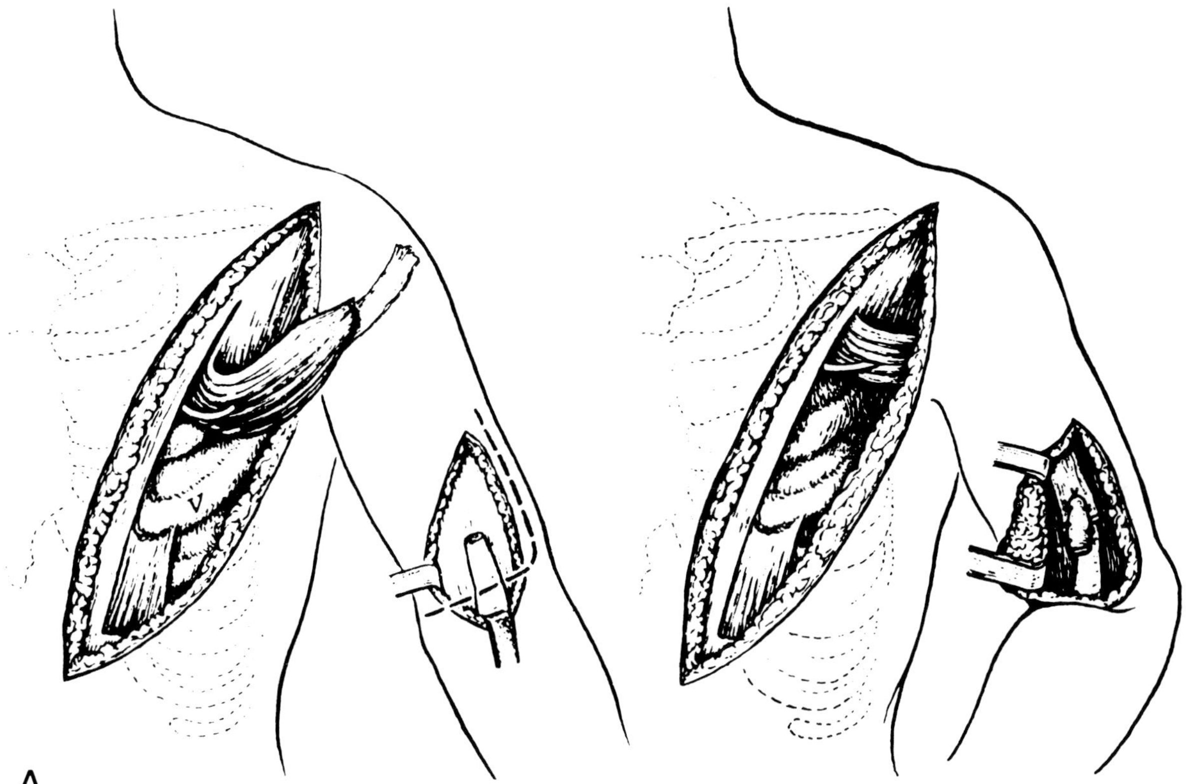

A

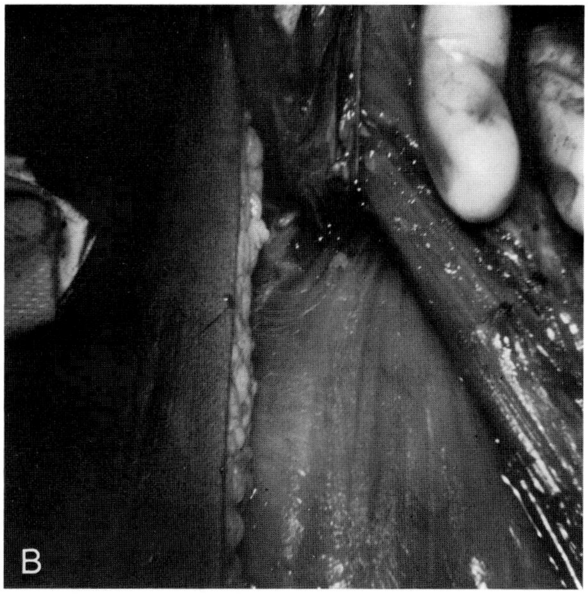

B

Fig. 11.21. **A**: The Clark's pectoral transfer. Note the preservation of the lateral pectoral branch to the pedicle. (Reproduced from Clark JMP: Reconstruction of biceps brachii by pectoral muscle transplantation. Br J Surg 34:180, 1946.) **B**: The pectoral nerve shown entering the pedicle after it has been raised. The remaining sternocostal pectoralis major is indicated by the gloved finger.

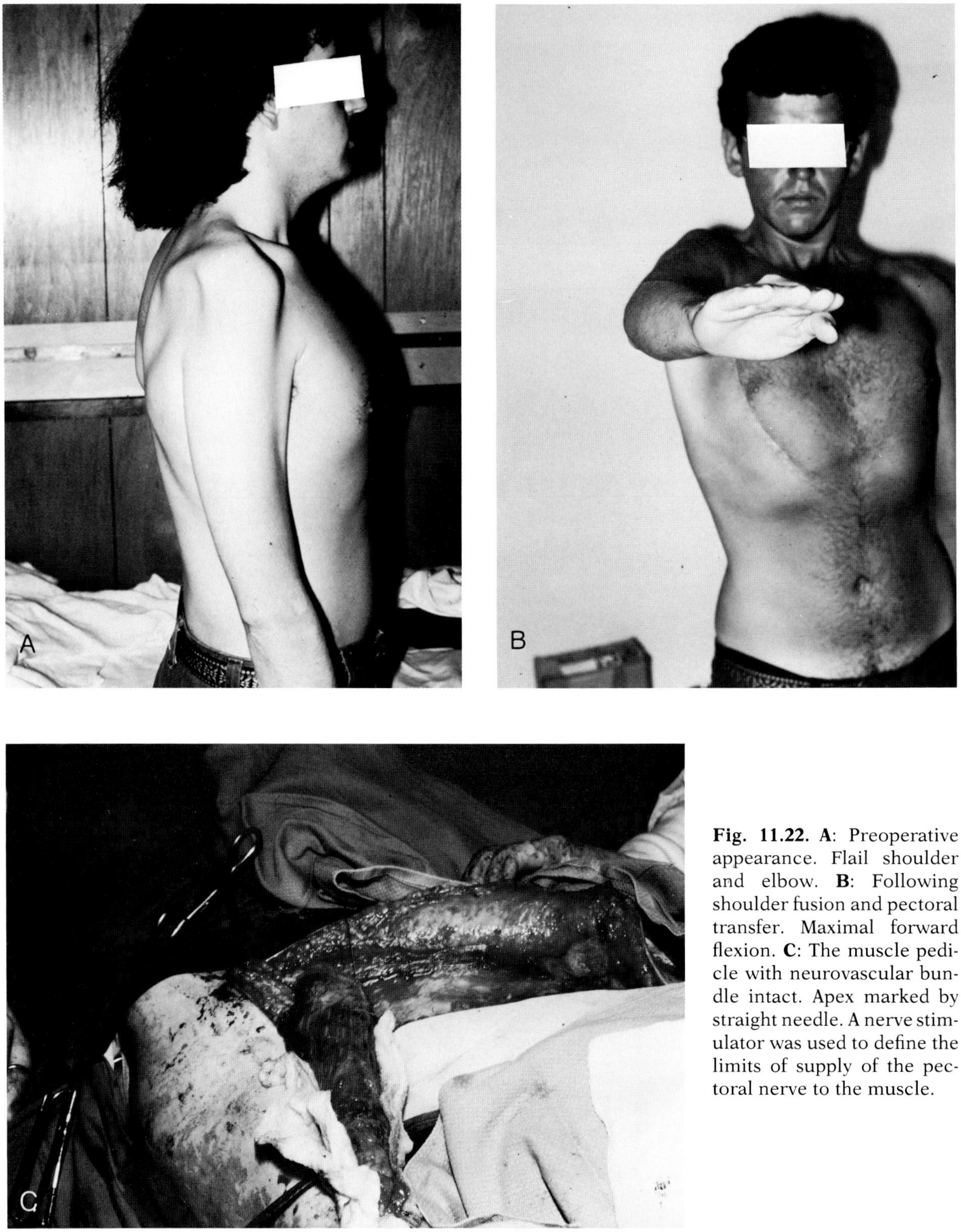

Fig. 11.22. A: Preoperative appearance. Flail shoulder and elbow. **B**: Following shoulder fusion and pectoral transfer. Maximal forward flexion. **C**: The muscle pedicle with neurovascular bundle intact. Apex marked by straight needle. A nerve stimulator was used to define the limits of supply of the pectoral nerve to the muscle.

Fig. 11.22 *(continued)* **D**: Subcutaneous tunnel created with a long clamp and muscle gently drawn down without kinking pedicle or neurovascular supply.

(Fig. continues on next page.)

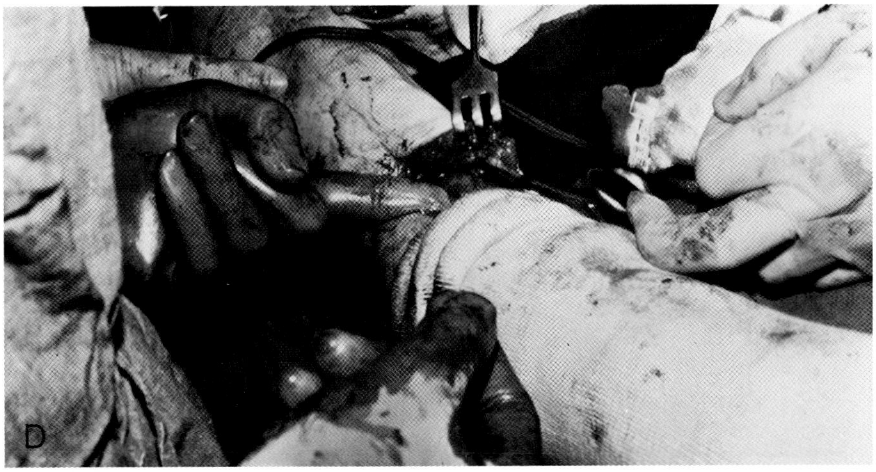

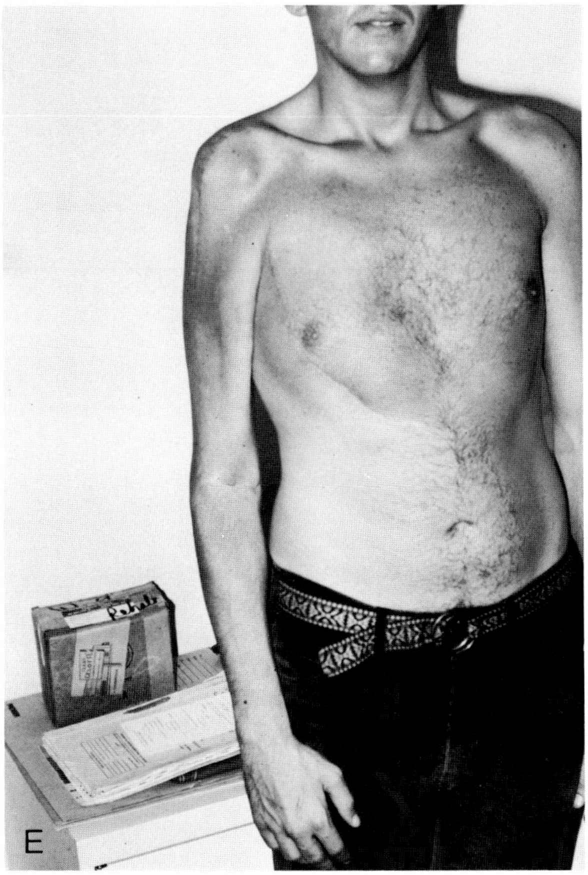

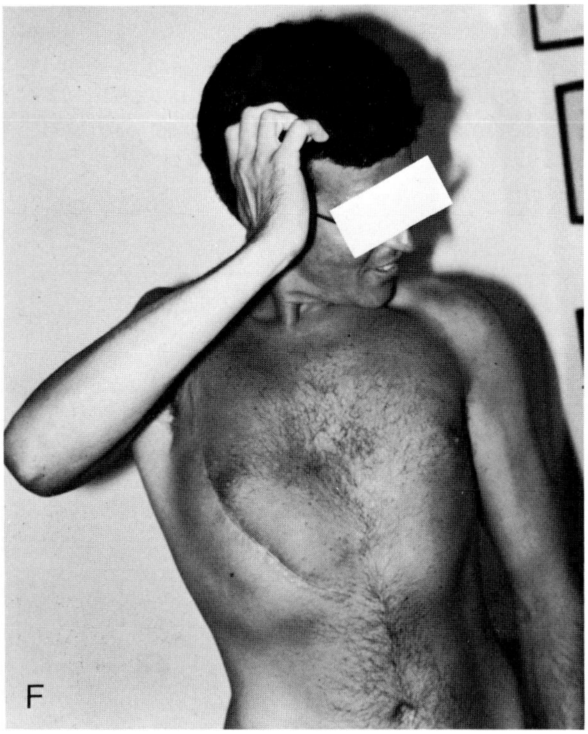

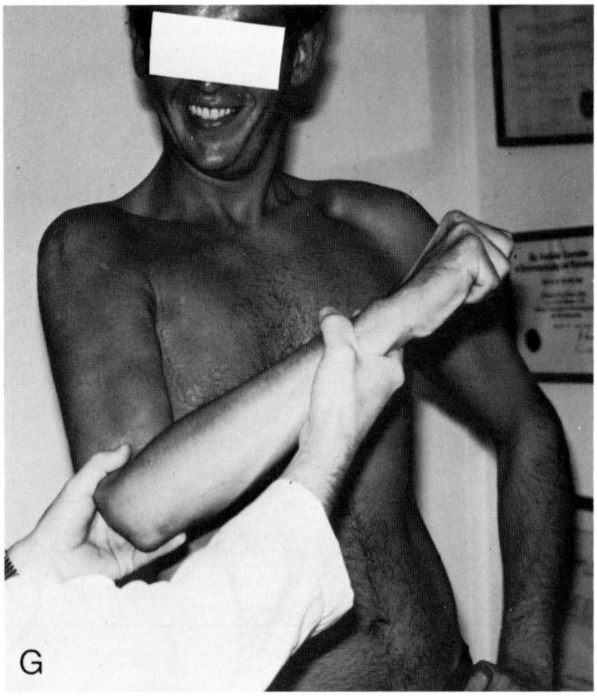

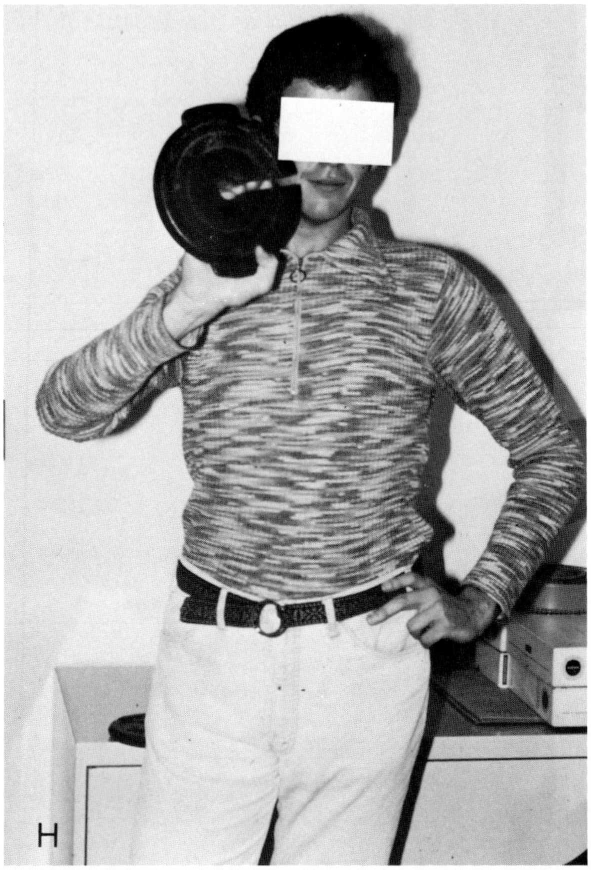

Fig. 11.22 *(continued)* **E–H**: Postoperative appearance and function. The 10-lb weight is comfortably supported.

Latissimus Transfer

The use of the latissimus dorsi as a transfer to restore active elbow extension was described in 1930 by Lange.[32] In 1955, in the same article in which the pectoral transfer was illustrated for elbow flexion, Schottstaedt, Larsen, and Bost[54] also described the latissimus transfer for either elbow extension or flexion. The next year, Hovnanian[28] reported on the use of latissimus for elbow flexion and recommended it. Zancolli and Mitre[65] have subsequently reported favorably on this transfer. The muscle is equivalent in power and excursion to the pectoralis major. Unfortunately, it is often paralyzed in patients whose anterior brachial musculature is denervated by injury to the brachial plexus.

Triceps Transfer

The transfer of the triceps around the lateral aspect of the humerus to the radius can restore active flexion to the paralyzed elbow. It was described by Bunnell[10,11] and then again in 1952 by Carroll,[13] who reported an excellent modification of the technique and in 1970 published its results in a series of 15 patients.[17] The procedure is extremely useful in patients in whom other alternatives of peripheral reconstruction are not available because of the extent or pattern of paralysis. We have already discussed some of the disadvantages to the triceps transfer. In 1970 Carroll[17] cautioned that bilateral transfers should never be done because one functional triceps is needed for toilet care and assistance when rising from a chair. Further, he stated that the procedure was generally contraindicated in patients who must use crutches. Nevertheless, within these restrictions, I have found the triceps transfer to be a reproducibly dependable operation. In terms of muscle mass and excursion as well as alignment, it is quite satisfactory. The theoretical objection on the basis of phasic incompatibility has proved groundless in my patients in whom conversion has not been a problem. In patients in whom confused reinnervation following brachial plexus injury has occurred, triceps transfer

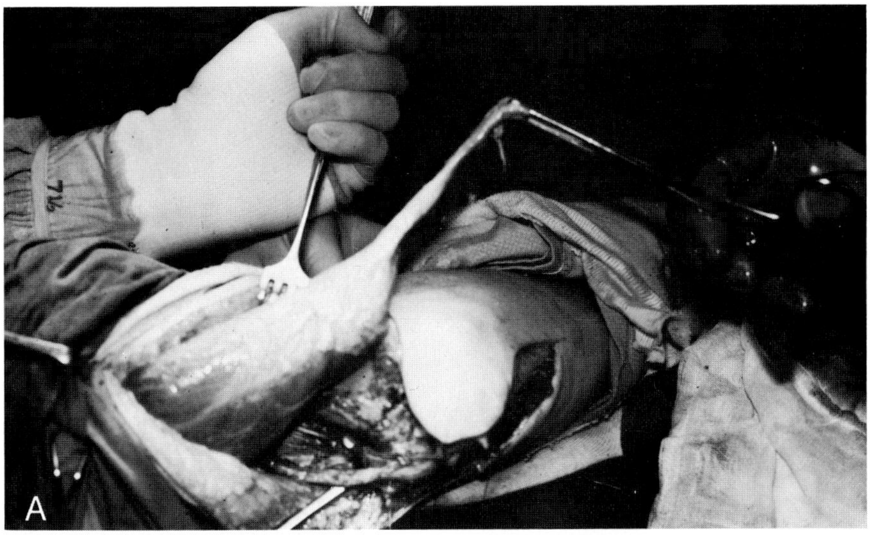

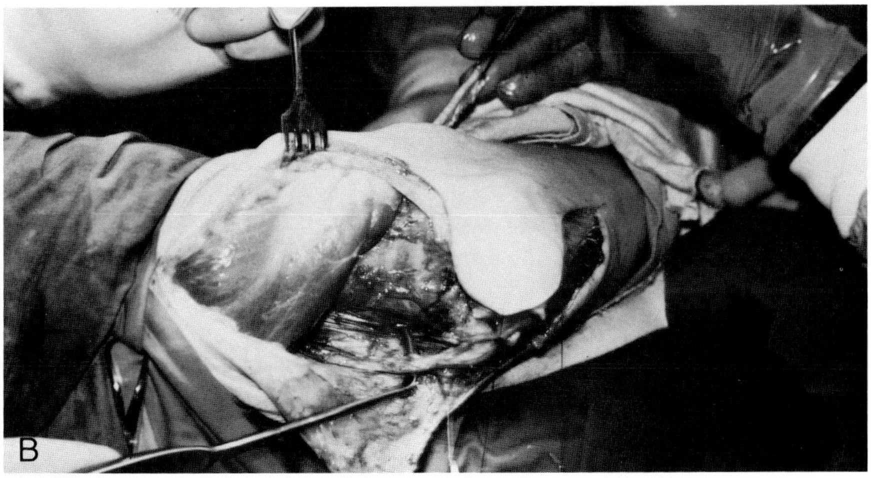

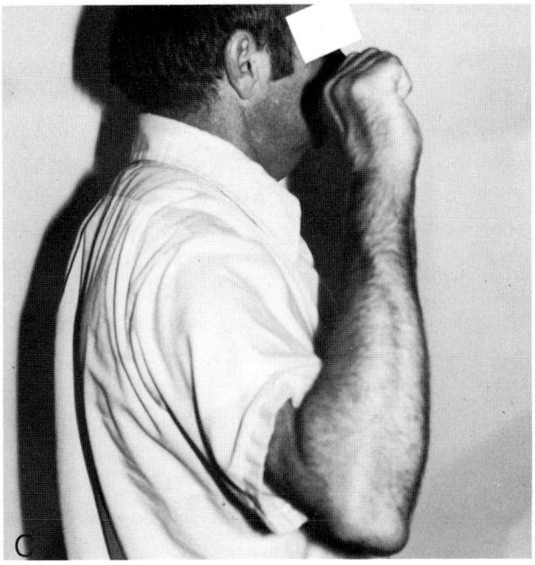

Fig. 11.23. **A**: The entire triceps has been mobilized along with contiguous periosteum and fascia. The ulnar nerve shown gently retracted. **B**: The pedicle is rerouted subcutaneously. Care must be taken to avoid injury to the radial nerve. **C**: Good elbow flexion which allows moderately heavy use of arm. Hand has also been reconstructed with tendon transfers.

can be extremely helpful. However, if there is a viable alternative to using the triceps for elbow flexion, I will not use it because it is an important stabilizer and antagonist in activities of daily living.

Technique of Triceps Transfer (after Carroll). The anesthetized patient is placed on the operating table in the lateral decubitus position and the involved arm is draped free (Fig. 11.23). If a pneumatic tourniquet is used, it must be a relatively narrow one (pediatric size is ideal) and placed as high in the axilla as possible to allow for a sufficient sterile field. In addition, it must be deflated after the dissection is completed and prior to final adjustment of the tension of the transfer. We have found that the midline incision beginning in the upper posterior part of the arm going lateral to the olecranon as advised by Carroll can be modified with benefit to an S-shaped one, which runs medially to the olecranon and affords direct access to the ulnar nerve in the olecranon groove as well as the radial nerve more proximally. It then curves distally over the shaft of the ulna as per Carroll. Obviously, the ulnar and radial nerves are the structures at greatest risk in the complete elevation of the triceps necessary for the transfer, and they must be handled with care. The bulk of the lower one third of the triceps is raised with the fibrous attachments to the olecranon and as long a tongue of periosteum from the subcutaneous surface of the ulna as possible, for this will obviate the necessity of the intercalated fascial graft used in the Bunnell procedure. The tongue of periosteum for about an inch is fashioned into a tube that will serve as a "tendon of insertion." The biceps tendon is exposed by a separate "L-shaped" incision in the antecubital fossa, with care to ligate and divide the radial recurrent vessels. A subcutaneous tunnel is then created by blunt dissection between the two incisions, and the transfer is routed anteriorly, superficial to the radial nerve, and attached to the biceps tendon under submaximal tension, with the elbow flexed to 90 degrees and the forearm supinated. If an interwoven method of attachment is used, I have not found it necessary to use additional attachment to the radius itself. The elbow is immobilized in this position for three weeks, following which gentle active mobilization is begun.

THE FOREARM

The dynamic imbalance in the paretic forearm of the brachial plexus-injured patient has been discussed in consideration of elbow flexorplasty. For the patient with a congenital palsy involving the lower segments (Klumpke) or one in whom paralysis is acquired early, during growth, the forearm will assume a fixed, fully supinated attitude, which is both unattractive and clumsy for function. Even if the hand has minimal function, correction of the deformity can contribute much to normalization of the individual's appearance.

Although several techniques, including osteotomy of the forearm bones, can be employed for this problem, the extensive release of the interosseous membrane and adjacent joints, supplemented by "Z" lengthening and rerouting of the biceps tendon around the neck of the radius described by Zancolli[64] has proved to be an extremely useful procedure. The biceps tendon becomes an active pronator rather than a supinator, and if not active, acts as a tenodesis against supination. The procedure involves an incision from elbow to wrist with release of all structures preventing pronation. Care must be taken to avoid injury to the posterior interosseous nerve and its branches, which are definitely at risk at several stages of the procedure (Figs. 11.24, 11.25, 11.26).

THE WRIST AND THE HAND

Consideration of control of the paretic or paralyzed wrist and hand in the brachial plexus-injured patient does not differ significantly from the problem presented by a patient with one or more peripheral nerve injuries, except that weakness is likely to be more extensive and often accompanied by loss of control of proximal parts of the limb. While the principles and techniques of reconstruction are identical, certain points deserve emphasis. Obviously, preservation or restoration of a mobile wrist under strong voluntary control is much to be desired. However, the paucity of available motors for both wrist and hand may force the sacrifice of wrist mobility to allow control of hand function. Only if there is no alternative should this compromise be made, since the excursion, and ultimate function of transfers done for the digits, will in almost all cases be enhanced by wrist motion. However, an unstable wrist will vitiate the effect of even the best tendon transfer that includes it in its kinetic chain.

There are numerous techniques that have been described for achieving solid arthrodesis of the wrist.[3,22,39,55] Use of any one of them with attention to detail will result in solid fusion. What is needed for the patient whose fusion is preliminary to tendon

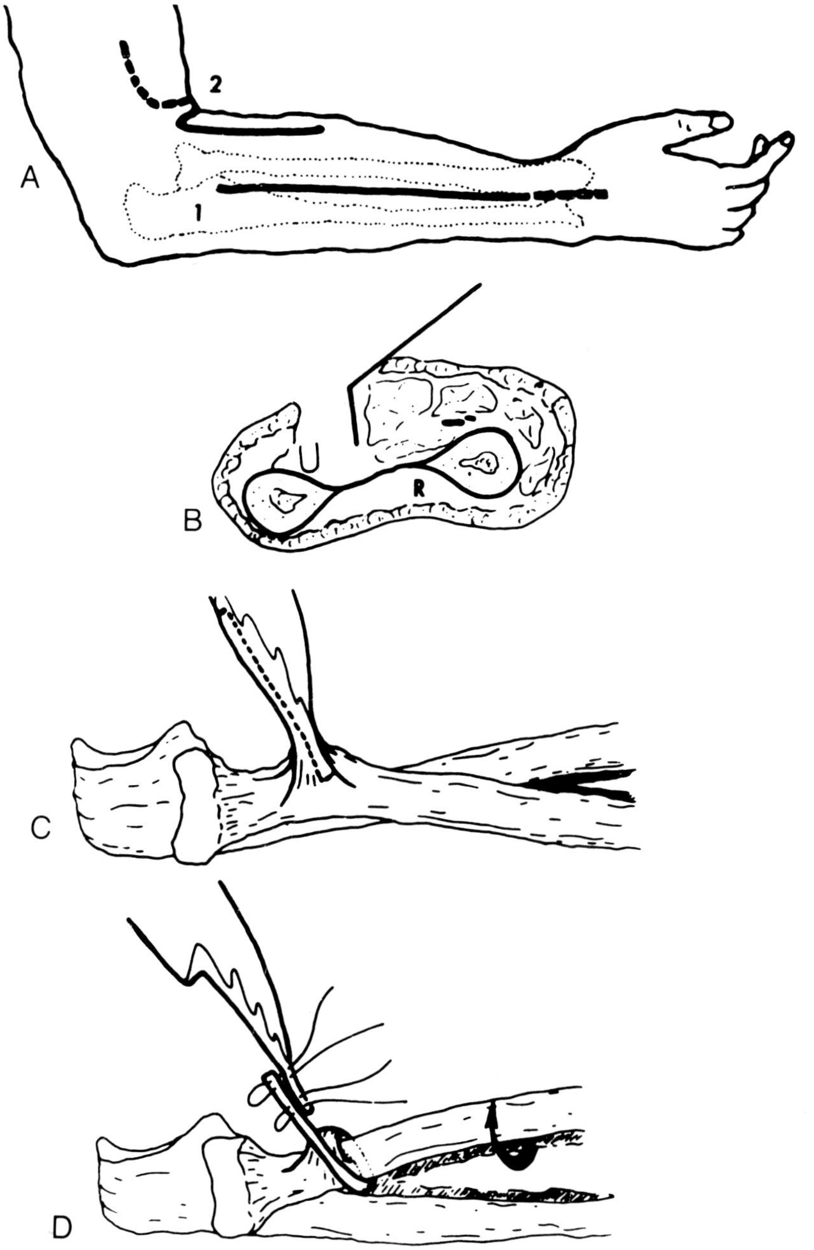

Fig. 11.24. A: The Zancolli procedure for correction of supination contracture of the forearm. The proximal and/or distal radioulnar joints may require release. **B:** Note that dissection begins on the ulna and that the entire extensor mass must be carefully mobilized toward the radius to avoid injury to the posterior interosseous nerve. **C**, **D**: When the biceps tendon is rerouted around the neck of the radius, it must again avoid impairing the interosseous nerve. (From Zancolli E: Paralytic supinator contracture of the forearm. J Bone Joint Surg 49A:1275, 1967.)

transfer, especially for finger and thumb extension, is essentially normal tissue on the dorsum of the wrist that will allow tendons to glide without compromise of their excursion. In my opinion, this requirement will eliminate the most commonly used dorsal approach to the joint in favor of one from the radial or ulnar side. The ulnar approach as described by Smith-Peterson[55] and later modified by Seddon,[52] uses the distal ulna as a radiocarpal graft, and, although it does spare the dorsum, it has the disadvantage of sacrificing the stability of the presumably normal distal radioulnar joint as well as producing a rather uncosmetically thin wrist due to the removal of the bone on its ulnar side. The Haddad-Riordan technique,[23] described in 1967, obviates these difficulties by using a radial approach through which an iliac bone graft is inlaid between the radius and the bases of the second and third metacarpals (Fig.

(Text continues on p. 228.)

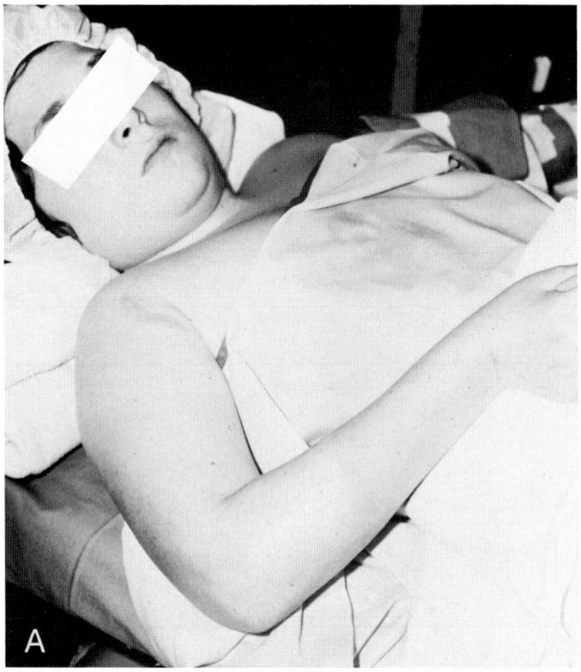

Fig. 11.25. **A**: Supination contracture as residual open injury to brachial plexus in childhood. **B**: The o erative field. **C**: The healed incision.

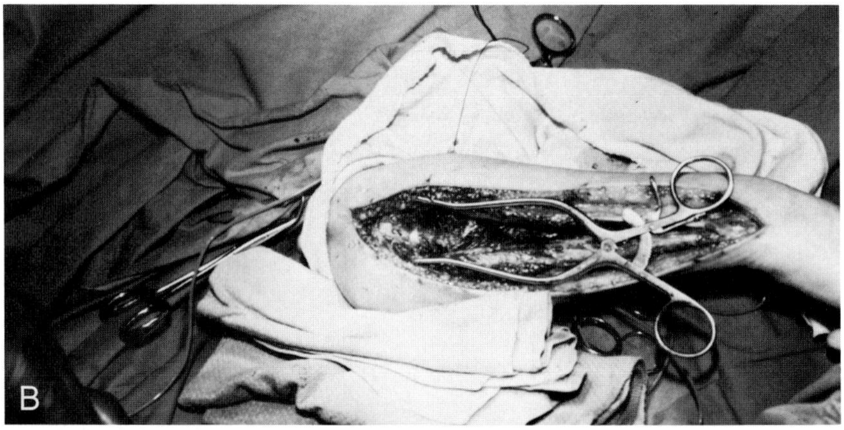

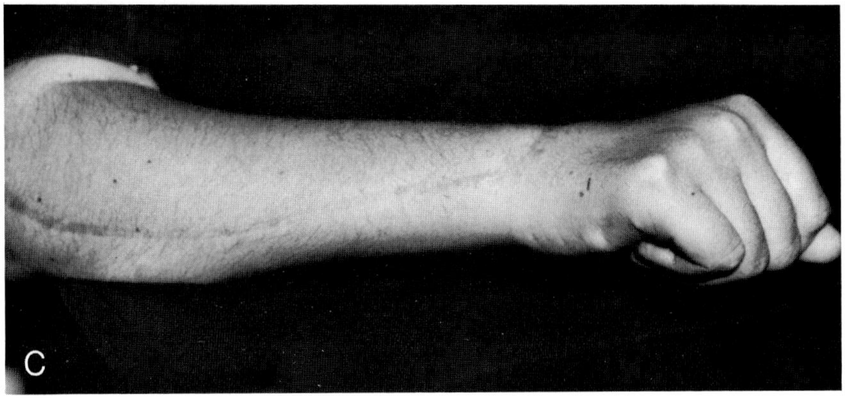

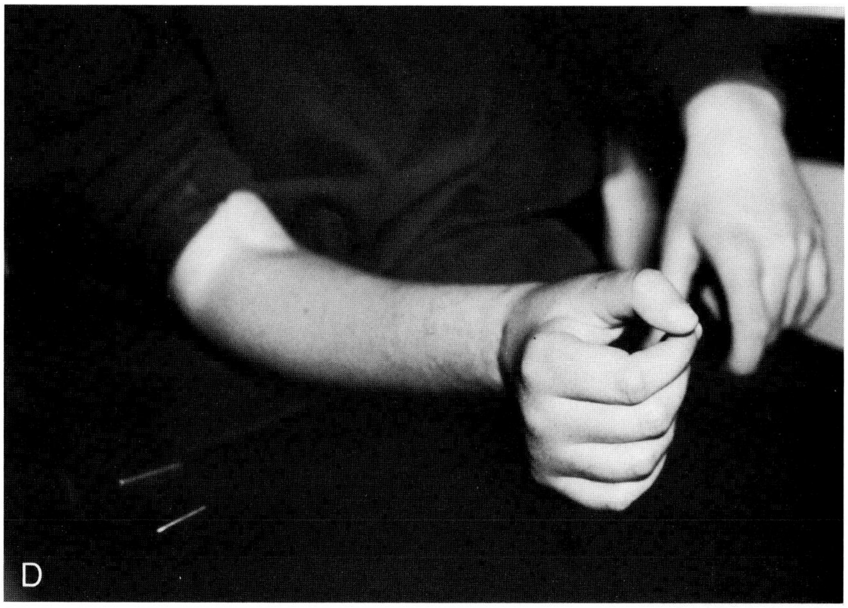

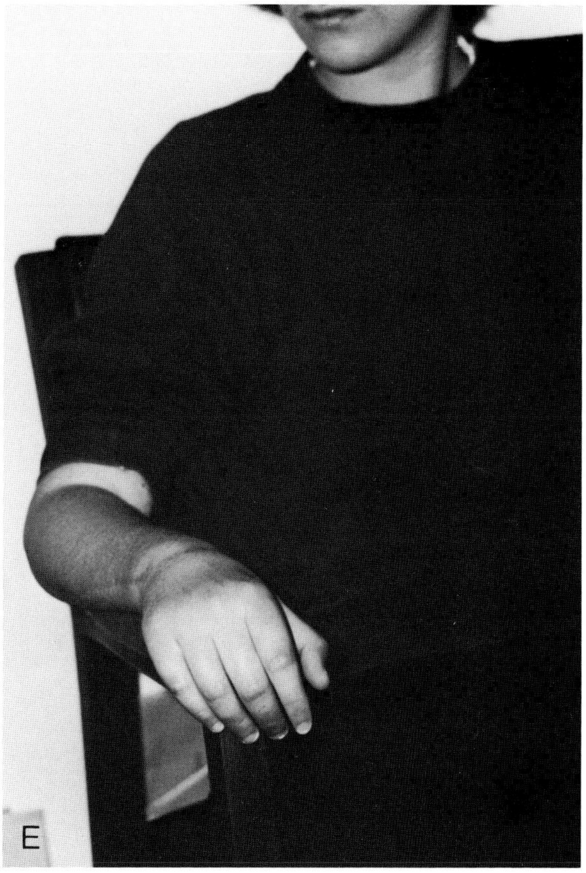

Fig. 11.25 *(continued)* **D**: Maximum active supination. **E**: Maximum active pronation.

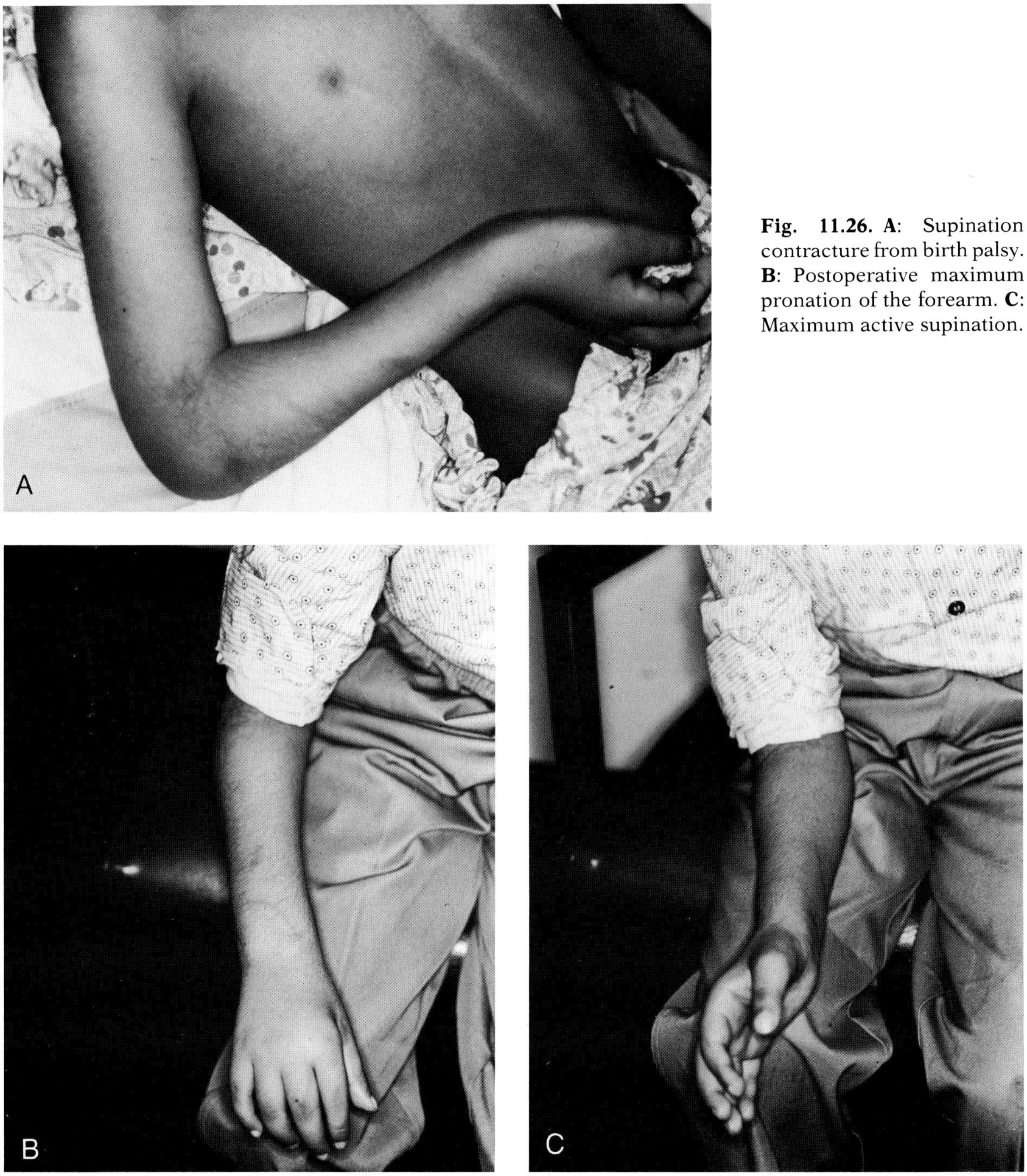

Fig. 11.26. A: Supination contracture from birth palsy. **B**: Postoperative maximum pronation of the forearm. **C**: Maximum active supination.

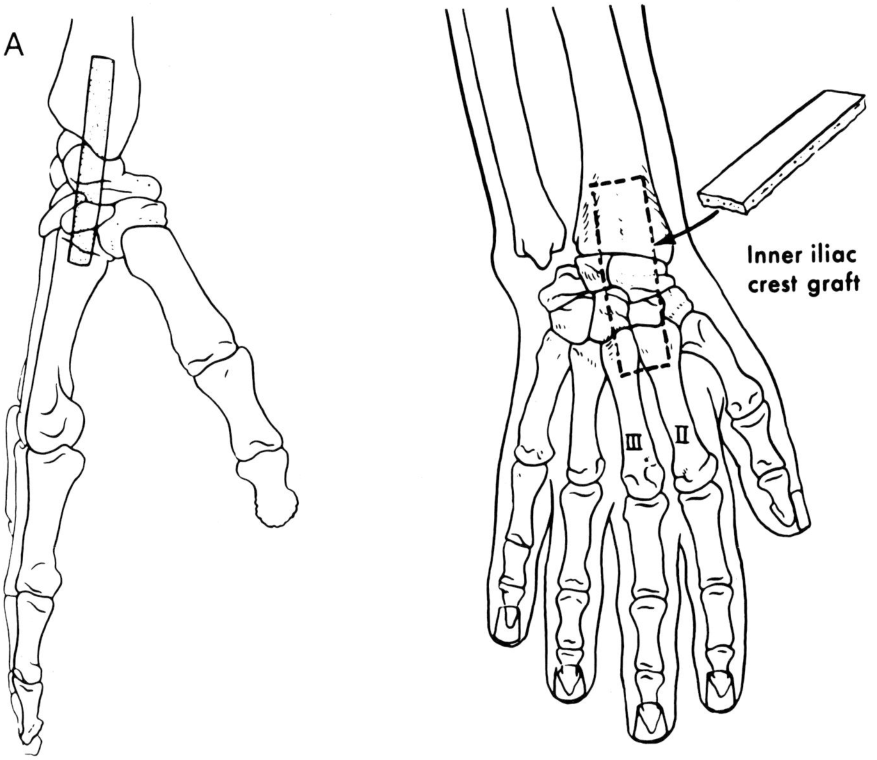

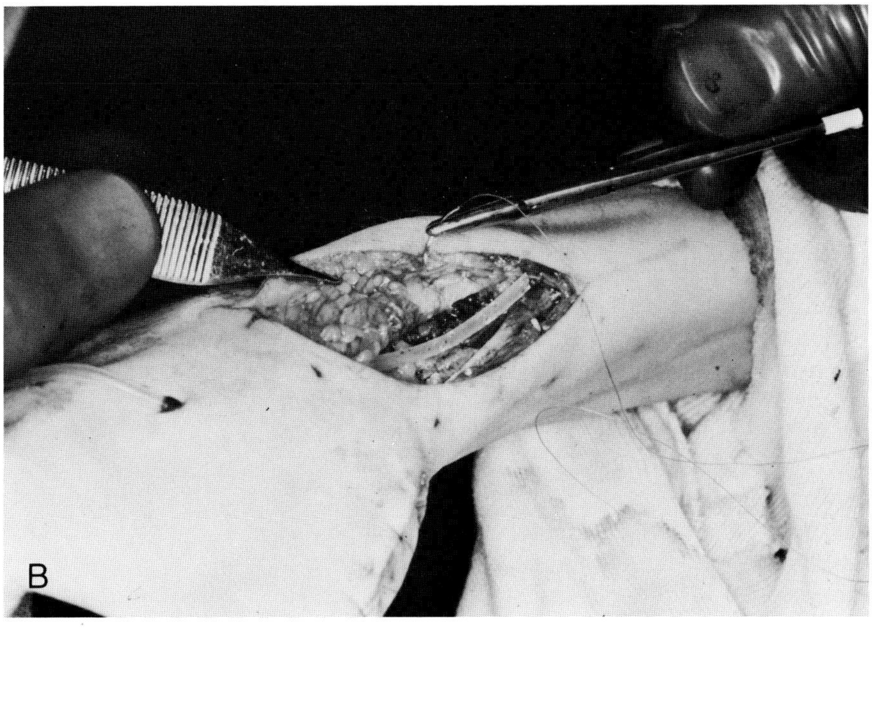

Fig. 11.27. A: The Haddad-Riordan wrist fusion. It is of advantage to decorticate and graft the intercarpal joints as well. (Reproduced from Haddad RJ, Riordan DC: Arthrodesis of the wrist. A surgical technique. J Bone Joint Surg 49A:950, 1917.) **B**: Closure over a soft suction drain. In this case, an osteotomy of the first metacarpal was also done to improve thumb position.

(Fig. continues on next page.)

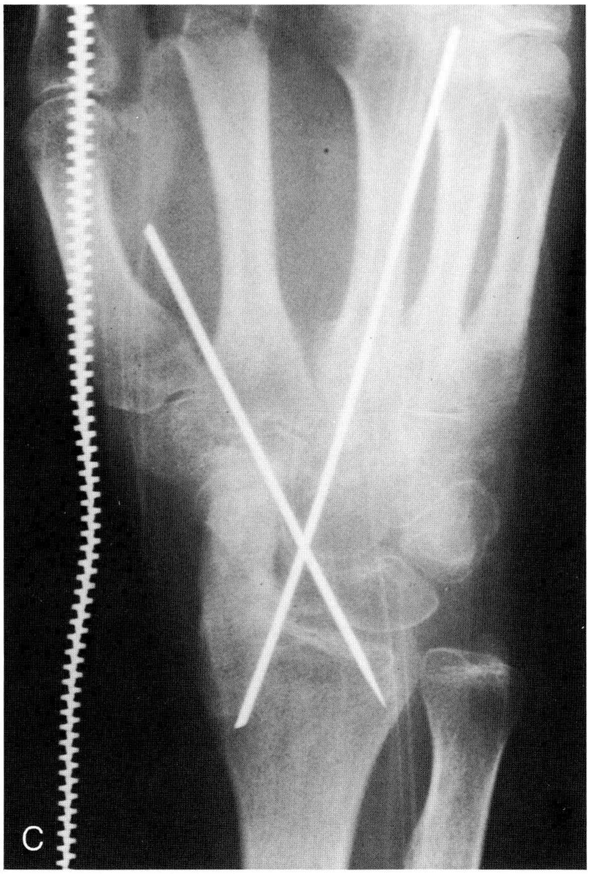

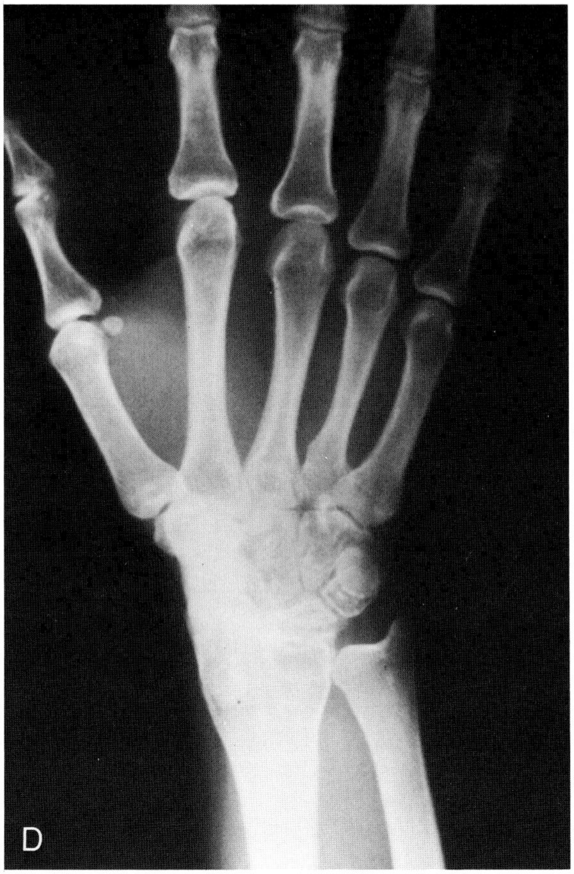

Fig. 11.27 *(continued)* **C**: Radiographs from another case showing wire fixation. **D**: Result shows solid fusion.

11.27A,B). The fusion site is reinforced by crossed Kirshner wires, usually removed in six to eight weeks, by which time the fusion is usually solid (Fig. 11.27C,D). My experience with this technique in two dozen cases has been uniformly favorable with no nonunions, but there have been three later fractures after fusion was solid (Fig. 11.28). These have all resulted from significant trauma, and one ultimately required bone grafting to achieve refusion. Since the incision crosses the superficial radial nerve at the wrist, care must be taken to avoid injury to it.

My preference for doing the hand reconstruction before the more proximal parts of the limb has already been commented upon. Certain circumstances, such as slow recovery of potential motors in the forearm, may make accurate assessment of their suitability for transfer difficult or impossible, and either suspension of the entire surgical rehabilitation program or switching attention more proximally may become necessary. In those cases, I would elect to work at the elbow, or if necessary the shoulder. For detailed consideration of reconstruction about the hand, the reader is directed to a number of excellent references pertaining to peripheral nerve injury, since they are identical to the problems encountered in the hands of patients with brachial plexus injuries.[5–8,10,12,42–44,62]

THE ROLE OF AMPUTATION IN TREATMENT OF BRACHIAL PLEXUS INJURY

Although the reader might think it odd to include a section on amputation in a chapter on reconstruction of the upper limb crippled by brachial plexus injury, it would be an omission that would not

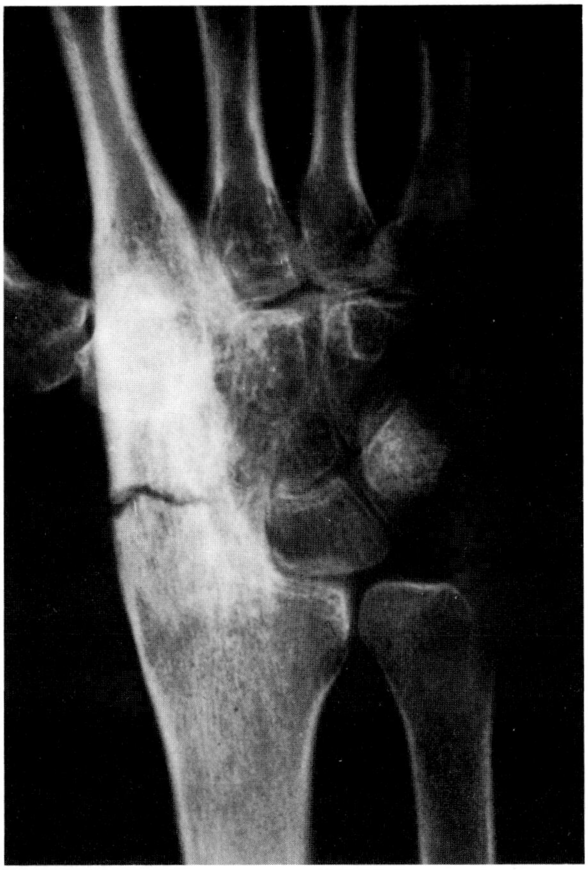

Fig. 11.28. This fracture of the fusion mass resulted from the hand being struck by a falling automobile hood. The patient continued to use the hand and a non-union developed. It ultimately required repair by means of bone graft, which again resulted in a solid and painless wrist.

serve the patients well.[40,46,49] Perhaps it is because amputation has such negative connotations and is so often equated with failure of treatment that today's reconstructive surgeons would prefer not to think about indications for and techniques of amputation and prosthetic fitting. Yet, despite the advances in technology of neurological reconstruction that allow for some restitution of sensory and motor function, the ultimate result in terms of hand function for the patient with a flail-anesthetic limb is far from normal. Some patients are not reconstructable (Fig. 11.29) or do not desire nerve surgery, some are seen too late, and some are plainly failures of reconstruction. For one reason or another, there remains a group of patients for whom amputation either with or without prosthetic fitting is a desirable and reasonable alternative.

Over the past twenty years, there has been a significant shift away from amputation, formerly the major option for a patient with a flail-anesthetic arm. In 1961 Yeoman and Seddon[61] published the results of their study of the two opposed methods of treatment, that of staged peripheral reconstruction, proposed by Hendry,[25] (1949) and simultaneous amputation through the arm and arthrodesis of the shoulder. They stressed the necessity for determination of the prognosis for recovery as early as possible (8 weeks) so that definitive treatment could be started and the patient could thereby avoid becoming "one-handed." Accordingly, after myelography and axon responses were performed, they would explore the plexus if they felt that some or all of the roots were damaged distal to the ganglia. If the roots were found to be ruptured, they considered repair impossible and proceeded with definitive treatment. Otherwise they awaited whatever recovery would occur. Ultimately, they studied 36 patients and compared the function after amputation-arthrodesis, so-called reconstructive procedures, and no operative treatment. The results of the reconstructions of flail-anesthetic arms were so disappointing that they urged that they not be done. They concluded that amputation of the arm with shoulder fusion provided a better result than either reconstruction or no operation (Fig. 11.30). They cautioned, however, that the procedure should not be done in patients more than two years after the injury, since they had essentially become "one-handed" and would be unlikely to use a prosthesis. Patients with severe pain in the limb were also considered to be poor candidates, as were those who were not mechanically minded or who had poor manual dexterity. At the meeting of the British Orthopaedic Association in London in 1965, Fletcher reported on 69 patients in whom amputation had been done for brachial plexus injury. He commented that below-elbow amputation was more advantageous than above if there was motor control of the elbow and that shoulder fusion improved function. Of the 449 amputees that he was able to trace, all were back at work and all were reported to be glad they had decided on amputation. Yeoman, in discussion, stated that in his experience, a third of his patients did not want amputation, and some were

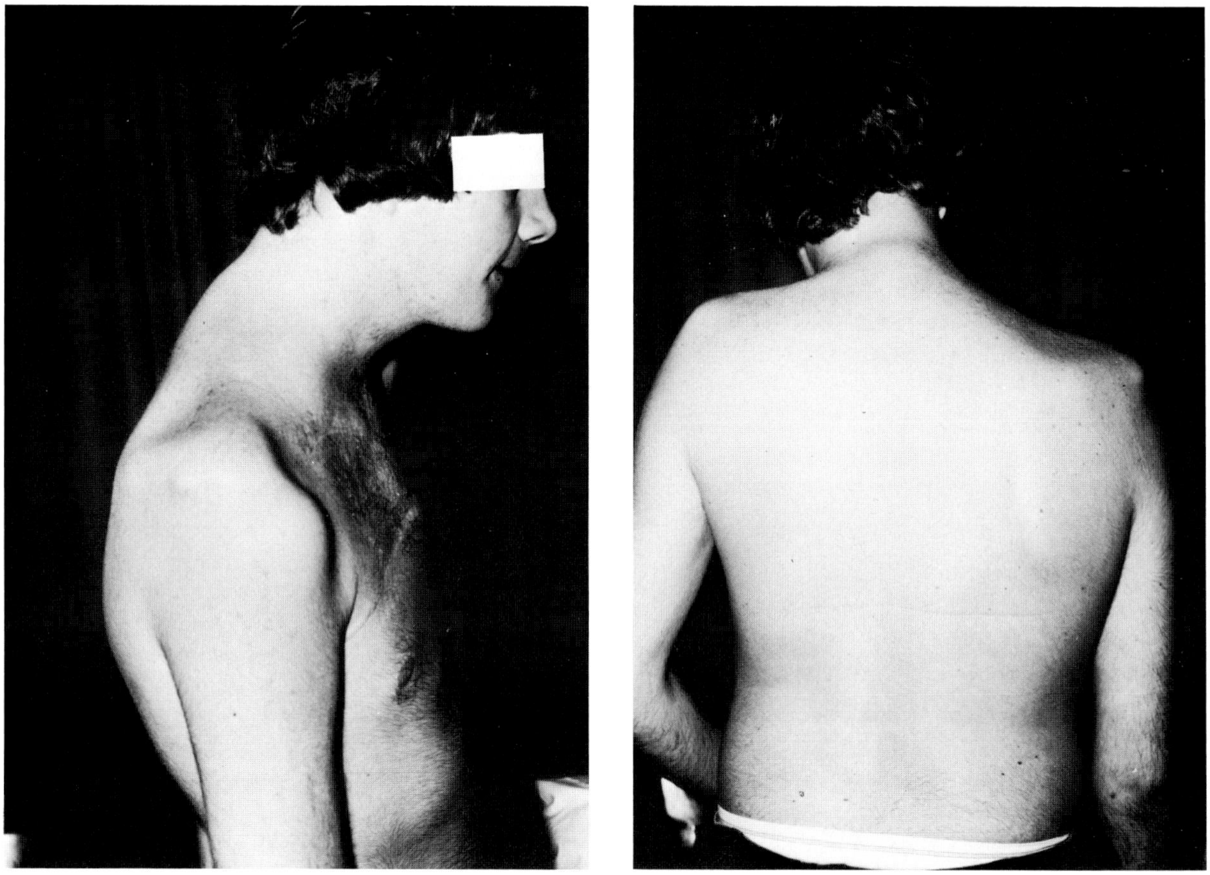

Fig. 11.29. This patient not only has a flail-anesthetic arm due to brachial plexus injury, but also has had a complete arterial occlusion and a traction injury to the spinal accessory nerve that has paralyzed his trapezius. No useful function will result from any combination of reconstructive operations. If amputation were to be done, it would be through the proximal humerus and no prosthetic fitting would be done.

worse with amputation. Both agreed that a flail-arm splint should be used as early as possible.

What then are the indications for amputation, and how should it be done? In some cases, the decisions is an easier one: the patient has had a flail-anesthetic arm for more than two years and wants to be unencumbered. As long as the patient's reason for desiring amputation is not to be relieved of pain of neurogenic character, the amputation can be done above the elbow at any length the surgeon and patient agree upon. Shoulder disarticulation is inadvisable, however, since it offers no advantage over high-humeral ablation and leaves a poorly padded stump. Obviously no functional prosthetic fitting is contemplated.

Patients with old brachial plexus injury and severe trophic changes in the hand and fingers due to lack of sensibility should be shown the prostheses before they undergo ablation, since the cosmetic gloves may prove very disappointing to them. Fortunately, recent improvements in design and manufacture of the cosmetic gloves by Pillet in Paris and Beasley in New York have improved their appearance tremendously, although they are expensive.

Some patients are seen soon after their injuries and have been advised amputation by physicians who are simply not aware of the possibilities for neurological reconstruction. Such patients must be realistically educated as to the potential benefits of the different approaches so that they can come to an informed and reasonable decision as to what to do with their arms. It may well be possible to provide

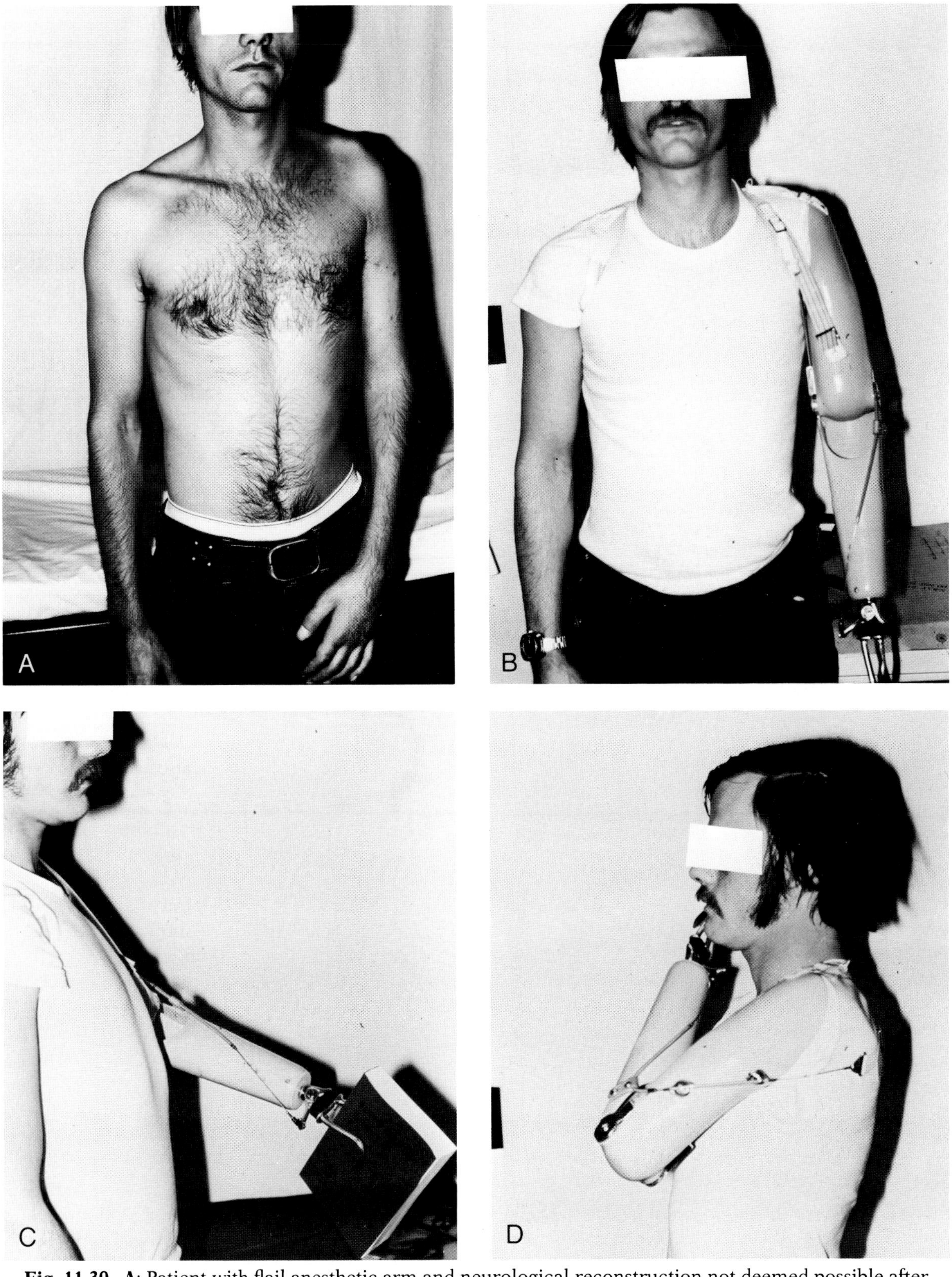

Fig. 11.30. A: Patient with flail-anesthetic arm and neurological reconstruction not deemed possible after myelography and supraclavicular exploration. **B**: Prosthetic fitting after above-elbow amputation and shoulder fusion. **C** and **D**: Function. This patient habitually used the prosthesis in his job in the "tool crib" of a factory.

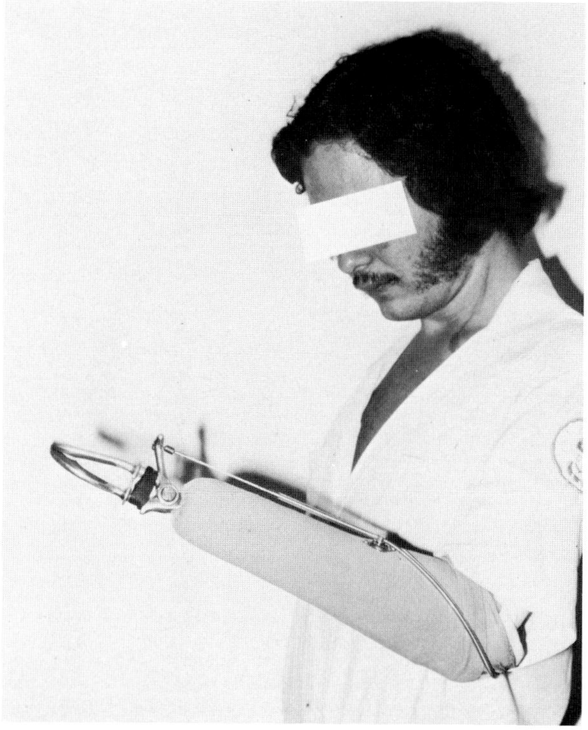

Fig. 11.31. This patient with avulsion at C8 and T1 and distal rupture at C5, C6, and C7 underwent grafting from upper trunk to lateral cord and regained excellent power of elbow flexion but nothing distally. A shoulder fusion and forearm amputation with prosthetic fitting resulted in a useful assistive member.

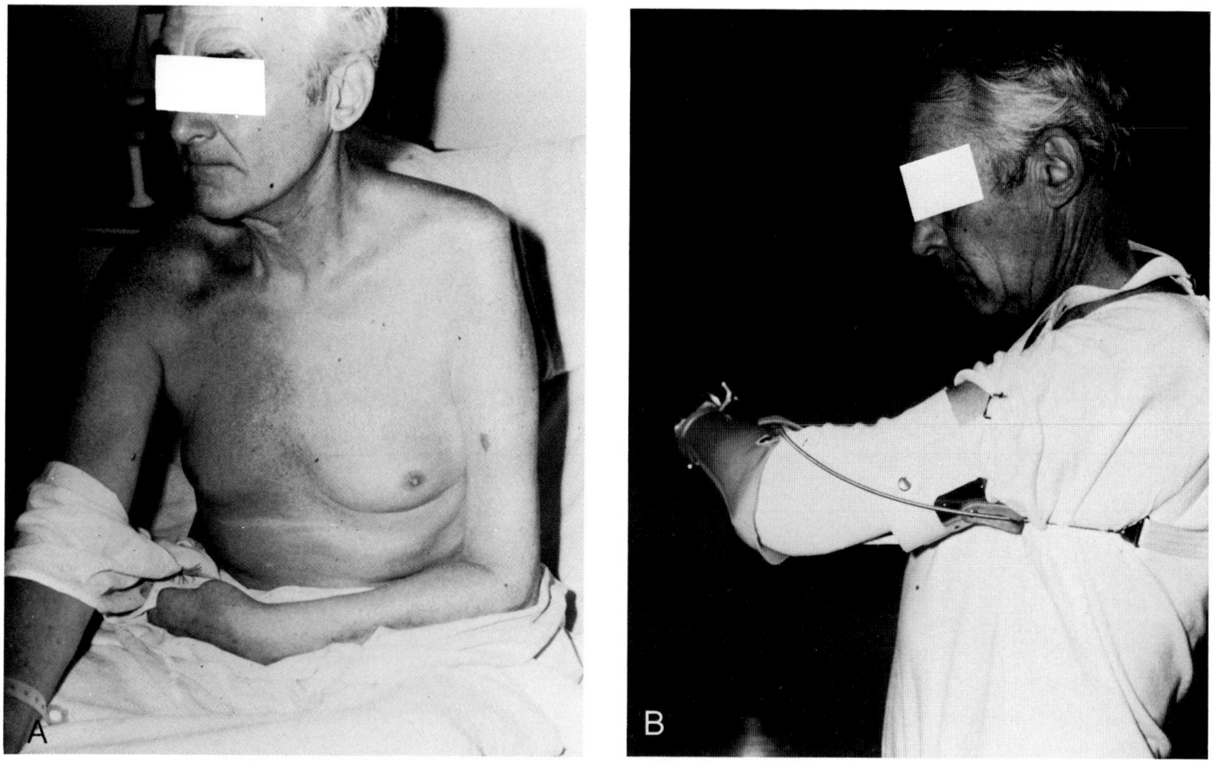

Fig. 11.32. **A** and **B**: An industrial accident produced a painful, mangled hand and a brachial plexus injury. Shoulder fusion and pectoral transfer were done prior to forearm amputation and prosthetic fitting. Pain due to the nerve injury interfered with use of the limb. A dorsal root entry zone radiofrequency lesion in the substantia gelatinosa of the spinal cord was produced by Dr. Nashold at Duke University. At three years the patient still has significant pain relief, which he estimates at 80%, and uses his prosthesis to advantage.

proximal function in the limb by a combination of shoulder fusion and neurologic reconstruction or tendon transfer (Fig. 11.32). The patient can be fitted with a functional splint that spares and protects the insensate hand. Then a decision can be made at leisure regarding whether or not an amputation and prosthetic fitting will be done. It is all-important to attempt to preserve the elbow if there is proprioceptive feedback from the joint, since the usefulness and degree of acceptability of the prosthesis will be much enhanced by it. Even if the elbow is flail and the skin over the proposed stump is insensate, proprioception may be intact and a useful prosthetic fitting may be obtained without stump breakdown.

For some patients, the decision for ablation will be because of a number of complicating factors such as nonunion of long bones, severe posttraumatic joint derangements, and vascular or soft-tissue deficits in addition to the brachial plexus injury. Such cases must obviously be considered on an individual basis (Fig. 11.32).

Whenever possible, patients with brachial plexus injuries contemplating amputation and prosthetic fitting should have the opportunity to see and talk with other patients who have already undergone the procedure. I believe that our high rate of habitual prosthetic use in this population can be largely attributed to this practice. Patients very often come with totally unrealistic ideas of "bionic arms" such as are seen on television. Unless they are disabused of these fantasies, they are unlikely to be satisfied with their results. On the basis of the last twenty years of experience in this area, I offer amputation far less often than I formerly did, but in carefully selected patients it may well be the most expeditious and desirable reconstructive procedure.

SUMMARY

Before leaving the subject of peripheral reconstruction, one point must be reemphasized. The techniques herein described should not be thought of only as alternatives to central reconstruction of the damaged nerves of the plexus, and designated as "palliative." While it is true that they cannot restore lost sensibility and are not intended to do so, there is no surgery that can restore normal motor and sensory function to a limb compromised by brachial plexus injury. Hence all surgery is "palliative" rather than "curative" in these patients. It remains for the imaginative and empathetic surgeon to advise the patient as to what alternatives, from all the techniques available, will best suit his needs. Whether those will include neurological reconstruction, peripheral reconstruction, or some combination will depend on the individual's requirements.

REFERENCES

1. American Academy of Orthopaedic Surgeons Committee on Prosthetics and Orthotics: Atlas of Limb Prosthetics. Mosby, St. Louis, Toronto, London, 1981
2. Ansart B: Die Myoplastik bei der Paralyse des Deltoideus. Z Orthrop Chir 48:57, 1927
3. Abbott LC, Saenders JB de CM, Bost FC: Arthrodesis of the wrist with the use of grafts of cancellous bone. J Bone Joint Surg 24:883, 1942
4. Barr JS, Freiberg JA, Colonna PC, Pemberton PA: A survey of end results on stabilization of the paralytic shoulder (report of the research committee of the American Orthopaedic Association). J Bone Joint Surg 24:699, 1942
5. Boyes JH: Tendon transfers for radial palsy. Bull Hosp Joint Dis 15:97, 1954
6. Boyes JH: Bunnell's Surgery of the Hand. 4th Ed. pp 12, 514. Lippincott, Philadelphia, 1964
7. Brand PW: Tendon transfers in the forearm. p 331. In Flynn JE (ed): Hand Surgery. Williams & Wilkins, Baltimore, 1966
8. Brand PW: Tendon transfers for median and ulnar paralysis. Orthop Clin North Am 1:447, 1970
9. Brooks DM, Seddon HJ: Pectoral transplantation for paralysis of the flexors of the elbow. A new technique. J Bone Joint Surg 41B:36, 1959
10. Bunnell S: Tendon transfers in the hand and forearm. American Academy of Orthopaedic Surgeons Instructional Course Lectures. Vol 6, Ann Arbor, MI, 1949
11. Bunnell S: Restoring flexion to the paralytic elbow. J Bone Joint Surg 33A:566, 1951
12. Burkhalter W: Tendon transfers in the hand in brachial plexus injury. Surg Clin North Am 5:259, 1974
13. Carroll RE: Restoration of flexor power to the flail elbow by transplantation of the triceps tendon. Surg Gynecol Obstet 95:685, 1952
14. Carroll RE, Gartland JJ: Flexorplasty of the elbow. An evaluation of a method. J Bone Joint Surg 35A:706, 1953
15. Carroll RE: Wire loop in arthrodesis of the shoulder. In DePalma AF (ed): Clinical Orthopaedics. Vol. 9. Lippincott, Philadelphia, 1957
16. Carroll RE: Restoration of elbow flexion by transplantation of the sternocleidomastoid muscle. Proceedings of the American Society for Surgery of the Hand. J Bone Joint Surg 44A:1039, 1962
17. Carroll RE, Hill NA: Triceps transfer to restore elbow flexion: A study of fifteen patients with paralytic le-

sions and arthrogryposis. J Bone Joint Surg 52A:239, 1970
18. Carroll RE, Kleinman WB: Pectoralis major transplantation to restore elbow flexion to the paralytic limb. J Hand Surg 4:501, 1979
19. Clark JMP: Reconstruction of biceps brachii by pectoral muscle transplantation. Br J Surg 34:180, 1946
20. D'Aubigne M, Benassy J, Ramadieu JO: Chirurgie orthopédique des paralysies. Masson, Paris, 1956
21. Fick R: Hanbuch der Anatomie und Mechanik der Gelenke, Vol 2. G. Fischer, Jena, 1911
22. Gill AB: Arthrodesis of the wrist. Orthop Corresp Club Lett, March 20, 1947
23. Haddad RJ, Riordan DC: Arthrodesis of the wrist. A surgical technique. J Bone Joint Surg 49A:950, 1971
24. Harmon PH: Surgical reconstruction of the paralytic shoulder by multiple muscle transplantation. J Bone Joint Surg 32A(3):583, 1950
25. Hendry AM: The treatment of residual paralysis after brachial plexus injuries. J Bone Joint Surg 31B:42, 1949
26. Hildebrand A: Über eine neue Methode der Muskeltransplantation. Arch Klin Chir 78:75, 1906
27. Hohmann G: Ersatz des gelähmten Biceps brachii durch den Pectoralis major. Münch Med Wochenschr 65:1240, 1918
28. Hovnanian AP: Latissimus dorsi transplantation for loss of flexion or extension at the elbow. A preliminary report on technique. Ann Surg 143:493, 1956
29. Inman VT, Saunders JB de CM, Abbott LC: Observations on the function of the shoulder. J Bone Joint Surg 26(1):1, 1944
30. Kettelkamp DB, Larson CB: Evaluation of the Steindler flexorplasty. J Bone Joint Surg 45A:513, 1963
31. Lange F: Die Entbindungslahmung der Arm. Münch Med Wochenschr, 1421, 1912
32. Lange F: Die epidemische Kinderlahmung. p 298. Lehmann, Munich, 1930
33. Lange M: Orthopaedisch-chirurgische Operationslehre. Bergmann, Munich, 1951
34. L'Episcopo JB: Restoration of muscle balance in the treatment of obstetrical paralysis. NY State J Med 39:357, 1939
35. Mau C: Kombinierte Muskelplastik bei Deltoideuslahmung. Verh Dtsch Orthop Ges 22:236, 1927
36. Mayer L: Transplantation of the trapezius for paralysis of the abductors of the arm. J Bone Joint Surg 9:412, 1927
37. Mayer L, Green W: Experiences with the Steindler flexorplasty at the elbow. J Bone Joint Surg 36A:775, 1954
38. Milgram JE: Discussion of Davis JB, Cottrell GW: A technique for shoulder arthrodesis. J Bone Joint Surg 44A:657, 1962
39. Muller ME, Allgower M, Willenegga H: Manual of Internal Fixation Technique Recommended by the AO-Group. Springer-Verlag, New York, Heidelberg, Berlin, 1970
40. New York University: Upper Limb Prosthetics. Revision 1979
41. Ober F: An operation to relieve paralysis of the deltoid. JAMA 99:2182, 1932
42. Omer GE Jr: The technique and timing of tendon transfers. Orthop Clin North Am 5:243, 1974
43. Omer GE Jr: Tendon transfers for reconstruction of the forearm and hand following peripheral nerve injuries. p 817. In Omer GE Jr, Spinner M (eds): Management of Peripheral Nerve Problems. Saunders, Philadelphia, 1980
44. Omer GE Jr: Combined nerve palsies. In Green DP (ed): Operative Hand Surgery. Churchill Livingstone, New York, 1982
45. Rivarola RA: Tratamiento de las paralisis definitivas del miembro superior. Bol Trabajos Soc Cir Buenos Aires 12:668 (reported in Sem Med, Buenos Aires, 2:294, 1928)
46. Robertson E: Rehabilitation of arm amputees and limb-deficient children. Baillière Tindall, London, 1978
47. Rowe CR: Reevaluation of the position of the arm in arthrodesis of the shoulder in the adult. J Bone Joint Surg 56A:913, 1974
48. Saha AK: Surgery of the paralyzed and flail shoulder. Acta Orthop Scand Suppl 97, 1967
49. Santschi WR (ed): Manual of Upper Extremity Prosthetics. 2nd Ed. Engineering Artificial Limbs Project, University of California at Los Angeles, 1958
50. Schulze-Berge: Ersatz der Beuger des Vorderarmes (Bizeps und Brachialis) durch den Pectoralis major. Dtsch Med Wochenschr 43:433, 1917
51. Seddon HJ: Transplantation of pectoralis major for paralysis of the flexors of the elbow. Proc R Soc Med 42:837, 1949
52. Seddon HJ: Reconstructive surgery of the upper extremity. In Poliomyelitis, Second International Poliomyelitis Congress. Lippincott, Philadelphia, 1952
53. Segal A, Seddon HJ, Brooks DM: Treatment of paralysis of the flexors of the elbow. J Bone Joint Surg 41B:44, 1959
54. Schottstaedt ER, Larsen LJ, Bost FG: Complete muscle transposition. J Bone Joint Surg 37A:897, 1955
55. Smith-Peterson MN: A new approach to the wrist joint. J Bone Joint Surg 22:122, 1940
56. Spitzy H: Aussprache zur Deltoideuslahmung, Muskelplastik. Verh Dtsch Orthop Ges 22:239, 1927
57. Stein I: Gill turnabout radial graft for wrist arthrodesis. Surg Gynecol Obstet 106:231, 1958
58. Steindler A: Reconstruction work on hand and forearm. NY Med J 108:117, 1918
59. Steindler A: Muscle and tendon transplantation at the

elbow. In Thomson JEM (ed): Instruction Course Lecture on Reconstructive Surgery. Vol. 2. American Academy of Orthopaedic Surgeons, Chicago, 1944
60. Steindler A: Kinesiology of the human body. Charles C Thomas, Springfield, IL, 1955
61. Yeoman PM, Seddon HJ: Brachial plexus injuries: Treatment of the flail arm. J Bone Joint Surg 43B:3, 1961
62. White WL: Restoration of function and balance of the wrist and hand by tendon transfers. Surg Clin North Am 40:427, 1960
63. Zachary RB: Tendon transplantation for radial paralysis. Br J Surg 33:358, 1946
64. Zancolli E: Paralytic supination contracture of the forearm. J Bone Joint Surg 49A:1275, 1967
65. Zancolli E and Mitre, H: Latissimus dorsi transfer to restore elbow flexion. An appraisal of eight cases. J Bone Joint Surg 55A:1265, 1973

Index

Page numbers followed by f represent figures; those followed by t represent tables.

A

B

C

D

E

F

G

H

I

J

K

L

M

N

O

P

R

S

T

U

V

W

X

Z